T...

...nalized
...h

Ryan Dradzynski Editor
Associate Aquisitions Editor
Sociology & Criminology

Lexington Books
An Imprint of Rowman & Littlefield

4501 Forbes Blvd., Suite 200 • Lanham, Maryland 20706
301.459.3366 ext. 5415 • fax 301.429.5749 • www.lexingtonbooks.com
301.459.3366 ext. 5415 • fax 301.429.5749
rdradzynski@rowman.com

The Marginalized in Death

A Forensic Anthropology of Intersectional Identity in the Modern Era

Edited by
Jennifer F. Byrnes and
Iván Sandoval-Cervantes

Foreword by
Zoë Crossland

LEXINGTON BOOKS
Lanham • Boulder • New York • London

Published by Lexington Books
An imprint of The Rowman & Littlefield Publishing Group, Inc.
4501 Forbes Boulevard, Suite 200, Lanham, Maryland 20706
www.rowman.com

86-90 Paul Street, London EC2A 4NE

Cover photo: Anthropologists recovering remains of a Camp Fire fatality, November 16, 2018. Dr. Eric Bartelink, Maghan Maberry, Dr. Alison Galloway, Mallory Peters (left to right).

British Library Cataloguing in Publication Information Available

Library of Congress Cataloging-in-Publication Data

Names: Byrnes, Jennifer F., editor. | Sandoval-Cervantes, Iván, editor.
Title: The marginalized in death : a forensic anthropology of intersectional identity in the modern era/edited by Jennifer F. Byrnes and Iván Sandoval-Cervantes; foreword by Zoë Crossland.
Description: Lanham : Lexington Books, [2022] | Includes bibliographical references and index.
Identifiers: LCCN 2022026687 (print) | LCCN 2022026688 (ebook) |
    ISBN 9781666923094 (cloth; alk. paper) | ISBN 9781666923100 (ebook)
Subjects: LCSH: Forensic anthropology—Social aspects. | Minorities—Mortality. |
    Minorities—Violence against. | Marginality, Social.
Classification: LCC GN70 .M37 2022 (print) | LCC GN70 (ebook) |
    DDC 599.9—dc23/eng/20220705
LC record available at https://lccn.loc.gov/2022026687
LC ebook record available at https://lccn.loc.gov/2022026688

♾™ The paper used in this publication meets the minimum requirements of American National Standard for Information Sciences—Permanence of Paper for Printed Library Materials, ANSI/NISO Z39.48-1992.

Contents

List of Figures and Tables

FIGURES

TABLES

Foreword

Reimagining Forensic Anthropology

Zoë Crossland

This collection of chapters represents a significant shift in forensic anthropology, initiated by a new generation of scholars who are as engaged with the literatures of medical anthropology, public health, and sociology as they are with the forensic anthropological subfield. The chapters in this volume are part of a broader set of changes, that on the one hand are taking a more critical orientation toward the baseline assumptions that have been caught up in forensic anthropological work, and on the other are reconsidering the scope and remit of forensic anthropology. This volume takes up questions of structural and intersectional violence, asking how forensic work might contribute to a better understanding of the different violent forces that are enacted upon the bodies of the most marginalized members of our society. This shift marks a major reorientation of the field, and is the result of a confluence of different strands in forensic anthropological work that have developed over the last thirty years, particularly the influence of medicolegal work in the field of human rights and humanitarian exhumation, and the mass movements of displaced people in recent years.

For most of the twentieth-century forensic anthropology was a small field in the United States, usually undertaken by university- or museum-based biological anthropologists, at the request of local law enforcement. The field expanded radically in the 1990s with the wide-scale recruitment of biological anthropologists and archaeologists to investigate human rights abuses in Rwanda and the former Yugoslavia. At around the same time, the Argentine Forensic Anthropology Team (EAAF), trained by American anthropologist Clyde Snow in the 1980s, was developing strategies for forensic investigation that moved the work away from a narrow medicolegal perspective, to emphasize the training of local investigators in forensic techniques, and the importance of working closely with family members in initiating and developing investigations (e.g., EAAF 1992; Rosenblatt 2015). They also positioned their work as historical inquiry that aimed to "contribute to the reconstruction of the recent past" (1992, 2). These dimensions of forensic practice were not part of established investigative techniques in the United States, which remained structured by the needs and expectations of law enforcement until relatively recently.

In medicolegal investigation, as established in the United States in conjunction with police inquiries, the corpse has figured primarily as an object of analysis, a "case" that is more or less divorced from wider social, political, and economic questions. The questions that are asked of the dead have been narrowly constrained to those of mode and manner of death and any identifying information, framed in terms of the biological profile. The site of inquiry for these questions is the body itself. Questions of why particular populations are overrepresented as murder victims, what kind of risk factors were involved, or how social conditions may have contributed to their deaths have not been a key focus of concern. This enacts a kind of separation of the dead from the living and their concerns, one in which death is individualized and particularized to a specific set of circumstances and little attention is given to the socioeconomic currents within which such deaths are positioned. This separation is reinscribed by the careful control of the body as evidence and its sequestration in dedicated space staffed by medicolegal professionals, where the chain of evidence is necessarily carefully maintained. Family members and funerary professionals enter into this space only at moments of identification and when remains are returned. This is to constitute the corpse as a "case" that can be solved and closed, relating to a singular set of conditions that led to a particular death. Any wider resonance of such medicolegal deaths has been understood primarily in terms of the expectations and loss of family and close friends, not in relation to wider society. The chapters in this volume demonstrate the necessity of placing the forensic dead back into society, both because forensic work can speak to broader anthropological questions of pressing concern, and because the particular conditions of society influence how people die, and how anthropologists make sense of their remains.

It is clear that, as the field has developed over the last decades, the forensic interpretation of violence has been framed differently depending on national context. Whereas in the context of Latin America for example, forensic investigation of deaths and disappearances has long been understood in systemic terms, first in relation to political violence, extending to narcoviolence (see DiGangi and Santamaria Vargas, this volume), and feminicide (e.g., Sanford 2008); in the United States violence has traditionally been treated as an individuated problem of particular bodies. It is only relatively recently that wider perspectives have opened up that situate interpersonal violence within sustained conversations and activism around forms of structural and slow violence (Nixon 2011; Schindel 2019; Beatrice et al. 2021), gender violence, and most recently racial violence, particularly in relation to the protests mobilized via the Black Lives Matter movement. Contributing to this widening perspective has been the increased awareness of the many deaths at the U.S.-Mexico border as a direct result of U.S. border policy, leading to changes in the ways that forensic anthropology is imagined and deployed in the United States (De León 2015; Anderson and Spradley 2016; Giordano and Spradley 2017; Kaplan et al., this volume). This has encouraged more nuanced attention toward the intersectional violence at play in the "silent mass disaster" constituted by the vast numbers of missing and unidentified persons recovered in the United States (Ritter 2007; also Bird and Bird, this volume) and elsewhere, as the chapters in this volume demonstrate.

Forensic anthropology has a great deal to offer to these conversations, not least in showing some of the ways in which forms of marginalization can be incorporated into the body, and demonstrating the visible effects of poverty and discrimination, whether through oral pathologies (Soler, Beatrice, and Martínez, this volume), or in the skeleton itself (Winburn et al., this volume). Moore and Kim's chapter on the osteology of poverty in Detroit shows how extreme poverty can be embodied in the skeleton. Biological anthropologists and archaeologists are used to seeing the evidence of unhealed disease lesions in the skeletons of people who lived in the time before modern medicine and antibiotics, including the extremely painful and profound changes to the skeleton that can be wrought by diseases such as syphilis or leprosy. It is disturbing in the extreme to see untreated conditions expressed in the bones of marginalized populations from the modern-day United States. Not only do Moore and Kim document the evidence of blunt and sharp force trauma, but they also lay out how the effects of frostbite, untreated dental pathologies, advanced rheumatoid arthritis, and nutritional deficiencies such as scurvy can be seen clearly in the skeletons that have been analyzed by them as part of forensic anthropology casework for Detroit, Michigan from 2014 to 2020. Forensic anthropology has a powerful capacity to make structural violence visible, in a way that is immediate and compelling, even shocking. This is the strength of the case study and one of the reasons why it has been so central in many popular forensic narratives (e.g., Bass and Jefferson 2003; Maples and Browning 1994). The case study makes structural violence personal and biographical—shifting it from something that is largely dispersed, downplayed, and ignored or hidden to something intensely personal and recognizable (cf. Farmer 1996). This evidence is essential for a full accounting of such forms of violence and can be mobilized toward potential future change. The chapters here show how much more can be said about and with the forensic evidence of the dead. They refuse to let these stories resolve into particular ungeneralizable histories, but insist that they remain embedded in a wider frame that sees the patterns and inequities that give rise to them. The research that is outlined in this book is doing vital work not only in shifting the forensic conversation toward these questions, but also in intervening into how state and local forensic investigations take place. This wider frame of research has implications for how forensic anthropologists are trained and will surely continue to encourage a more engaged perspective with wider debates in anthropology and elsewhere, and with policy implications for both the dead and the living.

Although there is increasing specialization within forensic anthropology, to the extent that some practitioners suggest it be recognized as its own discipline (Passalacqua, Pilloud, and Congram 2021), many of the chapters in this volume also show how generative and important it is to be in conversation with colleagues across the anthropological field, including medical anthropology and archaeology. The chapter by Winburn and colleagues draws forensic anthropology together with trends in medical anthropology and social epidemiology; New and colleagues mobilize structural vulnerability theory to examine class and racial disparities in genetic family reference samples for missing service members from the Korean War; Mijal and Willey usefully introduce insights from disability studies to inform their analysis of the demographic profile of those killed in the 2018 Camp Fire in northern California. Engagement with the medical anthropology literature leads Winburn and colleagues to explore the potential of a bioanthropological structural vulnerability profile as an additional element of the biological profile. This advocates a more regularized and consistently carried out analysis of factors that are likely to impact the skeletons of socially marginalized individuals, offering one potential route to highlight the relationships between particular case studies and broader structural issues. DiGangi and Santamaria Vargas draw on work by medical anthropologists Nancy Scheper-Hughes and Philippe Bourgois (2004) to note that structural violence itself is not homogenous but rather operates along a continuum that marks people and communities differentially at different times and places.

These differential effects are explored in Byrnes, Belcher, and Woollen's chapter, which takes up the widespread perception that marginalized groups are overrepresented in the forensic archive and looks to see whether and how this is substantiated demographically in their work for the City and County of Honolulu, Hawai'i. They draw upon Klinenberg's "social autopsy" method (2002) to show how the demographic profile of the decedents that they have examined for the Department of the Medical Examiner in Honolulu is shaped by social and political conditions, that themselves are embedded in Hawai'i's long history of settler colonialism. They note that "the whole archive tells us about social patterns that the individual reports miss." A demographic approach allows forensic anthropologists to address systemic failures in public health or law enforcement and offers powerful grounds for advocacy and activism. This is important work; allowing arguments to be built that cannot be easily dismissed. This kind of nuanced approach demands to be replicated across other cities to show how the effects of different risk factors play out among various populations to better understand what is shared among these different sites and how forms of structural violence both vary and alter according to local conditions.

One of the themes that comes through strongly in these chapters is the ways in which structural inequities endure in death, whether via vulnerabilities that make some individuals or communities more susceptible to state abandonment and/or violent death (Byrnes, Belcher, and Woollen; Moore and Kim; Mijal and Willey, this volume), discriminatory medicolegal practices themselves (e.g., Bird and Bird; Haug, this volume); in the lack of available information to aid identification (as outlined by New et al. for the Korean War dead); in forms of social marginalization and stigmatized conditions that obstruct efforts to properly identify the dead (as outlined by Winburn et al.; Andronowski and Depp). The chapters show that structural violence takes on new and different forms after death, and that there is value in paying attention to how postmortem violence persists and transmutes. The chapter by Kaplan and colleagues considers the impact of the so-called Prevention through Deterrence border enforcement strategies on the bodies of the dead at Tres Norias cemetery in South Texas. They describe how necropolitical violence is continuously enacted through practices around recovery and burial, particularly through the classificatory work that informs the burial of the most vulnerable and impoverished members of society. The bodies of those who die attempting to cross the border are buried together with the bodies of others positioned as marginal, and at the same time distinctions are made between them through mortuary treatment. This management of the dead is part of a long tradition of differential burial of the so-called unclaimed dead in Anglo-American legal traditions, dating back to the Anatomy Acts of the early to mid-nineteenth century (Richardson 1987; Sappol 2002; Blakely and Harrington 1997). Archaeologically we see a history of similar distinctions made in death even among the most marginal members of society. In the United Kingdom, a similar pattern is found historically among the bodies of the "unclaimed"; although buried in mass graves or with little distinction, they were generally laid out on their backs with hands placed carefully. In contrast, the criminal dead were deposited in the ground with little care as to how they lay, and sometimes, if they had been autopsied, no attempt to repair the bodies before disposal (Cherryson, Crossland, and Tarlow 2012; Crossland 2009). There is a kind of postmortem punishment of the dead going on here, something with a very long tradition in Euro-American anatomical practices—what is very clear in the treatment described by Kaplan and colleagues is the way in which these migrant bodies are similarly being positioned as criminal bodies even in death. This demonstrates the ways in which other more familiar forms of postmortem violence—such as the failure to search for relatives, or to properly document the missing—are accompanied by physical postmortem violence and dehumanized again through mortuary practice.

It is essential to attend to these persistent forms of postmortem violence, not only as a matter of equity and justice, but also because of the ways in which these conditions of violence impact forensic anthropological assessment and analysis. Winburn and colleagues make a strong case for the need to take better account of the ways in which the stressors involved in social marginalization are incorporated into the body, and how this can be expressed as apparent premature aging in elements of the skeleton. Similarly, Andronowski and Depp note that the negative judgments associated with risk factors such as "mental illness, poor health, substance abuse disorders, and traits that lead to social exclusion" can lead to a lack of attention to them in death. They show how these factors can interact with other aspects of life history to influence bone metabolism, potentially affecting the results of skeletal analyses, whether histological or macroscopic. For example, opioid use has the potential to depress osteon counts, and to increase porosity and pitting of bones, both effects that can influence age-at-death estimations, and are likely to be compounded by a range of other complicating factors. These chapters show that without further study to better understand this interplay of risk factors, the effects of extreme poverty, illness, and substance abuse will continue to contribute to the non- or mis-identification of human remains.

These questions of postmortem violence extend into the classificatory language and practices used by forensic practitioners around and of the dead. Bird and Bird observe the tension between the need for "purposeful, tactful and considerate labeling" to help in the identification of unknown persons and the reinscription of social marginalization in death through dehumanizing or disparaging terminology. Haug's thoughtful contribution explores how marginalized gender identities are approached (or not) by forensic anthropology. This contribution foregrounds an important and difficult question around the forensic ascription of sex and its relationship to gender. Haug notes that sex is generally treated as a binary in forensic contexts, so creating three categories, "male, female, or unknown." Gender is then understood to somehow float on top of this as a form of social elaboration of biological sex. Haug draws on Judith Butler's work to expand recognition of gender diversity (2004); in addition to her critique of the sex-gender distinction, her insistence on the performativity of sex itself is helpful (1993), both for thinking about how osteological practice around human remains normatively reinscribes sex through the process of sexing the skeleton, but also for putting the biological ground of binary sex into question. The issues around how to recognize gender-diverse individuals in a system where sex must always be rendered as a binary are reminiscent of the related issues around identifying race or ancestry (DiGangi and Bethard 2021); in both cases forensic anthropologists are forced into defining bodies in terms of dominant classifications of people as raced or as sexed. However, as human osteologists recognize, skeletons do not fall into a rigid binary of male and female but rather grade from one set of characteristics to another. This chapter, therefore, opens up a wider question of how sex itself is seen and conveyed in forensic work, as much as how that is understood to underwrite questions of gender. The question of how skeletons are sexed and placed within a gendered classificatory system would benefit from being considered together with the question of ancestry to think further about how both systems of analysis were developed in tandem, in the context of social formations and expectations that thankfully no longer hold the force that they once did, and are coming under more sustained critical examination (e.g., Watkins 2018).

This re-examining of established practices in forensic work also encompasses a careful questioning of the epistemological foundations that have long been understood to underpin the field, especially in the United States. Winburn and colleagues grapple with the question of "cognitive bias" and Bird and Bird note that "although those in the medicolegal community strive for pure objectivity, we are never separate from the social, historical, and political forces of the structures in which we operate." Following Winburn and Clemmons, they argue for an approach of "mitigated objectivity" which works to recognize and eliminate bias (2021). The question of objectivity also extends beyond issues of bias and the effects of social and historical context on categories of analysis. The forensic anthropological imagination of the mid- to late twentieth century was formed around an ethos of objectivity that tied the work of science to an affective demeanor that fostered a refusal or dampening down of strong emotions. This has been clung to and proclaimed in much of the popular literature on forensic anthropology (Crossland 2011, 2015), and yet it could be productively challenged and rethought. Research by historians of science Lorraine Daston and Peter Galison on objectivity is useful to think with here (2007). Tracing changes in the standards and expectations for scientific images, they show how concepts of objectivity have shifted across the centuries. The work of objectivity is not established through any historically stable set of standards, but rather in response to the changing conditions of scientific production. In this sense, we are in a moment where forensic objectivity may well be altering again, moving to take better account of the feelings that are caught up in forensic anthropological work, of the personhood of the dead that are examined, and of the potential role of forensic practitioners as advocates for the living and the dead. This is to reimagine the role of the forensic anthropologist, as mediators "between the deceased, their families, and the broader community" (Soler, Beatrice, and Martínez, this volume), and as involved in postmortem care for the dead (also Reineke 2019). There is sometimes some concern expressed that if forensic anthropologists are overly critical of concepts of objectivity that this will undermine the integrity of the evidence they produce for the courts. However, it is already clear that there are multiple evidential regimes in play in forensic work, and that courts and scientists also have divergent definitions of truth and its relationship to evidence (Crossland 2013). Not only does this provide wide scope to take a critical orientation to established notions of objectivity (e.g., Winburn 2018), but it has also opened the way for forensic anthropology in North America to follow the lead of humanitarian forensic work elsewhere in the world, to work more closely with families, interest groups, and activists. Rather than undermining their work, arguably this is instead shifting the way that objectivity is understood and deployed by forensic specialists.

All the chapters in this book touch on this interesting question of advocacy. New and colleagues build on their work with the Korean War dead to argue for more interdisciplinary engagement by forensic anthropologists with advocacy groups and/or non-governmental organizations (NGOs) as a way to work with and support living relatives and descendants. This book offers new ways to imagine forensic anthropology, showing how productive conversations with medical anthropology and other fields can be, and contributing to the ongoing critical interrogation of categories and practices that have long been part of forensic anthropological work. Moving away from the established pattern in the United States of focusing on individual forensic case studies enables practitioners to engage in wider anthropological debates and to have an impact on policymaking. It also brings U.S. domestic casework into more fluid conversation with anthropologists of all kinds working in contexts of mass violence and humanitarian investigation. The volume shows why forensic anthropology is important: it deals with people who, for a variety of reasons, die alone or violently and who were denied access to medical care or to public health systems. Similarly, it records those who are often positioned outside of regular mortuary practice. These are people whose circumstances are rarely recorded and whose conditions were relatively uncared for, in life and death. The chapters show the power of individual case histories to be seen in aggregate to identify and make visible wider forms of violence, and to be taken individually to narrate the personal and painful impacts of contemporary socioeconomic life. All the authors show in different ways how the absence of care is not an oversight. Rarely is it a simple failure to give care where care was due; rather a lack of care is made visible as a sustained and pervasive form of violence that is underpinned by policy and that reproduces deeply embedded attitudes around race, gender and class, attitudes that encode prejudice but that have been rarely queried or brought to notice. This volume opens the question of not only how forensic anthropology is imagined, but also what it might bring to the field of anthropology and to the humanities and social sciences more broadly. How might we think *from* forensic anthropology, not only to bring the bodies of the marginalized into view, but also to bring new questions and theoretical issues into view, and to act as advocates for the dead and the living? In this volume, I see great potential to broaden the reach of forensic anthropology—to reimagine its role in anthropology as a whole, as well as the work that it does in investigating conditions of structural violence in the world today.

REFERENCES

Anderson, Bruce E., and M. Kate Spradley. 2016. "The Role of the Anthropologist in the Identification of Migrant Remains in the American Southwest." *Academic Forensic Pathology* 6, no. 3: 432–38. doi: 10.23907/2016.044

Bass, William M., and Jon Jefferson. 2003. *Death's Acre: Inside the Legendary Forensic Lab the Body Farm, Where the Dead Do Tell Tales.* New York: Penguin.

Beatrice, Jared S., Angela Soler, Robin C. Reineke, and Daniel E. Martínez. 2021. "Skeletal Evidence of Structural Violence among Undocumented Migrants from Mexico and Central America." *American Journal of Physical Anthropology* 176, no. 4: 584–605. https://doi.org/10.1002/ajpa.24391

Blakely, Robert L., and Judith M. Harrington. 1997. *Bones in the Basement: Postmortem Racism in Nineteenth-Century Medical Training.* Washington: Smithsonian Institution Press.

Butler, Judith. 1993. *Bodies That Matter: On the Discursive Limits of "Sex."* New York: Routledge.

——— *Undoing Gender.* 2004. New York: Routledge.

Cherryson, Annia, Zoë Crossland, and Sarah Tarlow. 2012. *A Fine and Private Place: The Archaeology of Death and Burial in Post-Medieval Britain and Ireland.* Leicester: Leicester University Monographs.

Crossland, Zoë. 2009. "Acts of Estrangement: The Making of Self and Other through Exhumation." *Archaeological Dialogues* 16, no. 1: 102–25. doi:10.1017/S1380203809002827

——— 2011. "The Archaeology of Contemporary Conflict." In *The Oxford Handbook of the Archaeology of Ritual and Religion*, edited by Timothy Insoll, 285–306. Oxford: Oxford University Press. DOI: 10.1093/oxfordhb/9780199232444.013.0020

——— 2013. "Evidential Regimes of Forensic Archaeology." *Annual Review of Anthropology* 42: 121–37. https://doi.org/10.1146/annurev-anthro-092412-155513

——— 2015. "Writing Forensic Anthropology. Transgressive Representations." In *Disturbing Bodies: Perspectives on Forensic Anthropology*, edited by Zoë Crossland and Rosemary A. Joyce, 103–20. Santa Fe: School for Advanced Research Press.

Daston, Lorraine, and Peter Galison. *Objectivity*. 2007. Boston: Zone Books.

De León, Jason. 2015. *The Land of Open Graves*. Oakland: University of California Press.

DiGangi, Elizabeth A., and Jonathan D. Bethard. 2021. "Uncloaking a Lost Cause: Decolonizing Ancestry Estimation in the United States." *American Journal of Physical Anthropology* 175, no. 2: 422–36. https://doi.org/10.1002/ajpa.24212

EAAF. 1992. *Annual Summary of National and International Activities (January 1991-February 1992)*. Buenos Aires: Argentine Forensic Anthropology Team.

Farmer, Paul. 1996. "On Suffering and Structural Violence: A View from Below." *Daedalus* 125, no. 1: 261–83.

Giordano, Alberto, and M. Katherine Spradley. 2017. "Migrant Deaths at the Arizona–Mexico Border: Spatial Trends of a Mass Disaster." *Forensic Science International* 280: 200–12. doi: 10.1016/j.forsciint.2017.07.031

Klinenberg, Eric. 2002. *Heat Wave: A Social Autopsy of Disaster in Chicago*. Chicago: University of Chicago Press.

Maples, William R., and Michael Browning. 1994. *Dead Men Do Tell Tales: The Strange and Fascinating Cases of a Forensic Anthropologist*. New York: Doubleday.

Nixon, Rob. 2011. *Slow Violence and the Environmentalism of the Poor*. Cambridge: Harvard University Press.

Passalacqua, Nicholas V., Marin A. Pilloud, and Derek Congram. 2021. "Forensic Anthropology as a Discipline." *Biology* 10, no. 8: 691. https://doi.org/10.3390/biology10080691

Reineke, Robin. 2019. "Necroviolence and Postmortem Care along the US-México Border." In *The Border and its Bodies: The Embodiment of Risk along the U.S-México Line*, edited by Thomas E. Sheridan and Randall H. McGuire, 144–172. Tucson: University of Arizona Press.

Richardson, Ruth. 1987. *Death, Dissection and the Destitute*. London: Routledge and Kegan Paul.

Ritter, Nancy. 2007. "Missing Persons and Unidentified Remains: The Nation's Silent Mass Disaster." *National Institute of Justice Journal* 256, no. 7: 2–7.

Rosenblatt, Adam. 2015. *Digging for the Disappeared*. Redwood City: Stanford University Press.

Sanford, Victoria. 2008. "From Genocide to Feminicide: Impunity and Human Rights in Twenty-First Century Guatemala." *Journal of Human Rights* 7, no. 2: 104–22. https://doi.org/10.1080/14754830802070192

Sappol, Michael. 2002. *A Traffic of Dead Bodies: Anatomy and Embodied Social Identity in Nineteenth-Century America*. Princeton, N.J.: Princeton University Press.

Scheper-Hughes, Nancy, and Philippe Bourgois. 2004. "Introduction: Making Sense of Violence." In *Violence in War and Peace, An Anthology*, edited by Nancy Scheper Hughes and Phillipe Bourgois, 1–27. Oxford: Blackwell.

Schindel, Estela. 2019. "Death by 'Nature': The European Border Regime and the Spatial Production of Slow Violence." *Environment and Planning C: Politics and Space* 40, no. 2: 428–446. https://doi.org/10.1177%2F2399654419884948

Watkins, Rachel. 2018. "Anatomical Collections as the Anthropological Other: Some Considerations." In *Bioarchaeological Analyses and Bodies: New Ways of Knowing Anatomical and Archaeological Skeletal Collections*, edited by Pamela K. Stone, 27–47. Cham: Springer. https://doi.org/10.1007/978-3-319-71114-0_3

Winburn, Allysha P. 2018. "Subjective with a Capital S? Issues of Objectivity in Forensic Anthropology." In *Forensic Anthropology. Theoretical Framework and Scientific Basis*, edited by C. Clifford Boyd Jr. and Donna Boyd, 21–38. New York: Wiley. https://doi.org/10.1002/9781119226529.ch2

Winburn, Allysha P., and Chaunesey M.J. Clemmons. 2021. "Objectivity is a myth that harms the practice and diversity of forensic science." *Forensic Science International: Synergy* 3: 100196. doi: 10.1016/j.fsisyn.2021.100196

Acknowledgments

We would like to express deep gratitude to those who helped peer review the individual chapters in this volume (twenty-three peer reviewers in total!), helping to elevate the impact of the volume as a whole as well as the individual chapters' themes and importance. As well, multiple graduate students helped to review the formatting of the chapters during the developmental stages, including Taylor Flaherty, Heather Frigiola, and Katherine Gaddis.

This volume draws upon inspiration from our organized Executive podium session "Toward the Margins: Accounting for the Marginalized in Forensic Anthropology" presented at the 120th Annual Meetings of the American Anthropological Association in November 2021. Most of the presenters from that session also contributed chapters to this volume based on their podium. We are grateful to our colleagues who have contributed thought-provoking pieces to this volume, taking on our challenge wholeheartedly to engage with social theory to frame their work from a different perspective than the "normal" objective praxis of forensic anthropology.

JFB: I specifically recall thinking of my chapter's focus in 2018, and the impetus for this volume, after working on multiple forensic anthropology cases involving individuals who had experienced houselessness in Honolulu, HI. Because the Medical Examiner's Office in Honolulu is situated next to temporary houseless camps and a shelter, the houselessness crisis was not far from my mind while consulting on forensic cases. I began to wonder whether I may one day go to the Medical Examiner's Office to work with the anonymous remains of a person who, some months or years earlier, I had walked past at the same location. While resting in the shade outside the walls of the Medical Examiner's Office, did houseless people ever think that they may one day die alone and their remains would end up in earthly limbo, just inside those very same walls? Upon conducting a literature review of forensic anthropology casework publications, I realized the dearth that existed in our field and the opportunity to try to remedy this. Inviting scholars from diverse backgrounds and career stages has enhanced this volume's efforts to amplify the voices of the missing, unidentified, disappeared, or otherwise marginal-ized people who experienced untimely deaths. Recognizing that the marginal-ized represent the majority of forensic anthropology casework nationally and internationally not only allows us the opportunity to tell individual osteobio-graphical narratives, but also obligates us as scientists and practitioners to become public advocates of systemic societal reform.

ISC: This volume required unpaid work from many different scholars, who donated their time during a pandemic to make it possible. I am thankful to my colleague at UNLV, Jennifer Byrnes, who proposed we collaborated on this volume. Although interested in different forms of violence as a cultural anthropologist I had never fully engaged the work that forensic anthropolo-gists do, so I took this as an opportunity to learn about the important work they do, and to rethink in how cultural anthropologist think about violence and death. The volume has opened many possible paths of scholarly reflec-tion and action.

Introduction

Jennifer F. Byrnes and Iván Sandoval-Cervantes

John Donne, an English poet who was part of the metaphysical poetry movement, wrote, "Death comes equally to us all, and makes us all equal when it comes." Although the first part continues to be true, the second part does not. The chapters in this volume show that death, and what transpires after death, preserves socioeconomic differences and, in some cases, deepens the marginalization of some communities. Death, thus, does not make us equal, but actually presents opportunities to further dehumanize individuals and their communities as the lives and deaths of individuals continue going unnoticed, unmissed, and without proper social and/or cultural recognition. However, as this volume shows, this is a matter of justice, in which anthropologists, specifically forensic anthropologists, can intervene.

At the core of how these differences are preserved and furthered even after death lies the concept of structural violence. One of the central elements of structural violence, as elaborated by Galtung (1969) and Farmer (2004), is that it must pass unperceived by the subjects of such violence. Looking at structural violence "focuses attention on the often unnoticeable systems (legal, political, economic and sociocultural) and social relations that are part of the fabric of society and that shape individuals' experiences, including health and wellbeing" (Nandagiri, Coast, and Strong 2020).

One of the factors that complicates studying structural violence is its intentional invisibility; another important factor is that structural violence is often exerted from multiple sources. As the contributors in this volume show, structural violence originates from state actors, such as government agents; non-state actors, such as transnational corporations and well-meaning organizations; and even from the academic disciplines and professionals. Structural violence, thus, becomes particularly troublesome because it underlies many beliefs that often go unchallenged in multiple settings.

In fact, structural violence is woven into the fabric of how life itself is constituted and the categories that we use to describe, and act upon, the world. Analyzing and disentangling these different forms of oppression, which are structured through these almost invisible categories, also means taking a deeper look into the role that colonialism and capitalism have in the ongoing processes of marginalization that involve race, gender, sexual orientation, and class among other social identities (Crenshaw 1991). These factors contribute to the postmortem treatment and care of the deceased, evoking what Zoë Crossland (2000, 147) calls "the emotional relationship between the living and the dead." The ways in which the dead are created "as bodies and as people" is not only a commentary on the social status of the deceased, but mirrors the ongoing sociopolitical negotiation between the living and the dead. Here we understand that both categories of "the living" and "the dead" encompass a wide array of social communities with multiple fluid identities. When we talk about this constant (re)negotiation between the living and the dead, we situate the exercises of forensic anthropology in specific social, economic, and political contexts. In this way, aspects of structural violence become evident, especially when thinking about another form of structural violence: *necroviolence.*

Jason De León has called this particular form of dehumanization that occurs postmortem "necroviolence." For De León, necroviolence "[is] violence performed and produced through the specific treatment of corpses that is perceived to be offensive, sacrilegious, or inhumane by the perpetrator, the victim (and her or his cultural group), or both" (2015, 69). Throughout the volume, we see the ways in which social and personal identities are directly tied to corpses and, thus, the failure on the part of governments and other actors to recognize such identities is also a failure to see those individuals as part of larger communities. This might seem like an unintentional outcome of forensic science, but in fact it speaks to broader systemic issues that are often unacknowledged or overlooked by practices often considered "objective." Additionally, the failure to recognize and identify specific bodies, with social identities largely from marginalized groups, contributes to the erasure of those identities and the communities they represent.

The importance of the concept of necroviolence is that it extends the application of concepts such as biopower and necropower, advanced by Foucault and Mbembe respectively, beyond life and the living. For Foucault, power is exercised through the division and management of people and how they live through "governmentality," that is how individuals regulate their bodily behaviors. Building on this concept, Mbembe incorporated the idea that politics is the work of death and sovereignty is exercised as the state's right to kill (2003, 16–17), actively reconstituting the political order "as a form of organization of death" (2019, 7). Yet, when we return to the question posed by Mbembe himself: "What place is given to life, death, and the human body (in particular the wounded or slain body)? How are they inscribed in the order of power?" (2003, 12), we find that often the analysis of how power is operationalized on bodies is not analyzed beyond the moment of death. Thus, the concept of *necroviolence* moves the analysis of power forward by showing how human bodies, deceased bodies, are inscribed in the order of power in different ways and through different mechanisms.

This concept of *necroviolence* can be applied to numerous cases. For example, speaking about necroviolence in Palestina, Randa May Wahbee (2020) states that *racism* and *colonialism* are central in understanding how necroviolence further dehumanizes the deceased preserving racial hierarchies. However, as Hamdar (2018) shows in the case of Syria, the concept of "necroviolence" also helps to reflect on how corpses can, through their representations, become symbols of "post-mortem resistance."

Although not using the concept of necroviolence directly, Jonah Rubin (2020) shows how the exhumation of Spanish Civil War victims can allow for the reincorporation of the deceased into an alternative account of democracy by making their stories visible in context of historical opacity. In a similar way, the significance of forensic anthropology in other contexts of violence and democratic transitions, such as Latin America, shows that historical accountability in understanding how the deceased and the disappeared are treated have an impact in how societies, at large, conceptualize questions of truth, justice, and reconciliation (e.g., Theidon 2010).

In describing the current political situation in Mexico, Rosanna Reguillo (2021) also pays close attention to showing how, for example, Mbembe's necropolitics as the work of death continues to expand its reach. For Reguillo, Mbembe's necropolitics is no longer a metaphor, as shown by the ongoing massacres and acts of mass violence in Mexico. Instead, killing and dying are no longer sufficient to feed the necromachine that requires ever more brutal forms of extinguishing life. The treatment of dead bodies in specific ways responds not only to structural violence, discussed above, but also to what Rita Segato calls "expressive violence": that is, violence that has no objective but showcasing complete power over a population (2013). Violence over dead bodies is not only an expression of power but a way to exercise power itself; a form of necro-empowerment (see Valencia 2010, 15). In the case of Mexico, this sort of violence is deeply ingrained in how bureaucratic processes treat dead bodies and the disappeared. This is manifested in the "forensic crisis"— saturated morgues, a lack of information about the exact number of bodies and the miscarried processes of identification of such bodies, and the active discouragement of activists seeking their disappeared loved ones. Those who seek justice for the disappeared often become the embodiment of Agamben's "bare life" themselves (1998): existing liminally between the human and the animal, between culture and nature. However, the potential of forensic anthropologists is felt in Mexico, where they have played a key role in trying to attain some form of justice through the Equipo Mexicano de Antropología Forense A.C. (Mexican Team of Forensic Anthropology) a civil association led by Roxana Enríquez Farías (2020). Although not directly addressed in this volume, we bring up the case of Mexico as a way to bridge what many of the chapters in this volume demonstrate: the potential of forensic anthropology to tell politically relevant stories about how different populations are treated posthumously in different contexts.

ORGANIZATION OF THE VOLUME

This volume bridges the gap between forensic anthropology and cultural anthropology in how both disciplines describe and theorize the dead, highlighting the potential for interdisciplinary scholarship. We challenged contributors to interrogate their forensic anthropology work on how marginalization occurs in the postmortem treatment of human bodies. Presenting research from across the world, this volume emphasizes how forensic anthropologists engage with social theory to understand how marginalization influences forensic science and how forensic science can create marginalization. In addition, the chapters in this volume address how forensic anthropology can address larger ethical questions that cross disciplinary boundaries.

As applied disciplines dealing with some of the most marginalized people in our society, forensic anthropologists have the potential to shed light on important and persistent social issues that we face today. Over the last several decades, forensic anthropologists have successfully pursued research agendas primarily focused on the development of individual biological profiles (e.g., sex, age, ancestry), time since death, recovery, and identification. Few forensic anthropologists, however, have taken a step back from their lab bench to write about how and why people become forensic cases or place their work in a larger theoretical context. Thus, this volume challenges forensic anthropologists to consider how we can use our toolkit and databases to address larger social issues and quandaries that we face in a world where some are spared from becoming forensic anthropology cases and others are not. As witnesses to violence, crimes against humanity, and the embodied consequences of structural violence, we have the opportunity—and arguably, the responsibility—to transcend the traditional medicolegal confines of our small subdiscipline, by synthesizing forensic anthropology casework into theoretically grounded social science with potentially transformative potential. As ethical researchers, we must embrace our responsibility to reveal these truths, even if they go against the grain of mainstream forensic anthropology research. As anthropologists, we have the opportunity to go beyond case-specific description and analysis to understand what our work reveals about humanity.

Anecdotally, many forensic anthropologists probably have noticed certain demographic trends and speculated about the larger meaning, but statistics are hard to come by. For example, Indigenous, Black, and Brown bodies find their way into forensic anthropology casework in North America at disproportionately higher rates compared to white bodies (Kochanek et al. 2019). However, they are also far less likely to participate in body donation programs that contribute to the development of forensic anthropology methods used to determine biological profile and which make it harder to positively identify non-White people using forensic anthropology methods (Winburn et al. 2022). Thus, the colonial specters of racism and socioeconomic inequality not only increased the mortality rate of marginalized groups—hastening their lives—they continue to haunt them in death. How might forensic anthropologists advocate for the often anonymous people who become forensic anthropology cases? Moreover, women of color as well as transgender individuals contribute to forensic anthropology casework and missing persons databanks in North America at higher rates than these demographics exist in the general population (Human Rights Campaign 2021). Can increased awareness of this reality bring attention to the crises of femicide and transgender-directed violence? Can we move past binary sex determinations to recognize the embodied experience of people with trans- and non-binary gender identities? Verification of anecdotal observations with statistical evidence as well as osteobiographies will be an important step forward for forensic anthropologists becoming more than just expert technicians and witnesses, but advocates for the marginalized, persecuted, and voiceless. This volume is unique in that it incorporates and discusses multiple theoretical paradigms, investigating and questioning how we know what we know about marginalization. Meaningfully engaged with social theory, this volume looks at how marginalized populations can transform how we think about forensic science within larger conceptual debates.

Forensic anthropologists have only sporadically published their work leveraging social theory frameworks (e.g., Latham and O'Daniel 2018). Even though anecdotally many have expressed interest in sociocultural links to their work, few studies critically incorporate socially engaged theoretical frameworks (e.g., Beatrice et al. 2021; Goad 2020). The major theoretical foci of this volume are on paradigms applicable to marginalized peoples examined by forensic anthropologists. However, it will appeal to scholars across the humanities, social sciences, and medical professions interested in analyzing structural violence and power. As the United States struggles with social unrest related to issues involving people of color and systemic racism, other scholars will likely find the topics discussed in this volume of interest as they intersect with many of the social injustices seen and experienced by minoritized peoples. This volume is inherently interdisciplinary, and therefore those engaged in research in the fields of critical race theory, women's studies, the history of medicine, sociology, clinical medicine, public health, criminal justice, and anthropology will be interested in the volume. This socially contextualized understanding of how various social identities intersect to produce a marginalized experience in life and in death will serve to further interdisciplinary discussion on the topic and therefore appeal to a wide audience. Our volume demonstrates that in various geographical regions domestically and internationally an individual's intersectional identity plays a deciding role in who lives, dies, and who remains unidentified based on gender, disability, race, socioeconomic status, sexual orientation, and ethnicity.

Part I: At the Border: International and Domestic Efforts towards Identification

The chapters in the "At the Border" section provide international and domestic perspectives on those who become unidentified, disappeared, and/or missing. Chapter discussions engage with various social theoretical approaches to frame who goes missing and what systemic issues exist that contribute to their disappearance and ultimately their identification.

Soler, Beatrice, and Martínez (Chapter 1) focus geographically on the U.S.-Mexico border and those whose remains are, or presumed to be, undocumented migrants from Central America and Mexico. Utilizing the previously established biosocial approach (Anderson 2008), the authors use oral pathologies as visible lines of evidence to reveal the invisible structural violence inflicted upon migrant bodies. The authors' use of stigma is at the foundation of their argument that oral pathologies are visible signs of the lack of access to proper healthcare and thus an embodied and potentially visible sign of poverty.

Kaplan and colleagues (Chapter 2) present a unique situation in South Texas in which legal loopholes in death investigations have led to unidentified human remains from presumed undocumented migrants not being provided equitable postmortem care. Through the lens of biopower and structural violence, the authors use a case study from a cemetery that contained the remains of unidentified but presumed undocumented migrants and indigent local individuals. They argue that these two different groups of individuals have similarities in their postmortem treatment, in which they have been relegated to forgotten spaces and thus structurally disappeared due to their intersectional identities.

DiGangi and Santamaria Vargas (Chapter 3) present the complex history of violence and forensic anthropology work in Colombia. By providing fine-grained context to the geopolitical situation, they illuminate the structural groundwork laid over decades of conflict that come to a head via the violence experienced by impoverished rural villagers. The authors argue that capitalism has restricted living victims' agency, which is only exacerbated by the ongoing political unrest. Lastly, they draw attention to the blurred lines of victim and perpetrator, but make clear that the vast majority of the victims are those from low socioeconomic backgrounds who are disproportionately affected by both structural and direct violence.

Bird and Bird (Chapter 4) utilize the concept of stigma to frame how discriminatory language use within medicolegal death investigations adversely affects the identification of missing and unidentified remains of people across the United States. The authors make clear that the majority of those who comprise the missing and unidentified are derived mostly from vulnerable and at-risk communities, and thus there is a continuation of unequal treatment beyond the life of those individuals into their postmortem care. The identification disparities that the authors draw attention to are further exacerbated by depreciatory language choices from those in positions of power. Thus, the authors recommend that an equity-based approach to postmortem care be applied for the long-term missing and unidentified.

Part II: At the Intersection: Social Identities and Forensic Anthropology

The chapters in the "At the Intersection" section focus on the various ways that social identities intersect, creating unique identities that are differentially impacted and oppressed through structural violence and vulnerabilities. As with previous chapters, discussions engage with various social theoretical approaches to frame what systemic and structural issues exist that differentially impact marginalized groups in life and in death.

Winburn and colleagues (Chapter 5) propose a provocative theoretical framework from medical anthropology to help conceptualize the embodied forms of violence that forensic anthropologists encounter in their casework. They explore the various manifestations of violence that may become embodied, particularly by those of marginalized social identities, and how these physically embodied skeletal changes may impact the biological profile produced by a forensic anthropologist. They draw on the provocative "weathering hypothesis" to theoretically ask how this concept explains the development and application of specific forensic anthropology methods.

Mijal and Willey (Chapter 6) present a case study from the Camp Fire Communities, where the 2018 Northern California wildfire produced differential mortality among community members. By weaving disability theory as well as demography and disaster mortality concepts with their contextualized dataset, they lay out how the structural vulnerabilities of these communities that existed prior to the wildfire contributed to the disaster mortality profile of primarily elderly and/or impaired community members.

Haug (Chapter 7) provides a queer critique of sex determination, a key component of the biological profile. He argues that while it is widely acknowledged that sex and gender are fluid and non-binary, forensic anthropologists continue to perpetuate the male-female binary in their method developments and casework. This lack of recognition allows for the systemic erasure of marginalized gender identities by means of misidentification, higher rates of cold cases, as well as perpetuating violence via the postmortem treatment of these vulnerable individuals. While acknowledging the logistical difficulties and limitations, Haug calls for forensic anthropologists to take ownership of their work and become advocates and activists for people who are especially vulnerable due to their intersecting identities. He includes recommendations such as utilizing appropriate and accurate terminology, becoming familiar with gender identities and gender- or sex-affirming surgeries that may be observed skeletally, as well as increasing research efforts to include those of gender-diverse identities.

Moore and Kim (Chapter 8) use the biology of poverty model (Crooks 1998) to frame their forensic anthropology casework derived from Detroit, MI. The authors historically and socially situate Detroit, laying the foundation to make visible the invisible structural inequalities that exist and that are complexly entangled in the lives and deaths of those from socially marginalized groups. Moore and Kim further the biology of poverty model by incorporating embodiment of structural violence inscribed into human remains, referring to this as an osteology of poverty. They situate the cases further by discussing where and how they were deposited as well as their postmortem care (or lack thereof). They conclude by calling on forensic anthropologists to step forward to lead a humanitarian effort as advocates and activists to improve policies and services for the marginalized groups typically overrepresented in domestic casework so those who were made invisible in life are made visible in death.

Byrnes, Belcher, and Woollen (Chapter 9) use the concept of social autopsy to analyze how the houseless community on the Hawaiian Island of Oʻahu resists structural violence through the creation of resilient social networks, yet also how some houseless individuals remain detrimentally isolated from these social networks. By historically contextualizing the development and functioning of a "Local" Hawaiian culture and identity, they suggest that non-local White males who experienced houselessness at the time of their deaths were unlikely to be identified as Local during their life and therefore more likely to die alone. The authors show a paradox: while White individuals are underrepresented in the houseless communities, a disproportionate number of White male individuals who are unhoused experience a lonely death and thus become unmissed persons at higher rates than those who identify as Local and belong to effective social networks.

New and colleagues (Chapter 10) explore how structural vulnerabilities resulting from race and class impact the identification of the missing and unidentified of Korean War era military service members. By using genetic family reference sample (FRS) availability as a proxy for identification success, the authors identify a complex series of feedback cycles that contribute to and reinforce social inequities that exist and persist into the medicolegal realm. They specifically identify that FRSs are missing at double the rate for Black, Latin American, and Asian/Pacific Islander missing military service members compared to Whites. While this disparity has not created an imbalance in identification rates yet, the authors argue that the marked lack of FRSs may lead to inequitable identification distributions with hundreds of individuals remaining unidentifiable. Their work turns the lens of identification disparities toward FRS availability and identifies ways in which inequities experienced due to intersectional identities extend across individuals, families, and time.

Andronowski and Depp (Chapter 11) present some of the first forensic anthropological research and perspective on the impacts of opioid use on the biological profile and trauma assessment. By using a multidisciplinary approach, the authors walk through how the opioid epidemic has differentially affected various demographics within the United States and Canada, such as young to middle-aged males. They provide evidence via original research and case studies that substance abuse directly impacts the biological profile, subsequently affecting the identification process. They conclude by providing recommendations for practitioners that are working on known or suspected cases of chronic-drug users, and also highlight the need for additional research into this line of inquiry in spite of the societal stigma associated with these marginalized groups.

REFERENCES

Agamben, Giorgio. 1998. *Homo Sacer: Sovereign Power and Bare Life.* Stanford: Stanford University Press.
Anderson, Bruce E. 2008. "Identifying the Dead: Methods Utilized by the Pima County (Arizona) Office of the Medical Examiner for Undocumented Border Crossers: 2001-2006." *Journal of Forensic Sciences* 53, no. 1: 8–15. https://doi.org/10.1111/j.1556-4029.2007.00609.x

Beatrice, Jared S., Angela Soler, Robin C. Reineke, and Daniel E. Martínez. 2021. "Skeletal evidence of structural violence among undocumented migrants from Mexico and Central America." *American Journal of Physical Anthropology* 176, no. 4: 584–605.

Crenshaw, Kimberlé W. 1991. "Mapping the margins: Intersectionality, identity politics, and violence against women of color." *Stanford Law Review* 43, no. 6: 1241–99.

Crooks, Deborah L. 1995. "American children at risk: Poverty and its consequences for children's health, growth, and school achievement." *American Journal of Physical Anthropology* 38, no. S21: 57–86. https://doi.org/10.1002/ajpa.1330380605

Crossland, Zoë. 2000. "Buried Lives: Forensic Archaeology and the Disappeared in Argentina." *Archaeological Dialogues* 7, no. 2: 146–159. DOI:10.1017/S1380203800001707

De León, Jason. 2015. *The Land of Open Graves*. Oakland: University of California Press.

Enríquez Farias, Roxana. 2020. "Antropología forense: ritmos de cambio de una disciplina emergente en México." *IdentificaciónHumana.Mx* 4, no. 2:4–7

Farmer, Paul. 2004. "An anthropology of structural violence." *Current Anthropology* 45, no. 3: 305–25. https://doi.org/10.1086/382250

Galtung, Johan. 1969. "Violence, peace, and peace research." *Journal of Peace Research* 6, no. 3: 167–91.

Goad, Gennifer. 2020. "Expanding humanitarian forensic action: An approach to US cold cases." *Forensic Anthropology* 3, no. 1: 50.

Hamdar, Abir. 2018. "The Syrian corpse: the politics of dignity in visual and media representations of the Syrian revolution." *Journal for Cultural Research* 22, no. 1:73–89. DOI: 10.1080/14797585.2018.1429083

Human Rights Campaign. 2021. *Report: An Epidemic of Violence 2021: Fatal Violence Against Transgender and Gender Non-Confirming People in the United States in 2021* https://reports.hrc.org/an-epidemic-of-violence-fatal-violence-against-transgender-and-gender-non-confirming-people-in-the-united-states-in-2021

Kochanek KD, Murphy SL, Xu J, Arias E. 2019. "Deaths: Final data for 2017." *National Vital Statistics Reports* 68, no. 9: 1–77.

Latham, Krista E. and Alyson J. O'Daniel (editors). 2018. *Sociopolitics of Migrant Death and Repatriation: Perspectives from Forensic Science*. Cham: Springer.

Mbembé, Achille. 2003. "Necropolitics." *Public Culture* 15, no. 1: 11–40.

———. 2019. *Necropolitics*. Durham: Duke University Press.

Nandagiri, Rishita, Ernestina Coast, and Joe Strong. 2020. "COVID-19 and Abortion: Making Structural Violence Visible." *International Perspectives on Sexual and Reproductive Health* 46, no. 1: 83–89. https://doi.org/10.1363/46e1320

Reguillo, Rossana. 2021. *Necromáquina: Cuando morir no es suficiente*. NED Ediciones-ITESO Universidad Jesuita de Guadalajara.

Rubin, Jonah S. 2020. "Exhuming Dead Persons: Forensic Science and the Making of Post-Fascists Publics in Spain." *Cultural Anthropology* 35, no. 3: 345–73. https://doi.org/10.14506/ca35.3.01

Segato, Rita. 2013. *La escritura en el cuerpo de las mujeres asesinadas en Ciudad Juárez*. Buenos Aires, Argentina: Tinta Limón.

Theidon, Kimberly. 2010. "Histories of Innocence." In *Localizing Transitional Justice: Interventions and Priorities after Mass Violence,* edited by Rosalind Shaw and Lars Waldorf, with Pierre Hazan, 92–109. Stanford: Stanford University Press.

Valencia, Sayak. 2010. *Capitalismo Gore*. España: Editorial Medusa.

Wahbee, Randa May. 2020. "The Politics of Karameh: Palestinian Burial Rites under the Gun." *Critique of Anthropology* 40, no. 3: 323–40.

Winburn, Allysha P., Antaya Jennings, Dawnie W. Steadman, and Elizabeth A. DiGangi. 2022. "Ancestral diversity in skeletal collections: Perspectives on African American body donation." *Forensic Anthropology* 5, no. 2: 141–52. https://doi.org/10.5744/fa.2020.1023

Part I

AT THE BORDER

INTERNATIONAL AND DOMESTIC EFFORTS TOWARDS IDENTIFICATION

Chapter 1

Oral Pathologies as a Reflection of Structural Violence and Stigma among Undocumented Migrants from Mexico and Central America

Angela Soler, Jared S. Beatrice,
and Daniel E. Martínez

INTRODUCTION

Structural violence as a theoretical framework has recently received a great deal of attention from forensic anthropologists.[1] This is due in large part to the recognition that understanding structural vulnerabilities and the biosocial consequences of structural violence has important implications for forensic casework (Algee-Hewitt, Hughes, and Anderson 2018; Beatrice and Soler 2016; Beatrice et al. 2021; Hughes et al. 2017; Soler and Beatrice 2018; Soler et al. 2019, 2020; Goad 2020; Michael et al. 2021; Reineke and Anderson 2016; this volume). The advantages of an improved understanding of structural vulnerability in specific communities are two-fold: (1) it increases the chances of identification and repatriation of unknown individuals and (2) it provides additional perspective on the deaths—as well as the lives—of communities most represented in forensic casework. As intermediaries between the deceased, their families, and the broader community, forensic practitioners have obligations that extend to humanizing the individuals whose remains we examine through knowledge of, and sensitivity to, their lived experiences.

One important application of the structural violence framework by forensic anthropologists is the investigation of migrant deaths in the U.S.-Mexico borderlands. There is now a robust body of research demonstrating the ways in which structural violence impacts migrants in life, at death, and during the postmortem investigation (Soler et al. 2020). Examples of the effects of structural violence include embodied early life stress (Beatrice et al. 2021; Soler et al. 2019), the preventable deaths of migrants along the U.S.-Mexico border (De León 2015; Martínez et al. 2014; Slack et al. 2018), the difficulties of identifying undocumented individuals who die in the United States (Algee-Hewitt, Hughes, and Anderson 2018; Gocha, Spradley, and Strand 2018; Hughes et al. 2017; Reineke 2013, 2019; Reineke and Anderson 2016), and the embodied effects of ambiguous loss in migrant families searching for missing loved ones (Crocker, Reineke, and Ramos Tovar 2021). In this chapter, we contribute to an awareness of embodied structural violence in undocumented migrants through an examination of oral pathology and indicators of access to oral healthcare. We examine both the causes and consequences of this embodied structural violence through the lens of "stigmatized biologies" (Horton and Barker 2010), as dental pathologies can reveal much about structured access to care and the consequences of possible stigmatization due to visible oral health problems.

DENTAL PATHOLOGY, STRUCTURAL VIOLENCE, AND STIGMA

Pathological conditions of the teeth and jaws are often recorded by anthropologists interested in past behavior because they provide information on diet, nutrition, and subsistence (Lukacs 2012). However, many bioarchaeologists engaged in the clinical literature on the systemic effects of dental pathologies are interested in these conditions because of their potential influence on biological stress and elevated risk of death (DeWitte and Bekvalac 2010; Yaussy and DeWitte 2019). Clinically, oral health status is of broad concern because dental pathologies can lead to systemic inflammation and infection, either directly through bacterial invasion of the circulatory system or indirectly through immune response mechanisms (Cullinan, Ford, and Seymour 2009; Seymour et al. 2007). In living populations, dental disease is associated with a variety of systemic health problems including cardiovascular and respiratory diseases, and diabetes (Cullinan, Ford, and Seymour 2009; Maddi and Scannapieco 2013; Seymour et al. 2007).

When precipitated or exacerbated by factors such as poverty and systemic limitations on access to adequate care, dental pathologies may be viewed as embodied structural violence. As conceived by Galtung (1969, 171), structural violence occurs when power differentials create disparities in access to resources, ultimately resulting in "unequal life chances." In contrast to direct violence perpetrated by individual actors, structural violence creates harm when systemic inequalities structured along social "axes" of gender, ethnicity/race, or socioeconomic status place vulnerable individuals or groups at increased risk of adverse health outcomes, including death (Farmer 1996, 274). The process by which lived experiences of socio-structural factors such as racism and poverty are physically embodied as illness, injury, and death has received substantial attention from a range of scholars examining the impact of social forces on human biologies (Crooks 1995; Farmer 1996, 2004; Goodman 2013; Goodman and Leatherman 1998; Gravlee 2009; Holmes 2013; Klaus 2012; Krieger 1999, 2005; Schell 1997). Krieger (1994, 2012) in particular has developed a framework for understanding the embodiment of inequality, arguing that bodies are continuously shaped by interaction with their social and ecological contexts. Because human bodies reflect a life-long process of integration between individual biologies and their social worlds, forensic anthropologists who are attentive to skeletal and dental lesions are uniquely positioned to recognize embodied exposure to structural inequalities in decedents from marginalized groups.

A contextual examination of dental pathologies can reveal embodied structural violence in two primary ways. First, it may elucidate structural factors that are underlying causes of conditions such as caries, periapical lesions, and antemortem tooth loss. Those factors may include poverty, lack of access to potable water and fluoride, easy access to inexpensive processed and sugary foods, lower levels of education, and poor oral health literacy (Selwitz, Ismael, and Pitts 2007). Second, it may illustrate the consequences of structured access to adequate, affordable dental care. While the experience of dental disease is inevitable over the life course, its extent and progression are manageable with access to effective structures of care. Severe and/or numerous untreated lesions are thus suggestive of barriers to care that might include poverty, lack of dental insurance, geography, dominant language proficiency, racial or ethnic discrimination, or, in the case of undocumented migrants living in the United States, reluctance to seek treatment because of undocumented status. Additionally, because dental disease is age progressive, it is potentially informative about structural violence embodied throughout the life course. In this way, the present study augments previous work on skeletal and dental evidence of structural violence in migrants, which has to date focused almost exclusively on systemic early life stress (see Anderson et al. 2009 and Fancher 2018 for exceptions).

Importantly, the consequences of dental pathology may generate additional layers of indirect violence. Unlike skeletal indicators of systemic stress, untreated dental conditions are embodied inequalities that become visible features of living bodies. Horton and Barker (2010, 202) have deployed the concept of "stigmatized biologies" to describe the way in which oral pathologies function as "visible markers of disadvantage" among children of Mexican American farmworkers. They point out that having visibly healthy teeth is not only a social norm in the United

States, but also may shape perceptions of physical attributes associated with U.S. citizenship. Poor dentition, by contrast, is a marker of social vulnerability and difference—perhaps signaling foreign or undocumented status. Ethnographic work by Horton and Barker (2010, 2017) as well as Raskin (2017) makes clear that stigmatized dentition may constrain treatment options and cause a range of psychosocial stressors, in addition to having material consequences such as poor academic performance, lost school or work days, and decreased economic productivity noted by others (Hollister and Weintraub 1993). Even the fear that visible oral health problems may be obstacles to participation in social and professional life in the United State can generate stress, anxiety, and depression that may impact systemic health. As Raskin (2017, 201) demonstrates, the "embodied stress of dental stigma" can negatively interact with preexisting health conditions and in turn exacerbate the dental pathologies themselves. In short, dental pathologies can be a visible, stigmatizing embodiment of socioeconomic disadvantage in contexts where power relations structure resource access in ways that create oral health disparities. Furthermore, the biological, social, and economic consequences of dental stigma can reproduce those power relations in a cycle of structural vulnerability and embodied harm.

While structural violence can be a powerful explanatory framework, it is important to acknowledge its limitations. For example, it is possible to create deterministic interpretations of lived experiences that overlook the ways in which individuals respond to structural violence and the consequences of those responses (Bourgois and Scheper-Hughes 2004; Slack and Whiteford 2018). In a discussion of violence along the U.S.-Mexico border, Slack and Whiteford (2018) point out that an uncritical application of a structural violence framework may oversimplify or obscure more complex layers of violence and/or vulnerabilities that are created as individuals react to and attempt to navigate precarious circumstances. Additionally, because identities are intersectional and fluid over time and space, it is important to be mindful not to reduce individuals and their experiences based on membership within a single group. This note of caution extends to the process of embodiment itself. Krieger (2005, 2012) is careful to point out that the embodiment of inequality entails the cumulative integration of effects of social positions that are intersectional and variable, not disconnected and static. The process may also depend on factors that influence individual susceptibility and resistance to disease (Wood et al. 1992). With this in mind, we recognize that there is significant diversity among undocumented migrants in variables such as region and community of origin, socioeconomic status, and intersecting group membership. Understanding the diversity and complexity of migrant life experiences is therefore one of the primary goals of this study.

MIGRANT DEATHS ALONG THE
U.S.-MEXICO BORDER

Prior research has established an association between increased border enforcement and a corresponding increase in migrant deaths along the U.S.-Mexico border (Eschbach et al. 1999; Cornelius 2001; Rubio-Goldsmith et al. 2006; Martínez et al. 2013, 2021). Unfortunately, the true number of migrant deaths that have occurred since the escalation of federal border enforcement in the mid-1990s is unknown. Available estimates represent federally tracked cases rather than an exhaustive count of all deaths, and researchers typically use the term "recovered remains" rather than "migrant deaths" (see Martínez et al. 2021). To date, no border-wide system has been established to adequately track migrant deaths, which has led to notable discrepancies in estimates across the border. The U.S. Border Patrol (USBP), for example, recorded 7,805 migrant remains from 1998 to 2019, with 2,846 of these recoveries occurring within the Tucson Sector (USBP 2020). However, the Pima County Office of the Medical Examiner (PCOME), whose jurisdiction is largely within the USBP's Tucson Sector, investigated the deaths of 3,063 suspected migrants during that period, with the discrepancy between the two agencies widening after 2013 (Martínez et al. 2021).

Due to what appears to be a gross undercount by the USBP, researchers have urged caution when relying on the agency's estimates to draw conclusions about migrant deaths in southern Arizona and South Texas (Leutert, Lee, and Rossi 2020; Martínez et al. 2021). Nevertheless, the USBP estimates remain the only source available to examine trends in migrant deaths across geography and time. Though flawed, these data suggest that, on average, the remains of roughly 296 individuals have been recovered from the borderlands of Texas, Arizona, and California annually since 2013, when the discrepancy between USBP and PCOME estimates began to emerge. Researchers and forensic practitioners have produced more reliable data on migrant deaths within specific regions of the border. In southern Arizona, Martínez et al. (2021) found that the remains of 3,356 undocumented border crossers were investigated by PCOME from 1990 to 2020, averaging around 139 cases annually since 2013. In South Texas, Leutert, Lee, and Rossi (2020) recorded 2,655 migrant deaths from 1990 to 2019, averaging around 188 cases annually since 2013.

Given the clandestine nature of undocumented migration, as well as the precarious immigration statuses of undocumented migrants, investigating migrant deaths and identifying decedents presents a notable challenge. As such, practitioners at the PCOME adopted a biosocial approach to distinguish the remains of probable undocumented migrants to more accurately count the number of individuals dying while crossing the border, and to direct investigative efforts into more appropriate channels to increase identification rates (Anderson 2008; Birkby, Fenton, and Anderson 2008; Reineke and Anderson 2010; Soler et al. 2014). Through the examination and identification of thousands of individuals, a number of biological consequences of poverty were noted as important biosocial indicators of an undocumented migrant originating from Latin America. Embodied effects of developmental stress such as short stature, porotic cranial lesions, linear enamel hypoplasias, and cranial and vertebral neural canal asymmetry, have all been found to occur in higher frequencies in the remains of undocumented migrants (Beatrice and Soler 2016; Birkby, Fenton, and Anderson 2008; Koutlias et al. 2020; Weisensee and Spradley 2018; Znachko et al. 2020). Similarly, features of poor oral health status, such as prevalent caries, abscesses, antemortem tooth loss, and indicators of inadequate dental care, such as fewer restorations and poorly administered dental work, have also been noted (Anderson et al. 2009; Birkby, Fenton, and Anderson 2008; Fancher 2018; Soler et al. 2019). The current study builds upon previous findings of dental conditions utilized as part of the biosocial approach by comparing individuals recovered from the Arizona and Texas borders, as well as migrants from diverse regions and socioeconomic backgrounds.

MATERIALS

Full Dental Sample

The full dental sample includes 319 probable migrants from Mexico and Central America and a comparative sample of 66 U.S.-born individuals. A majority of the presumed migrants (*n*=236) were recovered from Arizona and examined at the PCOME. Another 83 presumed migrants were recovered from Texas and examined at forensic anthropology laboratories at Texas State University San Marcos, Baylor University, and the University of Indianapolis. The full sample of probable migrants includes 260 males, 57 females, and 2 individuals of indeterminate sex.

The comparative U.S.-born sample includes 11 individuals from the PCOME, 10 from the Texas State Donated Skeletal Collection, and 45 from the Maxwell Museum Donated Skeletal Collection. Individuals in this sample are predominantly of low-to-moderate socioeconomic status, and include those who were undomiciled, or of working and middle class. There are 47 males and 19 females in the comparative sample.

Biological profiles were either estimated by the first and second authors, collated from reports from each laboratory, or confirmed through known biological information for individuals who were subsequently identified. While the specific methods differed slightly depending on the laboratory, all biological profile estimations were made using standard osteological methods. In addition, DNA amelogenin results were utilized for all individuals examined at the PCOME to confirm the anthropological estimate or to estimate biological sex in cases where the remains were incomplete. Due to laboratory variation in aging methods and assigned age ranges, unidentified individuals were placed into broad, standardized age categories: <20, 20–35, 35–50, and 50+. When incompleteness or poor preservation precluded narrower estimates, individuals were placed into a generic adult category of 20+.

Identified Migrant Dental Subsample

Of the 319 probable migrants, 105 were positively identified after data collection. Anonymized information regarding age, sex, and town/city and/or country of birth was collected from missing persons reports and vital statistics from the consular offices, when available. Identified individuals had migrated from Mexico, Guatemala, Honduras, El Salvador, and Ecuador. Due to small sample sizes, all individuals from Central American countries, as well as a single individual from Ecuador, were combined into a group representing "Central America."

Additional contextual information on each individual's place of birth was collected from census information and other publicly available data (Instituto Nacional de Estadística y Geografía, México; Secretaría de Desarrollo Social, México; Instituto Nacional de Estadística, Guatemala; Instituto Nacional de Estadística, Honduras). Communities with fewer than 2,500 inhabitants were considered "rural" and communities with greater than 2,500 inhabitants were considered "urban" using the cutoff value from the Instituto Nacional de Estadística y Geografía, México. Information regarding indigeneity was also collected when available. Because death certificates do not indicate whether an individual self-identified as Indigenous or not, indigeneity was inferred based on place of birth. Individuals born in towns where a majority of the population (>50%) either self-identify as Indigenous or speak an Indigenous language were designated as originating from "Indigenous" communities. It is likely that the number of Indigenous individuals in this study is underestimated, as individuals who self-identified as Indigenous, but originated from towns where less than 50 percent of the population were Indigenous could not be counted. Furthermore, because complete information regarding the exact town or city of birth was not available for every identified individual, some individuals were designated as "unknown" for one or both parameters.

METHODS

Dental Analysis

Data on oral pathologies were collected by the first and second authors from 2012 to 2018 as part of a biosocial approach to the identification of presumed migrants who died while crossing the U.S.-Mexico border. A small subset of the oral pathology data ($n=11$) was collected by University of Indianapolis graduate students as part of the Beyond Borders program and was reviewed through photographs by the first and second authors. All individuals with an observable maxilla and/or mandible were examined for the presence of dental caries, periapical lesions, and antemortem tooth loss following the recommendations of Buikstra and Ubelaker (1994). An absent maxilla or mandible or areas with incomplete/damaged alveoli, as well as teeth that were broken or missing postmortem were marked as unobservable and excluded from analysis. All osseous and dental data were collected while individuals were unidentified and no destructive analyses were performed.

Caries and Dental Restorations

Caries refers to the progressive destruction of dental hard tissues caused by demineralizing acids produced by plaque bacteria (Kinaston et al. 2019). It is a complex disease process that is heavily dependent on disruptions in the stability of oral microbial communities due to refined carbohydrate consumption and a shift toward more acid-tolerant bacteria (Mira, Simon-Soro, and Curtis 2017). Additional extrinsic risk factors for caries include poor oral hygiene, inadequate access to fluoride and dental care, and poverty (Selwitz, Ismael, and Pitts 2007). Intrinsic risk factors for caries include genetics, hormones, and saliva composition and flow (Lukacs and Largaespada 2006; Selwitz, Ismael, and Pitts 2007). Untreated carious lesions may gradually increase in size, resulting in destruction of the dentin and pulp chamber.

Each complete, erupted tooth was assessed for the presence of dental caries and restorations. Teeth with extensive occlusal wear or postmortem damage were excluded from analysis unless carious destruction or a dental restoration was observable. Carious lesions were scored as present only when they penetrated the enamel surface, which was confirmed using a dental probe if unclear upon visual inspection. Dental radiographs were not available for all samples, and the total frequency of carious lesions may be somewhat under-reported, as incipient or poorly visualized caries could not be included. Each recorded lesion was assigned a severity score based on the amount of crown destruction: pinpoint caries, <50 percent crown destruction, >50 percent crown destruction, or destruction of the entire crown.

All observable teeth were also assessed for the presence of dental restora-tions, including fillings or crowns. Directed light and, when possible, a UV light, were utilized to assess the teeth for the presence of composite restora-tions, which can be difficult to visually discern. Some teeth had more than one restoration, however each restored tooth was counted only once, regard-less of how many restorations were present.

Other Dental Modifications

The maxillae and mandible were assessed for the presence of dental modifi-cations other than dental restorations to provide an alternative way of measur-ing how many individuals had access to some form of dental care. Removable full dentures and partial flippers, permanent bridges, and orthodontics were grouped into a single category of "other dental modifications." For the migrant sample, the presence of *cosmetic* dental modifications to the anterior teeth was assessed separately. Cosmetic dental modifications included white- or yellow-metal full or open-faced crowns, bars between the teeth, and shapes or letters applied to the tooth surface. Cosmetic dental restorations were assessed separately because they are often inherently cosmetic in nature and may not have been associated with intervention for a dental pathology. While inherent limitations to the inclusion of these other dental modifications (e.g., incomplete recovery of the maxilla/mandible or removable dentures and flip-pers) mean that they are likely undercounted, they are an important indicator of access to dental care.

Periapical Lesions and Antemortem Tooth Loss

Exposure of the pulp chamber through caries, attrition, or trauma can result in inflammation of the pulp and the alveolar bone, resulting in a periapical lesion (Hillson 2008; Kinaston et al. 2019). We follow Pilloud and Fancher (2019) and use the more general term periapical lesion as opposed to abscess, because the latter is one of several difficult to distinguish conditions that may cause a resorptive lesion around a root apex. Lesions are formed when the pulp is invaded by microorganisms, usually resulting in pulp death and subse-quent inflammation of the periapical tissues (Hillson 2008; Langlais, Miller, and Gehrig 2017). These destructive changes usually reflect advanced stages of longstanding dental disease that may contribute to severe systemic disease, oral and physical disability, and, in rare cases, death (Lypka and Hammoudeh 2011). Each observable tooth position was assessed for the presence or absence of periapical lesions. A periapical lesion was considered present when a channel perforated the alveolar bone associated with a root apex.

Antemortem tooth loss is another possible result of progressive caries, especially when tooth roots are exposed in periodontal disease (Kinaston et al. 2019). However, it is important to consider that teeth missing antemortem may have been intentionally extracted and may thus reflect intervention—even if done for the sake of economic expediency or as a last resort—to relieve discomfort. Because it is difficult to determine the cause of antemortem tooth loss (e.g., caries or periodontal disease vs. extraction), it is viewed by the authors as a general indicator of oral pathology with the caveat that it could reflect access to a rudimentary form of dental care. Each observable tooth position was assessed for the complete absence of the tooth, including the entire root(s), with partial or complete resorption of the alveolar process. Due to normal variation in extraction and agenesis, the third molars were excluded from calculations of antemortem tooth loss. When possible to discern, premolars extracted for the placement of orthodontics were also excluded from analysis.

STATISTICAL ANALYSIS

Prevalences and proportions were calculated for the aforementioned oral pathologies and indicators of dental care. Proportions were calculated for each individual based on the following observations:

—*Antemortem tooth loss*: number of missing teeth out of the total number of observable tooth positions;
—*Periapical lesions*: number of periapical lesions out of the total number of observable tooth positions;
—*Carious lesions*: number of teeth with a carious lesion out of the total number of complete observable teeth;
—*Dental restorations*: number of teeth with a dental restoration out of the total number of carious teeth;
—*Large unrestored caries*: number of unrestored teeth with a carious lesion larger than 50 percent of the tooth crown out of the total number of unrestored teeth with a carious lesion.

Crude prevalence rates (CPR) were calculated for other dental modifications and cosmetic dental modifications. A series of two-tailed proportions tests for unequal variances were used to compare the mean proportions for individuals based on recovery location (i.e., Arizona versus Texas) and membership within specific demographic groups (i.e., majority Indigenous versus non-Indigenous community, rural versus urban context, and Mexico versus Central America) among the identified migrant sample. We also compared the CPR and proportions of dental restorations and other dental modifications between the entire undocumented migrant sample and the U.S.-born sample to examine possible differences in access to dental care. All statistical analyses were conducted in Stata 16.

RESULTS

The CPR calculated by individual demonstrate that dental pathologies are extremely common in the migrant sample. Caries are the most prevalent condition, affecting 74 percent (222/300) of migrants with complete observable teeth. Despite the high prevalence of caries, only 26 percent (58/222) of individuals with carious teeth have at least one dental restoration. Nearly one half (48%; 149/312) of the migrant sample exhibits antemortem tooth loss excluding the third molars. Finally, 18 percent (56/311) of individuals in the migrant sample with observable tooth positions exhibit at least one periapical lesion.

Tables 1.1–1.5 report the CPR, proportions, standard deviations, range, 95 percent confidence intervals, and sample sizes for oral pathologies and indicators of dental care among each group. In the entire migrant sample (table 1.1), statistically significant differences were observed in the prevalence of large unrestored caries between migrants recovered in Arizona compared to those recovered in Texas. On average, 19.8 percent of observable teeth for individuals in the Arizona sample exhibit large unrestored caries compared to just 7.2 percent among the Texas sample. There were no statistically significant differences in the overall number of restored teeth; however, a comparison of prevalence rates of other dental modifications demonstrates a statistical difference between the two groups. Only 3.5 percent of individuals in the Arizona sample exhibit other dental modifications in comparison to 12.2 percent of individuals in the Texas sample. It is likely that the CPR of removable dentures and flippers in both Arizona and Texas is underestimated due to the outdoor postmortem contexts and probability for incomplete recovery of remains and personal effects.

We also found several significant differences between identified migrants from majority Indigenous communities and those from non-Indigenous communities (table 1.2). For example, migrants from mostly non-Indigenous communities on average exhibit periapical lesions at 1.7 percent of observable

Angela Soler et al.

Table 1.1 Descriptive Statistics and Proportions Tests among all Undocumented Migrants: Arizona vs. Texas

Trait	Individual Prevalence		Difference
	Arizona	Texas	
Periapical Lesion (% tooth positions among individuals)			
Proportion (%)	1.12	0.95	0.17
Std. Dev. (%)	2.71	2.98	
Range (%)	0.00–18.75	0.00–18.75	
95% CI (%)	0.77–1.48	0.30–1.61	
n	229	82	
AM Tooth Loss (% tooth positions among individuals)			
Proportion (%)	6.90	9.83	2.93
Std. Dev. (%)	13.87	16.89	
Range (%)	0.00–100.00	0.00–100.00	
95% CI (%)	5.09–8.70	6.14–13.52	
n	229	83	
Caries (% teeth among individuals)			
Proportion (%)	22.42	22.79	0.37
Std. Dev. (%)	25.16	21.74	
Range (%)	0.00–100.00	0.00–90.00	
95% CI (%)	19.09–25.75	17.89–27.69	
n	222	78	
Restored Teeth (% carious teeth among individuals)			
Proportion (%)	24.78	30.51	5.73
Std. Dev. (%)	39.83	41.87	
Range (%)	0.00–100.00	0.00–100.00	
95% CI (%)	18.54–31.02	19.96–41.05	
n	159	63	
Large Caries (% carious teeth among individuals)			
Proportion (%)	19.77	7.16	12.61**
Std. Dev. (%)	32.22	18.70	
Range (%)	0.00–100.00	0.00–100.00	
95% CI (%)	14.18–25.36	1.73–12.60	
n	130	48	
Other Dental Modifications (presence/absence among individuals)			
Prevalence (%)	3.49	12.20	8.70*
Std. Dev. (%)	18.40	32.92	
Range (%)	0.00–100.00	0.00–100.00	
95% CI (%)	1.10–5.90	4.96–19.43	
n	229	82	
Cosmetic Dental Modifications (presence/absence among individuals)			
Prevalence (%)	3.93	9.76	5.83
Std. Dev. (%)	19.47	29.85	
Range (%)	0.00–100.00	0.00–100.00	
95% CI (%)	1.39–6.47	3.20–16.32	
n	229	82	

Note: Two-tailed t-tests assuming unequal variance between samples.
*p < 0.05, **p < 0.01, ***p < 0.001

Table 1.2 Descriptive Statistics and Proportions Tests among Identified Undocumented Migrants: Indigenous vs. Non-Indigenous Communities

Trait	Individual Prevalence		Difference
	Indigenous	Non-Indigenous	
Periapical Lesion (% tooth positions among individuals)			
Proportion (%)	0.26	1.73	1.47**
Std. Dev. (%)	0.88	3.50	
Range (%)	0.00–3.13	0.00–18.75	
95% CI (%)	-0.11–0.63	0.88–2.58	
n	24	67	
AM Tooth Loss (% tooth positions among individuals)			
Proportion (%)	9.09	8.95	0.14
Std. Dev. (%)	16.65	18.04	
Range (%)	0.00–67.85	0.00–100.00	
95% CI (%)	2.06–16.12	4.55–13.35	
n	24	67	
Caries (% teeth among individuals)			
Proportion (%)	15.96	25.01	9.05*
Std. Dev. (%)	14.23	25.57	
Range (%)	0.00–40.91	0.00–100.00	
95% CI (%)	9.95–21.97	18.68–31.34	
n	24	65	
Restored Teeth (% carious teeth among individuals)			
Proportion (%)	22.22	23.74	1.52
Std. Dev. (%)	39.61	39.96	
Range (%)	0.00–100.00	0.00–100.00	
95% CI (%)	2.53–41.92	12.39–35.10	
n	18	50	
Large Caries (% carious teeth among individuals)			
Proportion (%)	1.67	17.72	16.05***
Std. Dev. (%)	6.45	24.78	
Range (%)	0.00–25.00	0.00–100.00	
95% CI (%)	-1.91–5.24	9.90–25.54	
n	15	41	
Other Dental Modifications (presence/absence among individuals)			
Prevalence (%)	4.17	8.96	4.79
Std. Dev. (%)	20.41	28.77	
Range (%)	0.00–100.00	0.00–100.00	
95% CI (%)	-4.45–12.79	1.94–15.97	
n	24	67	
Cosmetic Dental Modifications (presence/absence among individuals)			
Prevalence (%)	0.00	7.46	7.46*
Std. Dev. (%)	0.00	26.48	
Range (%)	0.00	0.00–100.00	
95% CI (%)	0.00	1.00–13.92	
n	24	67	

Note: Two-tailed t-tests assuming unequal variance between samples.
*p<0.05, **p<0.01, ***p<0.001

Angela Soler et al.

Table 1.3 Descriptive Statistics and Proportions Tests among Identified Undocumented Migrants: Rural vs. Urban

Trait	Individual Prevalence		Difference
	Rural	Urban	
Periapical Lesion (% tooth positions among individuals)			
Proportion (%)	1.14	1.62	0.48
Std. Dev. (%)	2.04	3.67	
Range (%)	0.00–6.25	0.00–18.75	
95% CI (%)	0.41–1.86	0.64–2.61	
n	33	56	
AM Tooth Loss (% tooth positions among individuals)			
Proportion (%)	11.04	7.52	3.52
Std. Dev. (%)	19.99	15.72	
Range (%)	0.00–100.00	0.00–78.57	
95% CI (%)	3.95–18.13	3.31–11.73	
n	33	56	
Caries (% teeth among individuals)			
Proportion (%)	23.11	22.32	0.79
Std. Dev. (%)	20.90	25.34	
Range (%)	0.00–75.00	0.00–100.00	
95% CI (%)	15.58–30.65	15.47–29.17	
n	32	55	
Restored Teeth (% carious teeth among individuals)			
Proportion (%)	8.65	29.80	21.15*
Std. Dev. (%)	27.33	41.91	
Range (%)	0.00–100.00	0.00–100.00	
95% CI (%)	-2.39–19.69	16.22–43.38	
n	26	39	
Large Caries (% carious teeth among individuals)			
Proportion (%)	12.29	17.95	5.66
Std. Dev. (%)	23.69	26.80	
Range (%)	0.00–100.00	0.00–100.00	
95% CI (%)	2.29–22.29	8.12–27.78	
n	24	31	
Other Dental Modifications (presence/absence among individuals)			
Prevalence (%)	12.12	5.36	6.76
Std. Dev. (%)	33.14	22.72	
Range (%)	0.00–100.00	0.00–100.00	
95% CI (%)	0.37–23.87	-0.72–11.44	
n	33	56	
Cosmetic Dental Modifications (presence/absence among individuals)			
Prevalence (%)	12.12	1.79	10.34
Std. Dev. (%)	33.14	13.36	
Range (%)	0.00–100.00	0.00–100.00	
95% CI (%)	0.37–23.87	-1.79–5.36	
n	33	56	

Note: Two-tailed t-tests assuming unequal variance between samples.
*p<0.05, **p<0.01, ***p<0.001

Table 1.4 Descriptive Statistics and Proportions Tests among Identified Undocumented Migrants: Mexico vs. Central America

Trait	Individual Prevalence		Difference
	Mexico	Central America	
Periapical Lesion (% tooth positions among individuals)			
Proportion (%)	1.59	0.74	0.85
Std. Dev. (%)	3.29	2.44	
Range (%)	0	18.75	
95% CI (%)	0.81–2.37	-0.12–1.59	
n	71	34	
AM Tooth Loss (% tooth positions among individuals)			
Proportion (%)	5.63	18.18	12.55*
Std. Dev. (%)	11.78	26.74	
Range (%)	0.00–67.86	0.00–100.00	
95% CI (%)	2.84–8.42	8.85–27.51	
n	71	34	
Caries (% teeth among individuals)			
Proportion (%)	21.52	29.29	7.77
Std. Dev. (%)	24.33	25.45	
Range (%)	0.00–100.00	0.00–100.00	
95% CI (%)	15.76–27.28	19.95–38.62	
n	71	31	
Restored Teeth (% carious teeth among individuals)			
Proportion (%)	22.86	36.33	13.47
Std. Dev. (%)	38.14	47.32	
Range (%)	0.00–100.00	0.00–100.00	
95% CI (%)	12.25–33.48	16.80–55.86	
n	52	25	
Large Caries (% carious teeth among individuals)			
Proportion (%)	17.06	12.55	4.51
Std. Dev. (%)	26.46	29.02	
Range (%)	0.00–100.00	0.00–100.00	
95% CI (%)	9.02–25.11	-2.92–28.01	
n	44	16	
Other Dental Modifications (presence/absence among individuals)			
Prevalence (%)	7.04	8.82	1.78
Std. Dev. (%)	25.77	28.79	
Range (%)	0.00–100.00	0.00–100.00	
95% CI (%)	0.94–13.14	-1.22–18.87	
n	71	34	
Cosmetic Dental Modifications (presence/absence among individuals)			
Prevalence (%)	5.63	2.94	2.69
Std. Dev. (%)	23.22	17.15	
Range (%)	0.00–100.00	0.00–100.00	
95% CI (%)	0.14–11.13	-3.04–8.93	
n	71	34	

Note: Two-tailed t-tests assuming unequal variance between samples.
*p<0.05, **p<0.01, ***p<0.001

Angela Soler et al.

Table 1.5 Descriptive Statistics and Proportion Tests: Undocumented Migrants vs. Non-Migrants

	Individual Prevalence		Difference
Trait	Undocumented Migrants	Non-Migrants	
Restored Teeth (% carious teeth among individuals)			
Proportion (%)	26.40	57.75	31.35***
Std. Dev. (%)	40.40	41.82	
Range (%)	0.00–100.00	0.00–100.00	
95% CI (%)	21.06–31.75	46.65–68.85	
n	222	57	
Other Dental Modifications (presence/absence among individuals)			
Prevalence (%)	5.79	6.06	0.27
Std. Dev. (%)	23.39	24.04	
Range (%)	0.00–100.00	0.00–100.00	
95% CI (%)	3.18–8.40	0.15–11.97	
n	311	66	
Cosmetic Dental Modifications (presence/absence among individuals)			
Prevalence (%)	5.47	0.00	5.47***
Std. Dev. (%)	22.77	0.00	
Range (%)	0.00–100.00	0.00	
95% CI (%)	2.93–8.01	0.00	
n	311	66	

Note: Two-tailed t-tests assuming unequal variance between samples.
*p<0.05, **p<0.01, ***p<0.001.

tooth positions, while migrants from mostly Indigenous communities exhibit periapical lesions at 0.3 percent of observable tooth positions. Similarly, individuals from non-Indigenous communities exhibit a significantly higher mean proportion of carious teeth (25.0%) and teeth with large unrestored lesions (17.7%) in comparison to those from mostly Indigenous communities (16% and 1.7%, respectively). Finally, the CPR indicates that 7.5 percent of migrants from majority non-Indigenous communities have cosmetic dental modification, whereas none of the migrants from Indigenous communities have such modifications. This likely indicates a difference in cultural preference for cosmetic dental modifications.

Comparisons of identified migrants from rural versus urban communities (table 1.3) found little empirical support for any differences between those two groups, with the exception of the proportion of restored teeth. On average 29.8 percent of observable teeth with a carious lesion exhibit dental restorations in individuals from urban communities compared to an average of 8.7 percent of observable teeth with a carious lesion in individuals from rural communities.

Similarly, we found no statistically significant differences between identified migrants from Mexico and those from Central America (table 1.4), with the exception of antemortem tooth loss (excluding the third molars).

An average of 18.2 percent of teeth was lost antemortem in the sample of migrants from Central America compared to an average of 5.6 percent of teeth in the sample from Mexico.

Due to differences in mean age, we did not compare the prevalence of age-dependent oral pathologies (i.e., caries, antemortem tooth loss, and periapical lesions) between the undocumented migrant and comparative U.S.-born samples. However, comparisons of restorations and modifications revealed some clear differences (table 1.5). We found that 57.8 percent of carious teeth among individuals in the U.S.-born sample exhibit dental restorations, compared to just 26.4 percent in the undocumented migrant sample. Additionally, 5.5 percent of the undocumented migrants have cosmetic dental modifications, compared to none of the individuals in the non-migrant sample. We failed to find a statistically significant difference between the migrant and U.S.-born sample in the proportion of individuals with other types of dental modifications.

DISCUSSION

Oral Pathologies as Embodied Structural Violence

Overall, the results of this study are relatively consistent with previous examinations of oral pathology in undocumented migrants who died while crossing the U.S.-Mexico border. Anderson et al. (2009) examined a sample of Mexican nationals recovered from the Arizona border and found that 44 percent of individuals exhibited caries and 66 percent exhibited antemortem tooth loss. Similarly, in a sample of 136 presumed migrants recovered from the Texas border, Fancher (2018) found that 58 percent of individuals exhibited active carious lesions and 21 percent exhibited moderate-to-severe periodontitis. While the CPR of caries in the present study is somewhat higher, all three studies indicate that caries is frequent in undocumented migrants crossing through both Arizona and Texas. Furthermore, the moderate prevalence of antemortem tooth loss in samples with a relatively young mean age—early thirties in both Anderson et al. (2009) and among identified individuals in the present study—indicates that antemortem tooth loss is not simply due to age-related changes.

Recurrent findings of oral pathology in undocumented migrant samples are not surprising given the clinical literature on oral health in the region. Studies indicate that caries are prevalent throughout Mexico and Central America, with rates ranging from 59 percent to more than 90 percent of study participants (Acuña et al. 2019; Archila et al. 2003; Molina-Frechero et al. 2009). Even with recent improvements in oral healthcare education and the implementation of salt fluoridation programs, caries continues to be a public health issue in Latin America and the Caribbean, especially among individuals of lower socioeconomic status (Gimenez et al. 2016). Similarly, regional studies of individuals in their thirties and forties have indicated that more than half experience antemortem tooth loss and that most have lost multiple teeth (Aguilar-Diáz, Borges-Yáñez, and de la Fuente-Hernández 2021; Minaya-Sánchez et al. 2010). While the loss of dentition with advanced age is expected, the incidence of tooth loss among individuals of a relatively young mean age is rather remarkable.

Researchers postulate a number of reasons for the high prevalence of caries and antemortem tooth loss in the region, many of which are driven by structural forces. Local-level influences include lack of access to clean drinking water, low levels of fluoride in drinking water, poor oral hygiene, tobacco use, and low socioeconomic status (Aguilar-Diáz, Borges-Yáñez, and de la Fuente-Hernández 2021; Aguilar-Zinser et al. 2008; Archila et al. 2003; Medina-Solís et al. 2006; Molina-Frechero et al. 2009; Villalobos-Rodello et al. 2007). There are also global political-economic processes that ultimately influence local biologies in ways that predispose individuals to dental disease. For example, cheap, highly processed starches and beverages with high sugar content are progressively replacing more balanced traditional diets, which have become more expensive and harder to maintain for middle- and working-class communities (Gálvez 2018). Many scholars link such changes to the implementation of free-trade agreements and the shift away from community agriculture to a monetized global corporate agriculture (Gálvez 2018; Day, Magaña-González, and Wilson 2021). Traditional diets are also less viable when all members of the household work long hours and there is little time to prepare more balanced meals (Day, Magaña-González, and Wilson 2021). Unfortunately, processed diets are not only high in sugar and sodium, but also extremely low in micronutrients, and this dietary transition has led to an increase in obesity and chronic metabolic diseases (Gálvez 2018; Marrón-Ponce et al. 2019) in addition to a chronic struggle with oral diseases.

Acknowledging that the causes of oral pathologies are numerous, intersecting, and occurring at levels from the individual to global, it is worth emphasizing that in Latin America they are associated with factors such as poverty, income inequality, educational attainment, and knowledge of factors that affect oral hygiene (Casanova-Rosado et al. 2021; Medina-Solís et al. 2006; Villalobos-Rodelo et al. 2007). Importantly, disparities in oral health based on socioeconomic status, level of education, and race/ethnicity persist north of the border as well (Horton and Barker 2009, 2010; Huang and Park 2014; Sabbah et al. 2009), and in that context may include the effects of undocumented status (Horton and Barker 2009, 2010; Wilson et al. 2018).

In addition to factors that contribute to their prevalence, oral pathologies in undocumented border crossers are frequently untreated because of socioeconomic or geographic limitations on access to dental care. The results of this study showing that individuals in a U.S.-born sample exhibit a significantly higher proportion of treated teeth than individuals in the migrant sample (see table 1.5) provide evidence for this basic disparity. Similar results were obtained by Anderson et al. (2009), who found significantly lower rates of restorations in a Mexican foreign national sample (36%), in comparison to a Mexican American sample (78%). Anderson et al. (2009) also found a correlation between frequent oral pathologies, lower rates of restorations, and shorter stature in the Mexican foreign national group, which they argue reflects comparatively poor diets and higher levels of poverty.

In Mexico and Central America, lack of access to dental care may be predicated on a number of structural factors, including socioeconomic status, education, dental insurance, and cost (Jiménez-Gayosso et al. 2015; Pérez-Núñez et al. 2006, 2007). While low-cost dental clinics exist, most are located in urban areas which may add geographic barriers of transportation and the need to miss work to travel for care, especially among individuals living in rural areas (Masuoka, Komabayashi, and Reyes-Vela 2014; Maupomé et al. 2013). For example, overall estimates for Mexico and Guatemala indicate that there are only two to three dentists for every 10,000 inhabitants, with most concentrated in urban centers (Masuoka, Komabayashi, and Reyes-Vela 2014; PAHO 2012).

Furthermore, access to dental intervention does not necessarily correspond to quality or even adequate dental care. Tooth extraction, for example, may be considered a last resort in terms of standard dental care, but in many contexts, it has been utilized as a frequent and affordable way to reduce oral pain. A study of a low-cost dental clinic in Hidalgo, Mexico indicates that the most frequent reason for the extraction of permanent teeth included caries (43.1%), periodontal disease (27.9%), or for the placement of prosthetics (21.5%) (Medina-Solís et al. 2013). Further, individuals who attended just one appointment at the clinic (as opposed to multiple appointments) were more likely to have teeth extracted due to caries. In many instances, a delay in dental intervention resulted in caries severe enough that tooth extraction was the only option. Additionally, extraction does not require the travel, time off work, or costs of additional office visits required for dental restorations. At a more basic level, Hunter and Arbona (1995, 1217) indicate that untrained "tooth-pullers" may visit rural areas without access to a dentist to ease oral pain associated with caries and periodontal disease and to fit people with cheap prosthetics.

Lack of access and substandard dental care can be an issue for those living north of the border as well. Many discrepancies in access to quality dental care are the product of economics and inequities that are structured on whether or not an individual is an undocumented migrant. This includes fear and discrimination due to undocumented status, dominant language proficiency, lack of insurance and the high costs of dental care, issues related to transportation, and previous unsatisfactory experience when receiving dental care (Cristancho et al. 2008; Fuentes-Afflick and Hessol 2009; Velez et al. 2017). Wilson et al. (2016) indicate that non-citizen and naturalized migrants living in the United States are not only less likely to access dental services or receive a full preventative dental examination, but are also more likely to have teeth extracted than U.S.-born citizens. These disparities in access also impact the non-citizen and citizen children of undocumented migrant parents (Horton and Barker 2009, 2010, 2017; Maserejian et al. 2007). Among children of migrant farmworkers in the United States, Horton and Barker (2010) indicate that dentists accepting California state dental insurance are more inclined to extract teeth than provide dental restorations for low-income patients, as restorations are more time consuming and reimbursed at a lower rate. Unfortunately, these low-cost dental interventions in childhood can cause long-term dental problems that persist into adulthood (Horton and Barker 2010). While these individuals are receiving some form of dental intervention, none are gaining access to a level of care likely to prevent further deterioration of the dentition.

Dental Stigma as an Additional Layer of Violence

As outlined above, frequent and untreated oral pathologies in undocumented migrants can be viewed as a product of structural violence because they reflect biological harm caused indirectly by inequalities that negatively affect dental health. The visibility of inequalities embodied in the dentition, however, is a layer added to the already complex biosocial interactions that characterize indirect violence. Individuals with visible oral pathology, including carious destruction and antemortem tooth loss (especially of anterior teeth), may be perceived as impoverished, uneducated, or foreign—even marked as undocumented—simply due to their oral presentation. This type of harm was recognized by Farmer (2004), who included stigmatization in a list of adverse outcomes associated with structural violence. In the present study, the remote outdoor postmortem context resulted in the incomplete recovery of crania and mandibles and a high incidence of postmortem loss of anterior teeth, precluding a representative calculation of the CPR of unrestored caries and antemortem loss of anterior teeth. However, it is important to consider the possibility that dental pathologies recorded in this study—which were somewhat commonly observed on anterior teeth—were a locus of stigma, with consequences that could perpetuate inequalities.

Again, the ethnographic studies of Horton and Barker (2010, 2017) poignantly illustrate this dynamic among children of Mexican American farmworkers. They show that older individuals who desire social and economic integration into U.S. society experience barriers when constrained dental treatment options leave them with life-long oral health problems. In a cultural context where the absence of visible oral pathologies is a social norm—perhaps even indicative of U.S. citizenship—their bodies are marked as different and unequal. Other researchers have shown that the stigmatization of oral health status can create impediments to upward social mobility by eliciting feelings of embarrassment, anxiety, and depression (Coles et al. 2011; Hollister and Weintraub 1993; Raskin 2017; Rouxel et al. 2018). Finally, dental pathologies have important implications for overall health status. This is not only because they have been implicated in the causes of systemic diseases through traditional biological pathways, but also because biosocial processes such as stigmatization can generate psychosocial stress that may interact with and worsen preexisting health conditions (Raskin 2017; Vered et al. 2011; Watt 2007).

While the present study cannot incorporate ethnographic accounts to connect dental lesions with the process and effects of stigmatization, it nevertheless demonstrates that severe and, in many cases, visible oral pathologies are prevalent in the remains of individuals who died crossing the border. As forensic scientists working to identify and repatriate the remains of individuals who may have experienced structural violence and stigmatization in life, we must also recognize how these structured harms may continue to influence individuals – and their surviving family—in death (see also Bird and Bird; Byrnes, Belcher, and Woollen; Moore and Kim; Kaplan et al.; Winburn et al., this volume). In the border context, there is a paradox of how visible oral conditions were potentially the cause and consequence of structured inequities experienced during life, and after death they have also become features that may help distinguish the unidentified skeletal remains of probable undocumented migrants. The distinction here is that the recognition of oral pathologies and, crucially, an awareness of their broader implications, can be considered an important component of the system of postmortem care (see Reineke 2019). Collectively, the presence of these oral pathologies along with other biosocial features (e.g., recovery location, culturally specific body modifications and personal effects, and skeletal evidence of embodied poverty and marginalization) are a critical means to adequately count the number of migrants unnecessarily dying along our southern border, but also to assist in the identification of migrants and ultimately ease the suffering of their families (see also Bird and Bird, this volume). However, engaging in postmortem care also means being cognizant that biological indicators of marginalization are not exclusive to undocumented migrants (Moore and Kim, this volume) or any individual who crosses the border, nor are they static over time.

Contextualizing Oral Pathologies and Sociodemographic Variables

While examining oral pathologies within a structural violence framework reveals visibly embodied inequalities in the full migrant sample, comparisons of oral pathologies between sociodemographic groups in the identified migrant subsample provide a glimpse of the diversity of lived experiences among migrants of various backgrounds. For example, the finding that presumed migrants recovered from the Texas border exhibited significantly fewer large unrestored carious teeth and more dental modifications is interesting, as it could indicate that migrants recovered in Texas had increased access to oral healthcare. While there is no inherent relationship between recovery location and access to a dentist, this could reflect greater socioeconomic diversity in the undocumented migrants from the Texas sample. This hypothesis is supported by data that show a greater incidence of probable nutritional stress in the group of migrants crossing through Arizona, who were 3.76 times more likely to exhibit porotic hyperostosis than those crossing through Texas (Beatrice et al. 2021). Indicators of childhood nutritional stress and inadequate access to dental care in adulthood together reflect socioeconomic instability throughout the life course and could also indicate potential differences in the economic and/or social capital required to cross through Texas versus Arizona. If the route through Texas is longer, farther, and potentially more prohibitively expensive, then individuals with less economic or social capital may attempt to cross through Arizona instead.

Border Patrol apprehension statistics also indicate more variation in the demographics of migrants who cross through Texas compared to those who cross through Arizona. Historically, and in the years of data collection for this study, individuals crossing through Arizona were overwhelmingly from Mexico, whereas those crossing through Texas were more equally divided between individuals originating from Mexico and those originating from Central America (USBP 2020). The composition of the present sample reflects these Border Patrol trends, with approximately 73 percent of the identified individuals recovered in Arizona originating from Mexico and 69.2 percent of the identified individuals recovered from Texas originating from Central America.

Despite regional trends in migration routes, it is unclear if there is a true difference in access to oral healthcare between individuals from Mexico versus those from Central America. While it appears that Central Americans may exhibit more restorations and other dental modifications, we failed to find a statistically significant difference in these indicators of oral care between the two groups. The only significant difference was the higher prevalence of antemortem tooth loss in the Central American group. There are a number of possibilities, however it could potentially indicate an increased incidence of dental extractions to more easily and affordably mitigate dental pathologies or place prosthetics. This may indicate at least some perfunctory oral healthcare in the form of extractions of affected teeth among the Central American migrants, either through traveling home remedy "tooth pullers" or in low-income dental clinics.

A comparison of individuals coming from mostly Indigenous versus non-Indigenous identifying communities revealed a number of statistically significant differences. Individuals from non-Indigenous communities exhibited significantly more carious lesions, large unrestored caries, and periapical lesions. These differences are perhaps unsurprising as clinical studies have found a lower incidence of caries within more remote and traditional Indigenous communities throughout Mexico and Central America. According to Vega Lizama and Cucina (2014), a more balanced traditional Indigenous diet, even with heavy consumption of maize, is likely to be less cariogenic than the highly processed foods and sugary beverages more easily accessible in some communities. For example, Levin et al. (2017) found that Ecuadorian Indigenous communities that were more geographically remote and that more heavily harvested and consumed their own locally grown foods were less susceptible to caries than communities whose proximity to highways and stores made them more prone to consumption of processed foods. The exposure to and need for these processed foods is increasing with globalization and the encroachment of large-scale agricultural industry into Indigenous communities throughout Mexico and Central America (Day, Magaña-González, and Wilson 2021). Without proper intervention, this could lead to a host of health problems including increased rates of oral pathologies.

The only significant difference between the subsamples of individuals originating from urban versus rural communities is the prevalence of dental restorations. Despite exhibiting the same overall prevalence of caries, individuals from urban locales exhibit significantly more dental restorations than those originating from rural communities. This is understandable in part because of the concentration of dentists in urban centers rather than rural communities, as discussed above (Masuoka, Komabayashi, and Reyes-Vela 2014; PAHO 2012). A study by Maupomé et al. (2013) found a significant increase in the prevalence of filled teeth among Mexicans who resided in communities with paved roads and piped potable water, indicating that rural communities without this kind of infrastructure had even less access to dental care. Further, there is a correlation between dental coverage, higher levels of education and socioeconomic status, and access to health insurance in Mexico, all of which are more likely to be concentrated in urban areas (Pérez-Núñez et al. 2006). It is worth noting that while individuals in the urban group appear to have more access to dental care, on average only 29.5 percent of carious teeth in individuals from the urban locales were restored. This indicates that regular access to dental care was relatively infrequent regardless of urban or rural residence.

CONCLUSION

This study assessed the prevalence of oral pathologies and indicators of access to dental care in a skeletal sample of undocumented migrants recovered from the Texas and Arizona borderlands. High prevalences of caries and antemortem tooth loss and a moderate prevalence of periapical lesions are suggestive of marginal oral health status, while an exceptionally low mean number of restored teeth suggests insufficient access to oral healthcare. While untreated oral pathologies are not unique to the undocumented migrant community in the United States, a comparison of the prevalence of restored teeth between the undocumented migrant sample and a sample of U.S.-born individuals of low-to-moderate socioeconomic status also suggests a marked disparity in dental care. When taken together with previous studies of developmental stress in the skeletal remains of Latin American migrants, the prevalence of untreated dental pathologies demonstrates that differential exposure to systemic stress and inadequate access to healthcare are continuously embodied throughout the life course. The results of this research may also suggest that the experience of dental stigma recorded in ethnographic studies of migrants and their children are a common occurrence. The remains of migrants examined here frequently exhibit the same extensive and untreated dental pathologies interpreted by Horton and Barker (2010) as visible markers of social vulnerability. While it was beyond the scope of this research to directly access the lived experiences of the individuals in this sample, their dental conditions serve as evidence of the biological consequences of structural violence and could potentially reflect elements of stigma—a biosocial outcome that may reproduce socioeconomic and health inequalities.

Importantly, however, this study did not uncover evidence of a uniform experience of structured risk of dental pathologies and barriers to oral healthcare. Rather, the results of comparisons of dental conditions between sociodemographic groups reveal critical differences in the experiences of individuals crossing the border, reflective of the diversity of migrants from Mexico and Central America. Certain patterns were anticipated to some extent, such as a greater proportion of restored teeth in migrants from urban communities and a greater proportion of carious teeth in migrants from non-Indigenous communities. This could be related to better access to dental care in the former and a more cariogenic diet in the latter. Other findings point to areas where additional research is needed to better understand the use of different migration routes. For example, the interesting possibility that migrants crossing through Texas exhibit greater socioeconomic diversity dovetails with the results of a previous comparison of skeletal indicators of stress (Beatrice et al. 2021). The present findings thus provide a glimpse of diverse individuals and communities navigating risk of adverse socioeconomic and health outcomes in personal and localized ways. Therefore, as we consider the causes and consequences of embodied stress, structural vulnerabilities, and the possibility of stigma—in both the antemortem and postmortem contexts—it must be acknowledged that these experiences are also individual, intersectional, and may change over time.

NOTE

1. Acknowledgments: We thank Dr. Robin Reineke for suggestions regarding the theoretical framing of this paper. A special acknowledgment to the PCOME, including Drs. Bruce Anderson, Jennifer Vollner, Caitlin Vogelsberg, and Gregory Hess, and former postdoctoral fellows, Drs. Traci Van Deest and Cate Bird, for assistance with data collection, expert input, and institutional support. In addition, thanks to Dr. Krista Latham and her Master's students for assistance with data collection at the University of Indianapolis, and Drs. Kate Spradley and Lori Baker for access to collect data at Texas State and Baylor University. This research was supported in part by a SOSA grant from The College of New Jersey. Disclaimer: The views and opinions expressed in this paper are the author's own and do not reflect the opinions of the New York City Office of Chief Medical Examiner or the City of New York.

REFERENCES

Acuña, Jenny E., Karina M. Freitas, Rafael P. Henriques, Emerson F. Cruz, Maria C. Binz Ordoñez, Ghenna E. Arias, and Guillermo M. Balseca. 2019. "Prevalence of Early Childhood Caries in Children Aged 1 to 5 Years in the City of Quito, Ecuador." *The Open Dentistry Journal* 13: 242–48. https://doi.org/10.2174/1874210601913010242

Aguilar-Díaz, Fatima del Carmen, Socorro Aída Borges-Yáñez, and Javier de la Fuente-Hernández. 2021. "Risk Indicators of Tooth Loss among Mexican Adult Population: A Cross-Sectional Study." *International Dental Journal* 71 (5): 414–19. https://doi.org/10.1016/j.identj.2020.12.016

Aguilar-Zinser, V., M.E. Irigoyen, G. Rivera, G. Maupomé, L. Sánchez-Pérez, and C. Velázquez. 2008. "Cigarette Smoking and Dental Caries among Professional Truck Drivers in Mexico." *Caries Research* 42: 255–62. https://doi.org/10.1159/000135670

Algee-Hewitt, Bridget F.B., Cris E. Hughes, and Bruce E. Anderson. 2018. "Temporal, Geographic and Identification Trends in Craniometric Estimates of Ancestry for Persons of Latin American Origin." *Forensic Anthropology* 1 (1): 4–17. https://doi.org/10.5744/fa.2018.0002

Anderson, Bruce E. 2008. "Identifying the Dead: Methods Utilized by the Pima County (Arizona) Office of the Medical Examiner for Undocumented Border Crossers: 2001–2006." *Journal of Forensic Sciences* 53 (1): 8–15. https://doi.org/10.1111/j.1556-4029.2007.00609.x

Anderson, Bruce E., T.R. Smith, Walter H. Birkby, Todd W. Fenton, Carolyn V. Hurst, and Claire C. Gordon. 2009. "Differentiating Between Foreign National Hispanics and US Hispanics in the Southwest: The Influence of Socioeconomic

Status on Dental Health and Stature." Poster presented at the 61st annual meeting of the American Academy of Forensic Sciences, Denver, CO.

Archila, Luis, Robert D. Bartizek, Robert W. Gerlach, Steven A. Jacobs, and Aaron R. Biesbrock. 2003. "Dental Caries in School-Age Children in Five Guatemalan Communities." *The Journal of Clinical Dentistry* 14 (3): 53–58.

Beatrice, Jared S., and Angela Soler. 2016. "Skeletal Indicators of Stress: A Component of the Biocultural Profile of Undocumented Migrants in Southern Arizona." *Journal of Forensic Sciences* 61 (5): 1164–72. https://doi.org/10.1111/1556-4029.13131

Beatrice, Jared S., Angela Soler, Robin C. Reineke, and Daniel E. Martínez. 2021. "Skeletal Evidence of Structural Violence among Undocumented Migrants from Mexico and Central America." *American Journal of Physical Anthropology* 176 (4): 1–22. https://doi.org/10.1002/ajpa.24391

Birkby, Walter H., Todd W. Fenton, and Bruce E. Anderson. 2008. "Identifying Southwest Hispanics Using Nonmetric Traits and the Cultural Profile." *Journal of Forensic Sciences* 53 (1): 29–33. https://doi.org/10.1111/j.1556-4029.2007.00611.x

Bourgois, Philippe, and Nancy Scheper-Hughes. 2004. "Response to: Farmer, Paul. An Anthropology of Structural Violence." *Current Anthropology* 45 (3): 317–18. https://doi.org/10.1086/382250

Buikstra, Jane E., and Douglas H. Ubelaker. 1994. *Standards for Data Collection from Human Skeletal Remains*. Fayetteville: Arkansas Archeological Survey Research Series No. 44. https://doi.org/10.1002/ajhb.1310070519

Casanova-Rosado, J.F., A.J. Casanova-Rosado, M. Minaya-Sánchez, J.A. Casanova-Sarmiento, J.L. Robles-Minaya, S. Márquez-Rodríguez, M. Mora-Acosta, et al. 2021. "Self-Reported Dental Caries by Mexican Elementary and Middle-School Schoolchildren in the Context of Socioeconomic Indicators: A National Ecological Study." *Children* 8 (4): 289. https://doi.org/10.3390/children8040289

Coles, Emma, Karen Chan, Jennifer Collins, Gerry M. Humphris, Derek Richards, Brian Williams, and Ruth Freeman. 2011. "Decayed and Missing Teeth and Oral-Health-Related Factors: Predicting Depression in Homeless People." *Journal of Psychosomatic Research* 71 (2): 108–12. https://doi.org/10.1016/j.jpsychores.2011.01.004

Cornelius, Wayne A. 2001. "Deaths at the Border: Efficacy and Unintended Consequences of US Immigration Control Policy." *Population and Development Review* 27 (4): 661–85. https://doi.org/10.1111/j.1728-4457.2001.00661.x

Cristancho, Sergio, D. Marcela Garces, Karen E. Peters, and Benjamin C. Mueller. 2008. "Listening to Rural Hispanic Immigrants in the Midwest: A Community-based Participatory Assessment of Major Barriers to Health Care Access and Use." *Qualitative Health Research* 18 (5): 633–46. https://doi.org/10.1177/1049732308316669

Crocker, Rebecca M., Robin C. Reineke, and María Elena Ramos Tovar. 2021. "Ambiguous Loss and Embodied Grief Related to Mexican Migrant Disappearances." *Medical Anthropology* 40 (7): 598–11. https://doi.org/10.1080/01459740.2020.1860962

Crooks, Deborah L. 1995. "American Children at Risk: Poverty and its Consequences for Children's Health, Growth, and School Achievement." *Yearbook of Physical Anthropology* 38 (S21): 57–86. https://doi.org/10.1002/ajpa.1330380605

Cullinan, Mary P., Pauline J. Ford, and Gregory J. Seymour. 2009. "Periodontal Disease and Systemic Health: Current Status." *Australian Dental Journal* 54 (s1): S62–S69. https://doi.org/10.1111/j.1834-7819.2009.01144.x

Day, Angela, Claudia R. Magaña-González, and Kathi Wilson. 2021. "Examining Indigenous Perspectives on the Health Implications of Large-Scale Agriculture in Jalisco, Mexico." *The Canadian Geographer* 65 (1): 36–49. https://doi.org/10.1111/cag.12642

De León, Jason. 2015. *The Land of Open Graves: Living and Dying on the Migrant Trail.* Oakland: University of California Press.

DeWitte, Sharon N., and Jelena Bekvalac. 2010. "Oral Health and Frailty in the Medieval English Cemetery of St Mary Graces." *American Journal of Physical Anthropology* 142: 341–54. https://doi.org/10.1002/ajpa.21228

Eschbach, Karl, Jacquelin M. Hagan, Nestor Rodriguez, Ruben Hernandez-Leon, and Stanley Bailey. 1999. "Death at the Border." *International Migration Review* 33 (2): 430–54. https://doi.org/10.2307/2547703

Fancher, James P. 2018. "Overview of Dental Disease and Differential Diagnosis Based on Detectable Artifacts of Disease." Poster presented at the 87th annual meeting of the American Association of Physical Anthropologists, Austin, TX.

Farmer, Paul. 1996. "On Suffering and Structural Violence: A View from Below." *Daedalus* 125 (1): 261–83. https://www.jstor.org/stable/20027362

———— 2004. "An Anthropology of Structural Violence." *Current Anthropology* 45: 305–25. https://doi.org/10.1086/382250

Fuentes-Afflick, Elena, and Nancy A. Hessol. 2009. "Immigration Status and Use of Health Services Among Latina Women in the San Francisco Bay Area." *Journal of Women's Health* 18 (8): 1275–80. https://doi.org/10.1089/jwh.2008.1241

Galtung, Johan. 1969. "Violence, Peace, and Peace Research." *Journal of Peace Research* 6: 167–91. https://www.jstor.org/stable/422690

Gálvez, Alyshia. 2018. *Eating NAFTA: Trade, Food Policies, and the Destruction of Mexico.* Oakland: University of California Press.

Gimenez, Thais, Beatriz Albuquerque Bispo, Daniela Pereira Souza, Maria Eduarda Viganó, Marcia Turolla Wanderley, Fausto Medeiros Mendes, Marcelo Bönecker, and Mariana Minatel Braga. 2016. "Does the Decline in Caries Prevalence of Latin American and Caribbean Children Continue in the New Century? Evidence from Systemic Review with Meta-Analysis." *PLoS ONE* 11 (10): e0164903. https://doi.org/10.1371/journal.pone.0164903

Goad, Gennifer. 2020. "Expanding Humanitarian Forensic Action: An approach to US Cold Cases." *Forensic Anthropology* 3 (1): 50–59. https://doi.org/10.5744/fa.2020.1006

Gocha, Timothy P., M. Katherine Spradley, and Ryan Strand. 2018. "Bodies in Limbo: Issues in Identification and Repatriation of Migrant Remains in South Texas." In *Sociopolitics of Migrant Death and Repatriation: Perspectives from Forensic Science,* edited by Krista E. Latham and Allison J. O'Daniel, 143–56. Cham: Springer. https://doi.org/10.1007/978-3-319-61866-1_11

Goodman, Alan H. 2013. "Bringing Culture into Human Biology and Biology Back into Anthropology." *American Anthropologist* 115 (3): 359–73. https://doi.org/10.1111/aman.12022

Goodman, Alan H., and Thomas L. Leatherman. 1998. *Building a New Biocultural Synthesis: Political-Economic Perspectives on Human Biology.* Ann Arbor: University of Michigan Press. https://doi.org/10.3998/mpub.10398

Gravlee, Clarence C. 2009. "How Race Becomes Biology: Embodiment of Social Inequality." *American Journal of Physical Anthropology* 139 (1): 47–57. https://doi.org/10.1002/ajpa.20983

Hillson, Simon. 2008. "Dental Pathology." In *Biological Anthropology of the Human Skeleton, Second Edition*, edited by M. Anne Katzenberg and Shelley R. Saunders, 301–40. Hoboken: Wiley-Liss. https://doi.org/10.1002/9780470245842

Hollister, M.C., and Jane A. Weintraub. 1993. "The Association of Oral Health Status with Systemic Health, Quality of Life, and Economic Productivity." *Journal of Dental Education* 57 (12): 901–12. https://doi.org/10.1002/j.0022-0337.1993.57.12.tb02821.x

Holmes, Seth M. 2013. *Fresh Fruit, Broken Bodies: Migrant Farmworkers in the United States.* Berkeley: University of California Press.

Horton, Sarah, and Judith C. Barker. 2009. "'Stains' on their Self-Discipline: Public Health, Hygiene, and the Disciplining of Undocumented Immigrant Parents in the Nation's Internal Borderlands." *American Ethnologist* 36 (4): 784–98. https://doi.org/10.1111/j.1548-1425.2009.01210.x

———. 2010. "Stigmatized Biologies: Examining the Cumulative Effects of Oral Health Disparities for Mexican American Farmwork Children." *Medical Anthropology Quarterly* 24 (2): 199–219. https://doi.org/10.1111/j.1548-1387.2010.01097.x

———. 2017. "Oral Health as a Citizen-Making Project: Immigrant Parents' Contestations of Dental Public Health Campaigns." In *Thinking through Resistance: A Study of Public Oppositions to Contemporary Global Health Practice*, edited by Nicola Bulled, 112–27. New York: Routledge. https://doi.org/10.4324/9781315209685

Huang, Deborah L., and Mijung Park. 2014. "Socioeconomic and Racial/Ethnic Oral Health Disparities among US Older Adults: Oral Health Quality of Life and Dentition." *Journal of Public Health Dentistry* 75 (2): 85–92. https://doi.org/10.1111/jphd.12072

Hughes, Cris E., Bridget F.B. Algee-Hewitt, Robin Reineke, Elizabeth Clausing, and Bruce E. Anderson. 2017. "Temporal Patterns of Mexican Migrant Genetic Ancestry: Implications for Identification." *American Anthropologist* 119 (2): 193–208. https://doi.org/10.1111/aman.12845

Hunter, John M., and Sonia Arbona. 1995. "The Tooth as a Marker of Developing World Quality of Life: A Field study in Guatemala." *Social Science & Medicine* 41 (9): 1217–40. https://doi.org/10.1016/0277-9536(95)00011-U

Jiménez-Gayosso, Sandra I., Carlo E. Medina-Solís, Edith Lara-Carillo, Rogelio J. Scougal-Vilchis, Rubén de la Rosa-Santillana, Sonia Márquez-Rodríguez, Martha Mendoza-Rodríguez, and José de J. Navarette-Hernández. 2015. "Socioeconomic

Inequalities in Oral Health Service Utilization Any Time in Their Lives for Mexican Schoolchildren 6 to 12 Years Old." *Gaceta Médica de México* 151 (1): 27–33.

Kinaston, Rebecca, Anna Willis, Justyna J. Miszkiewicz, Monica Tromp, and Marc F. Oxenham. 2019. "The Dentition: Development, Disturbances, Disease, Diet, and Chemistry." In *Ortner's Identification of Pathological Conditions in Human Skeletal Remains*, third edition, edited by Jane E. Buikstra, 749–98. San Diego: Academic Press. https://doi.org/10.1016/B978-0-12-809738-0.00021-1

Klaus, Haagen D. 2012. "The Bioarchaeology of Structural Violence: A Theoretical Model and a Case Study." In *The Bioarchaeology of Violence*, edited by Debra L. Martin, Ryan P. Harrod, and Ventura R. Pérez, 29–62. Gainesville: University of Florida Press. https://doi.org/10.5744/florida/9780813041506.003.0003

Koutlias, Lauren G., Michelle D. Hamilton, Diana Newberry, Nicholas P. Herrmann, and Kate Spradley. 2020. "Comparing Dental Indicators of Developmental Stress in Unidentified Migrant Remains to Narratives from Living Migrants: A Cross-Disciplinary Approach." Paper presented at the 72nd annual meeting of the American Academy of Forensic Sciences, Anaheim, CA.

Krieger, Nancy. 1994. "Epidemiology and the Web of Causation: Has Anyone Seen the Spider?" *Social Science & Medicine* 39 (7): 887–903. https://doi.org/10.1016/0277-9536(94)90202-X

———. 1999. "Embodying Inequality: A Review of Concepts, Measures, and Methods for Studying Health Consequences of Discrimination." *International Journal of Health Services* 29 (2): 295–352. https://doi.org/10.2190/M11W-VWXE-KQM9-G97Q

———. 2005. "Embodiment: A Conceptual Glossary for Epidemiology." *Journal of Epidemiology and Community Health* 59 (5): 350–55. https://doi.org/10.1136/jech.2004.024562

———. 2012. "Methods for the Scientific Study of Discrimination and Health: An Ecosocial Approach." *American Journal of Public Health* 102 (5): 936–45. https://doi.org/10.2105/AJPH.2011.300544

Langlais, Robert P., Craig S. Miller, and Jill S. Gehrig. 2017. *Color Atlas of Common Oral Diseases*, Fifth Edition. Philadelphia: Wolters Kluwer.

Leutert, Stephanie, Sam Lee, and Victoria Rossi. 2020. "Migrant Deaths in South Texas." Strauss Center for International Security and Law, The University of Texas at Austin Report. https://www.strausscenter.org/wp-content/uploads/Migrant_Deaths_South_Texas-1.pdf

Levin, Anna, Karen Sokal-Gutierrez, Anita Hargrave, Elizabeth Funsch, and Kristin S. Hoeft. 2017. "Maintaining Traditions: A Qualitative Study of Early Childhood Caries Risk and Protective Factors in an Indigenous Community." *International Journal of Environmental Research and Public Health* 14 (8): 907. https://doi.org/10.3390/ijerph14080907

Lukacs, John R. 2012. "Oral Health in Past Populations: Context, Concepts, and Controversies." In *A Companion to Paleopathology*, edited by Anne L. Grauer, 553–81. Malden: Blackwell.

Lukacs, John R., and Leah L. Largaespada. 2006. "Explaining Sex Differences in Dental Caries Prevalence: Saliva, Hormones, and 'Life History' Etiologies."

32   *Angela Soler et al.*

American Journal of Human Biology 18 (4): 540–55. https://doi.org/10.1002/ajhb .20530

Lypka, Michael, and Jeffrey Hammoudeh. 2011. "Dentoalveolar Infections." *Oral and Maxillofacial Surgery Clinics of North America* 23 (3): 415–24. https://doi.org /10.1016/j.coms.2011.04.010

Maddi, Abhiran and Frank A. Scannapieco. 2013. "Oral Biofilms, Oral and Periodontal Infections, and Systemic Disease." *American Journal of Dentistry* 26 (5): 249–54.

Marrón-Ponce, Joaquín, Mario Flores, Gustavo Cediel, Carlos A. Monteiro, and Carolina Batis. 2019. "Associations between Consumption of Ultra Processed Foods and Intake of Nutrients Related to Chronic Non-Communicable Diseases in Mexico." *Journal of the Academy of Nutrition and Diet* 119 (11): 1852–65. https:// doi.org/10.1016/j.jand.2019.04.020

Martínez, Daniel E., Robin C. Reineke, Raquel Rubio-Goldsmith, Bruce E. Anderson, Gregory L. Hess, and Bruce O. Parks. 2013. "A Continued Humanitarian Crisis at the Border: Undocumented Border Crosser Deaths Recorded by the Pima County Office of the Medical Examiner, 1990–2012." Report. Binational Migration Institute, University of Arizona.

Martínez, Daniel E., Robin C. Reineke, Raquel Rubio-Goldsmith, and Bruce O. Parks. 2014. "Structural Violence and Migrant Deaths in Southern Arizona: Data from the Pima County Office of the Medical Examiner, 1990–2013." *Journal on Migration and Human Security* 2 (4): 257–86. https://doi.org/10.1177 /233150241400200401

Martínez, Daniel E., Robin C. Reineke, G. Boyce, S.N. Chambers, Bruce E. Anderson, Gregory L. Hess, Jennifer M. Vollner, Bruce O. Parks, Caitlin M.C. Vogelsberg, Gabriella Soto, Michael Kreyche, and Racquel Rubio-Goldsmith. 2021. "Migrant Deaths in Southern Arizona: Recovered Undocumented Border Crosser Remains Investigated by the Pima County Office of the Medical Examiner, 1990–2020." Report. Binational Migration Institute, University of Arizona.

Maserejian, Nancy N., Felicia Trachtenberg, Catherine Hayes, and Mary Tavares. 2007. "Oral Health Disparities in Children of Immigrants: Dental Caries Experience at Enrollment and Follow-up in the New England Children's Amalgam Trial." *Journal of Public Health Dentistry* 68 (1): 14–21. https://doi.org/10.1111/j.1752 -7325.2007.00060.x

Masuoka, David, Takashi Komabayashi, and Enrique Reyes-Vela. 2014. "Dental Education in Mexico." *Journal of Oral Health and Dental Management* 13 (2): 279–84.

Maupomé, Gerardo, E. Angeles Martínez-Mier, Alanna Holt, Carlo E. Medina-Solís, Andrés Mantilla-Rodríguez, and Brittany Carlton. 2013. "The Association Between Geographical Factors and Dental Caries in a Rural Area in Mexico." *Cadernos de Saúde Pública, Rio de Janeiro* 29 (7): 1407–14. https://doi.org/10 .1590/s0102-311x2013000700014

Medina-Solís, Carlo E., Ricardo Pérez-Núñez, Gerardo Maupomé, and Juan F. Casanova-Rosado. 2006. "Edentulism Among Mexican Adults Aged 35 Years and Older and Associated Factors." *American Journal of Public Health* 96 (9): 1578–81. https://doi.org/10.2105/AJPH.2005.071209

Medina-Solís, Carlo E., A.P. Pontigo-Loyola, E. Pérez-Campos, P. Hernández-Cruz, R. De la Rosa-Santillana, J.J. Navarrete-Hernández, and Gerardo E. Maupomé. 2013. "Principal Reasons for Extraction of Permanent Teeth in a Sample of Mexican Adults." *Revista Investigación Clínica* 65 (2): 141–49.

Michael, Amy, Mariyam I. Isa, Lee Redgrave, and Anthony Redgrave. 2021. "Structural Vulnerability in Transgender and Non-Binary Decedent Populations: Analytical Considerations and Harm Reduction Strategies." Paper presented at the 73rd Annual Meeting of the American Academy of Forensic Sciences, Virtual Conference.

Minaya-Sánchez, Mirna, Carlo E. Medina-Solís, Juan F. Casanova-Rosado, Alejandro J. Casanova-Rosado, Ma. De Lourdes Márquez-Corona, Horacio Islas-Granillo, and Arturo J. Islas-Márquez. 2010. "Tooth Loss and Periodontal Status Variables among Policemen from Campeche, Mexico." *Gaceta Médica de México* 146 (4): 264–68. https://europepmc.org/article/med/20964069

Mira, Alex, A. Simon-Soro, and M.A. Curtis. 2017. "Role of Microbial Communities in the Pathogenesis of Periodontal Diseases and Caries." *Journal of Clinical Periodontology* 44 (Suppl. 18): S23–S38. https://doi.org/10.1111/jcpe.12671

Molina-Frechero, Nelly, Enrique Castañeda-Castaneira, María José Marques-Dos-Santos, Alejandra Soria-Hernández, and Ronell Bologna-Molina. 2009. "Dental Caries and Risk Factors in Adolescents of Ecatepec in the State of Mexico." *Revista de Investigación Clínica* 61 (4): 300–5.

Pan American Health Organization (PAHO). 2012. "Health in the Americas." 2012 Edition, Country Volume, Guatemala. Pan American Health Organization, Washington, DC.

Pérez-Núñez, Ricardo, Carlo Eduardo Medina-Solís, Gerardo Maupomé, and Armando Vargas-Palacios. 2006. "Factors Associated with Dental Health Care Covered in Mexico: Findings from the National Performance Evaluation Survey 2002–2003." *Community Dentistry and Oral Epidemiology* 34 (5): 387–97. https://doi.org/10.1111/j.1600-0528.2006.00289.x

Pérez-Núñez, Ricardo, Armando Vargas-Palacios, Ivan Ochoa-Morena, and Carlo Eduardo Medina-Solís. 2007. "Household Expenditure in Dental Health Care: National Estimations in Mexico for 2000, 2002, 2004." *Journal of Public Health Dentistry* 67 (4): 234–42. https:///doi.org/10.1111/j.1752-7325.2007.00035.x

Pilloud, Marin A., and James P. Fancher. 2019. "Outlining a Definition of Oral Health within the Study of Human Skeletal Remains." *Dental Anthropology* 32 (2): 3–11. https://doi.org/10.26575/daj.v32i2.297

Raskin, Sarah. 2017. "'Toothless Maw-Maw Can't Eat No More': Stigma and Synergies of Dental Disease, Diabetes, and Psychosocial Stress among Low-Income Rural Appalachians." In *Stigma Syndemics: New Directions in Biosocial Health*, edited by Bayla Ostrach, Shir Lerman, and Merrill Singer, 193–215. Lanham: Lexington.

Reineke, Robin C. 2013. "Lost in the System: Unidentified Bodies on the Border." *NACLA Report on the Americas* 46 (2): 50–53. https://doi.org/10.1080/10714839.2013.11721998

————. 2019. "Necroviolence and Postmortem Care Along the U.S.-Mexico Border." In *The Border and its Bodies: The Embodiment of Risk Along the U.S.-México Line*, edited by Thomas E. Sheridan and Randall H. McGuire, 144–72. Tucson: University of Arizona Press. https://openresearchlibrary.org/viewer/565fd311 -5b90-423d-9084-d8fec00fbc67

Reineke, Robin C., and Bruce E. Anderson. 2010. "Sociocultural Factors in the Identification of Undocumented Migrants." Poster presented at the 61st annual meeting of the American Academy of Forensic Sciences, Seattle, WA.

————. 2016. "Missing in the U.S.-Mexico Borderlands." In *Missing Persons: Multidisciplinary Perspectives on the Missing and Deceased*, edited by Derek Congram, 249–68. Toronto: Canadian Scholars Press.

Rouxel, Patrick, Georgios Tsakos, Tarani Chandola, and Richard G. Watt. 2018. "Oral Health – A Neglected Aspect of Subjective Well-Being in Later Life." *The Journals of Gerontology Series B: Psychological Sciences and Social Sciences* 73 (3): 382–86. https://doi.org/10.1093/geronb/gbw024

Rubio-Goldsmith, Raquel, M. Melissa McCormick, Daniel Martínez, and Inez Magdalena Duarte. 2006. "The 'Funnel Effect' and Recovered Bodies of Unauthorized Migrants Processed by the Pima County Office of the Medical Examiner, 1990–2005." Report submitted to the Pima County Board of Supervisors. Tucson: Binational Migration Institute.

Sabbah, Wael, Georgios Tsakos, Aubrey Sheiham, and Richard G. Watt. 2009. "The Effects of Income and Education on Ethnic Differences in Oral Health: A Study in US Adults." *Journal of Epidemiology and Community Health* 63 (7): 516–20. https://doi.org/10.1136/jech.2008.082313

Schell, Lawrence M. 1997. "Culture as a Stressor: A Revised Model of Biocultural Interaction." *American Journal of Physical Anthropology* 102 (1): 67–77. https://doi.org/10.1002/(SICI)1096-8644(199701)102:1<67:: AID-AJPA6>3.0.CO;2-A

Selwitz, Robert H., Amid I. Ismail, and Nigel B Pitts. 2007. "Dental Caries." *The Lancet* 369 (9555): 51–59. https://doi.org/10.1016/S0140-6736(07)60031-2

Seymour, Gregory J., Pauline J. Ford, Mary P. Cullinan, Shaneen Leishman, and K. Yamazaki. 2007. "Relationship Between Periodontal Infections and Systemic Disease." *Clinical Microbiology and Infection* 13 (S4): 3–10. https://doi.org/10 .1111/j.1469-0691.2007.01798.x

Slack, Jeremy, and Scott Whiteford. 2018. "Violence and Migration on the Arizona-Sonora Border." In *The Shadow of the Wall: Violence and Migration along the U.S.-Mexico Border*, edited by Jeremy Slack, Daniel E. Martínez, and Scott Whiteford, 43–62. Tucson: University of Arizona Press.

Slack, Jeremy, Daniel E. Martínez, Alison E. Lee, and Scott Whiteford. 2018. "The Geography of Border Militarization: Violence, Death, and Health in Mexico and the United States." In *The Shadow of the Wall: Violence and Migration along the U.S.-Mexico Border*, edited by Jeremy Slack, Daniel E. Martínez, and Scott Whiteford, 94–119. Tucson: University of Arizona Press.

Soler, Angela, Robin C. Reineke, Jared S. Beatrice, and Bruce E. Anderson. 2014. "An Integrated Approach to the Identification of Human Remains: The Biocultural

Profile of Undocumented Migrants." Paper presented at the 66th annual meeting of the American Academy of Forensic Sciences, Seattle, WA.

Soler, Angela, and Jared S. Beatrice. 2018. "Expanding the Role of Forensic Anthropology in a Humanitarian Crisis: An Example from the United States-Mexico Border." In *Sociopolitics of Migrant Death and Repatriation: Perspectives from Forensic Science*, edited by Krista E. Latham and Alyson J. O'Daniel, 115–28. Cham, Switzerland: Springer. https://doi.org/10.1007/978-3 -319-61866-1_9

Soler, Angela, Robin C. Reineke, Jared S. Beatrice, and Bruce E. Anderson. 2019. "Etched in Bone: Embodied Suffering in the Remains of Undocumented Migrants." In *The Border and its Bodies: The Embodiment of Risk Along the U.S.-México Line*, edited by Thomas E. Sheridan and Randall H. McGuire, 173–207. Tucson: University of Arizona Press. https://openresearchlibrary.org/viewer/565fd311 -5b90-423d-9084-d8fec00fbc67

Soler, Angela, Jared S. Beatrice, Robin C. Reineke, and Daniel E. Martínez. 2020. "Beyond Identification: Structural Vulnerability and the Investigation of Migrant Deaths." Paper presented at the 72nd annual meeting of the American Academy of Forensic Sciences, Anaheim, CA.

US Border Patrol. 2020. "Southwest Border Sectors: Southwest Border Deaths by Fiscal Year." Washington, DC. https://www.cbp.gov/sites/default/files/assets/doc-uments/2020-Jan/U.S.%20Border%20Patrol%20Fiscal%20Year%20Southwest %20Border%20Sector%20Deaths%20%28FY%201998%20-%20FY%202019 %29_0.pdf

Vega Lizama, Elma Maria, and Andrea Cucina. 2014. "Maize Dependence or Market Integration? Caries Prevalence among Indigenous Maya Communities with Maize-Based Versus Globalized Economies." *American Journal of Physical Anthropology* 153 (2): 190–202. https://doi.org/10.1002/ajpa.22418

Velez, Diane, Ana Palomo-Zerfas, Arcela Nunez-Alvarez, Guadalupe X. Ayala, and Tracy L. Finlayson. 2017. "Facilitators and Barriers to Dental Care among Mexican Migrant Women and Their Families in North San Diego County." *Journal of Immigrant and Minority Health* 19 (5): 1216–26. https://doi.org/10.1007/s10903 -016-0467-2

Vered, Yuval, Varda Soskolne, Avi Zini, Alon Livny, and Harold D. Sgan-Cohen. 2011. "Psychological Distress and Social Support are Determinants of Changing Oral Health Status among an Immigrant Population from Ethiopia." *Community Dentistry and Oral Epidemiology* 39 (2): 145–53. https://doi.org/10.1111/j.1600 -0528.2010.00581.x

Villalobos-Rodelo, Juan J., Carlo E. Medina-Solís, Gerardo Maupomé, América P. Pontigo-Loyola, Laura Lau-Rojo, and Lourdes Verdugo-Barraza. 2007. "Caries Dental en Escolares de una Comunidad del Noroeste de México con Dentición Mixta y su Asociación con Algunas Variables Clínicas, Socioeconómicas y Sociodemográficas." *Revista de Investigación Clínica* 59 (4): 256–67.

Watt, Richard Geddie. 2007. "From Victim Blaming to Upstream Action: Tackling the Social Determinants of Oral Health." *Community Dentistry and Oral Epidemiology* 35 (1): 1–11. https://doi.org/10.1111/j.1600-0528.2007.00348.x

Weisensee, Katherine E., and M. Katherine Spradley. 2018. "Craniofacial Asymmetry as a Marker of Socioeconomic Status among Undocumented Mexican Immigrants in the United States." *Economics and Human Biology* 29: 122–27. https://doi.org /10.1016/j.ehb.2018.02.007

Wilson, Fernando A., Yang Wang, Jim P. Stimpson, Kimberly K. McFarland, and Karan P. Singh. 2016. "Use of Dental Services by Immigration Status in the United States." *Journal of the American Dental Association* 147 (3): 162–69.e4. https://doi .org/10.1016/j.adaj.2015.08.009

Wilson, Fernando A., Yang Wang, Luisa N. Borrell, Sejong Bae, and Jim P. Stimpson. 2018. "Disparities in Oral Health by Immigration Status in the United States." *Journal of the American Dental Association* 149 (6): 414–21.e3. https://doi .org/10.1016/j.adaj.2018.01.024

Wood, James W., George R. Milner, Henry C. Harpending, and Kenneth M. Weiss. 1992. "The Osteological Paradox: Problems of Inferring Prehistoric Health from Skeletal Samples." *Current Anthropology* 33 (4): 343–70. https://www.jstor.org/ stable/2743861

Yaussy, Samantha L., and Sharon N. DeWitte. 2019. "Calculus and Survivorship in Medieval London: The Association between Dental Disease and a Demographic Measure of General Health." *American Journal of Physical Anthropology* 168: 552–65. https://doi.org/10.1002/ajpa.23772

Znachko, Caroline L., Michelle D. Hamilton, Bruce E. Anderson, M. Katherine Spradley, and James T. Watson. 2020. "Impacts of Biosocial Environment on Developmental Plasticity among Unidentified Presumed Migrant Skeletal Remains Recovered along the United States-Mexico Border." Paper presented at the 72nd annual meeting of the American Academy of Forensic Sciences, Anaheim, CA.

Chapter 2

Forgotten Spaces

The Structural Disappearance of Migrants in South Texas

Molly A. Kaplan, Courtney C. Siegert, Mariah
E. Moe, Chloe P. McDaneld, and M. Kate Spradley

INTRODUCTION

Since the implementation of the Prevention through Deterrence policy, thousands of migrants have died crossing the U.S.-Mexico border, as increased militarization and surveillance have funneled these individuals seeking refuge and opportunity into desolate and dangerous terrain.[1] While this strategy intends to deter migration by increasing the risk of detention and bodily harm, migration has not slowed (Hiemstra 2019; Meyers 2006). Coinciding with the ongoing U.S. denial of asylum and refugee claims (Hiemstra 2019), clandestine migration through hazardous landscapes to avoid apprehension has increased. These expanded border security strategies have produced the chronic mass disaster at the U.S.-Mexico border, characterized by missing migrants and migrant deaths (Martínez et al. 2014; Rubio-Goldsmith et al. 2006; Spradley et al. 2019; Slack and Martínez 2019; Slack 2019).

Since 1998, over 7,800 deaths along the southwest border have been recorded by the U.S. Customs and Border Patrol (USCBP) (U.S. Customs and Border Protection 2020). However, these numbers are likely a gross underestimate due to the difficulty of recovering decedents from remote landscapes as well as systemic failures in documentation and records keeping (Ortega 2018). Especially in the expansive desert and ranchland environments in which migrants often perish, natural processes, such as extreme temperatures and animal scavenging can quickly decompose and scatter an individual's remains, greatly reducing their chances of being discovered or identified (Beck et al. 2015; Spradley, Hamilton, and Giordano 2012; De León 2015).

Exacerbating this difficulty in Texas is that the majority of shared borderland is privately owned and cannot be searched without permission (Kovic 2013; Spradley et al. 2016). While these processes of death and disappearance in the desert are a known and desired outcome of current U.S. immigration strategies, this chapter will focus on a second dimension of disappearance for deceased migrants: entry into the fragmented Justice of the Peace medicolegal system in South Texas.

Even though international human rights and humanitarian standards mandate that it is the state's responsibility to identify deceased individuals, in the United States there is no national system of death investigation, so this responsibility falls to the level of the state and often the county (Hanzlick 2007; International Committee of the Red Cross 2003). In South Texas, the burden to identify decedents is typically placed on local jurisdictions that are overwhelmed with high numbers of deaths and limited access to resources to carry out transnational investigations. With thirty-two Texas border counties that are each responsible for their own death investigations, fragmentation is inherent to the medicolegal system throughout the region. Although this fragmented system was in place before the extreme spikes in migrant deaths of the past two decades, the continued lack of state or national infrastructure, protocols, and personnel to deal with migrant deaths in Texas have created and perpetuated systems of inaction that leave both identified and unidentified cases in limbo without a clear trajectory for resolution (Davies, Isakjee, and Dhesi 2017; Kovic 2013; Reineke 2019). The outcome of this strained system is the large-scale burial of migrant decedents in unmarked graves and the inability to track cases over time and space. Limited access to medical examiners or forensic pathologists also means that most unidentified migrant remains are not sampled for DNA as required by law and are thus not afforded the opportunity for identification. This systemic investigative neglect and often-undignified treatment of migrant decedents is what this chapter argues constitutes the structural postmortem disappearance of migrants along the South Texas-Mexico border.

Expanding on the concept of *los nuevos desaparecidos*, or "the new disappeared" developed by Lynn Stephen and Christine Kovic, structural disappearance of unidentified migrants refers to the violent, systemic failings that serve to hinder the counting and identification of unknown decedents (Kovic 2013; Stephen 2008). Although related to enforced disappearances carried out by state actors and military regimes, what distinguishes *los nuevos desaparecidos* from those who have been kidnapped or directly murdered by the state is the seemingly passive and institutional nature of their erasure. Rather than being disposed of in mass graves, clandestine burials, or cremations, the remains of *los nuevos desaparecidos* are instead willfully concealed by the natural processes of the desert, and—in this case—the Texas medicolegal system itself.

Whereas Stephen and Kovic eloquently describe examples of nation states' marginalization and erasure of indigenous and migrant populations via economic disenfranchisement, rape and feminicide, the commodification of smuggling, and America's militarized border policies, the current chapter extends this discussion to the death management and postmortem treatment of unidentified migrant remains in South Texas (Kovic 2013; Stephen 2008). In addition to the denial of migrant life inherent to Prevention through Deterrence strategies, the concealment of migrant death and denial of identity being exercised through an underfunded and fragmented Texas death management system are uniquely complex processes that are violent, intentional, systemic, and indirect.

This chapter focuses on the complexity of the structural postmortem disappearance of migrant individuals in South Texas and explores the hierarchical impacts that these violent systems have on local communities and other marginalized populations. After first reviewing international and U.S. state laws for handling unidentified remains, the chapter describes the realities of jurisdictional death investigation in South Texas and the ways this under-capacitated system is particularly overwhelmed by staggering rates of migrant death. A discussion of the biopolitical and structurally violent mechanisms of Prevention through Deterrence then provides a framework for understanding the willful political neglect toward changing or improving the region's medicolegal system. Finally, the chapter presents the archaeological evidence of *los nuevos desaparecidos* through examples encountered by Operation Identification (OpID), a humanitarian project whose mission is to locate, recover, and identify unidentified, presumed migrants to return them to their families. Here, case studies are presented from forensic excavations at the Tres Norias Cemetery, located in Willacy County, TX approximately 35 miles north of the U.S.-Mexico border, where both unidentified migrants and other marginalized groups were encountered. As a microcosm of the pervasive consequences of violent inaction, these case studies highlight the patterned ways in which decedent groups are treated. While indigent community members are also being allowed to disappear in South Texas cemeteries, marked differences in the care with which the burials of migrants and non-migrants were handled speaks to the biopolitical processes of disappearance at work. All names have been changed to maintain the privacy of the individuals involved.

INTERNATIONAL HUMANITARIAN AND HUMAN RIGHTS LAW AS COMPARED TO THE UNITED STATES

Before describing the disappearance of migrant decedents in South Texas cemeteries, understanding international human rights and humanitarian laws is critical to appreciate how the rights of decedents and their families are currently being violated. Reviewing U.S. federal and Texas state laws on handling unidentified remains also illuminates how county practices are often non-compliant and demonstrates the overall lack of governmental will for reform. While new legislation offers some hope for improved death investigation, there is still much work to be done.

INTERNATIONAL HUMANITARIAN STANDARDS

The United Nations Declaration of Human Rights (1948) continues to serve as the foundation for modern international human rights law as it stipulates the basic, fundamental rights that are inherent to all individuals in every society regardless of nationality, language, gender, or any other classification. While these declarations were meant to apply to all human beings, the Geneva Conventions of 1949 and the Additional Protocols of 1977 served specifically to protect individuals in the context of international armed conflict (Gaggioli 2018). As a result, International Humanitarian Law (IHL) was developed to protect the victims of armed conflict and to reduce the savagery of war by requiring the dead to be managed with dignity and respect (International Committee of the Red Cross 2003). These statutes were the only standardized procedural documents at the time to address those who had perished on foreign land and set the standard for best practices for handling unidentified human remains (Gaggioli 2018). Not only are the countries involved in the armed conflict obligated to search for and retrieve the dead, but they are also expected to make efforts toward the identification and repatriation of their counterparts. If identifications or repatriations are not possible or delayed, all individuals, unidentified or otherwise, are required to be interred respectfully with explicit documentation of their burial location. Finally, Objective 8 of the UN Global Compact on Safe Orderly and Regular Migration expresses a commitment to "identify those who have died or gone missing, and to facilitate communication with affected families," in addition to specifying the need to "centralize and systematize data regarding corpses and ensure traceability after burial" (United Nations 2018, 16). Despite marking an important milestone in the visibility of migrant death, the 2018 Global Compact lacks any legal authority to ensure that investigations are being carried out and does not address the regional challenges faced along each migration corridor around the world. However, this document provides a roadmap with recommendations that could be adopted on a national level and implemented locally. Under both international humanitarian and human rights laws, nation-states are responsible for maintaining the *Right to Know* regarding families and the fate of their missing loved ones (International Committee of the Red Cross

2003; Reineke 2013). These laws should be considered the minimum accept-able engagement with the management of the unidentified dead; however, these standards remain in stark contrast to the realities experienced along the U.S.-Mexico border.

THE TEXAS CRIMINAL CODE OF PROCEDURE (TCCP) AND NEW FEDERAL LAW

Echoes of the international standards described above are found in the Texas Criminal Code of Procedure (TCCP), which requires investigation into all unidentified deaths occurring within the state, including collecting and submitting a DNA sample, and maintaining records of the disposition of all remains for a minimum of ten years (Texas Constitution and Statutes 2020a and b). Considering that both Texas law and international human rights accords call for dignified treatment of the dead, swift identification of unknown remains, and efforts to track and preserve evidence for unresolved cases, the current death management practices in South Texas can be char-acterized as legally non-compliant and impeding the rights of unidentified migrant decedents and their families (Texas Constitution and Statutes 2020b; Interpol General Assembly 1996; United Nations 2018). As counties are cur-rently left on their own, overwhelmed beyond capacity and without supervi-sion, those most in need of assistance have been relegated to unmarked graves in cemeteries throughout the region.

At the federal level, there is hope for future intervention with the recent passing of the *Missing Persons and Unidentified Remains Act* (S.2174) in December 2020. This Act will allow state and local units of government, crime laboratories, forensic anthropology centers, and non-governmental organizations to apply for grant funding to assist with the identification of missing persons. The bill was proposed by Congressman Vicente Gonzalez from the 15th District in Texas to help local jurisdictions within border states and was passed through Congress with recent political momentum. Most notable about the bill is that it provides privacy protections for DNA samples from families of the missing, allows funds to be used to increase staff at laboratories working with unidentified human remains, covers costs for transportation, processing, and identification efforts, and requires reporting to the National Missing and Unidentified Persons System (NamUs) and the National Crime Information Center (NCIC). The bill further requires addi-tional reporting efforts for U.S. Customs and Border Patrol for unidentified human remains.

While this bill will hopefully provide funding to the jurisdictions and agen-cies that are currently overwhelmed with unidentified human remains, it does little to address the systemic problems of jurisdictional fragmentation and the transnational barriers related to identification. It is also currently unknown whether local jurisdictions have the capacity to write grants and administer the funds from this bill. However, this bill is a major step forward as it is the first acknowledgment by the federal government of the loss of life and the mass disaster at the border.

THE EFFECTS OF PREVENTION THROUGH DETERRENCE IN SOUTH TEXAS

Migrant deaths continue at disastrous proportions along the Texas southern border, with the true numbers remaining impossible to know. Particularly throughout the past decade, influxes of migration from Central America coupled with ever-increasing border militarization has led to shifting routes and increased deaths of more diverse groups of people throughout South Texas. Although migration from Central America, and particularly the "Northern Triangle" of Guatemala, El Salvador, and Honduras, has occurred since the 1980s, driven by civil wars, natural disasters, and economic hardships, recent increases in homicide rates, gang violence, and corruption in these countries has sparked even higher numbers of Central Americans seeking asylum in the United States (O'Connor, Batalova, and Bolter 2019). This demographic shift is reflected both in the record number of families and unaccompanied minors apprehended by U.S. Customs and Border Protection (USCBP) since 2011, as well as in the spikes of deaths occurring in South Texas since 2012 (O'Connor, Batalova, and Bolter 2019; U.S. Customs and Border Protection 2020). This is particularly evident in the Rio Grande Valley which has had approximately 1,000 additional migrant fatalities documented since then. These rates in death, however, are the direct result of expanding USCBP checkpoints in the region, such as that in Brooks County, which push migrants to traverse farther on foot through increasingly remote ranchland in extreme temperatures as far as 60 miles north of the border (Frey 2015; Spradley et al. 2019). Despite these increasing death rates in South Texas, the region remains one of the financially poorest and most sparsely populated in the country with local capacity utterly overburdened and underequipped to handle proper investigations.

While both Texas and Arizona have county-based medical examiner systems, Arizona has fewer counties, providing a higher ratio of medical examiners to counties, which creates a death investigation system that is accessible and streamlined, even for remote jurisdictions. The county-based system in Texas, however, is quite the opposite. The extremely low ratio of counties serviced by medical examiners relegates most death investigation along the

Texas border to Justices of the Peace, local sheriff's offices, and even funeral homes (Spradley et al. 2019; Gocha, Spradley, and Strand 2018). Although traditionally underfunded and under-developed, this jurisdictional system in South Texas was designed to handle only a few deaths per year and even fewer unidentified cases. Yet, despite the thousands of migrant deaths that have characterized the southern border throughout the past decade, nothing has been done at the state or federal level to reform or capacitate death investigation in Texas (Spradley et al. 2019; Gocha, Spradley, and Strand 2018). With only 14 of the 254 counties having medical examiners, and only one medical examiner in all of the Rio Grande Valley, counties continue to lack the necessary funding to transport decedents to forensic practitioners, pay for autopsies, and maintain proper storage (Spradley et al. 2019; Gocha, Spradley, and Strand 2018). Additionally, without access to transnational mechanisms to facilitate the comparison of antemortem and postmortem data, even counties with access to forensic services are unable to reconcile most migrant death cases, and, as such, put forth minimal efforts to do so. The majority of unidentified migrants found in South Texas are therefore buried in local cemeteries without having been forensically examined or genetically sampled. The manner in which these individuals are buried, including the marking of graves and tracking of cases, not only affects the preservation of evidence and the ability to re-locate burials for identification, but also greatly reflects the differential postmortem dignity afforded to these undocumented persons.

In response to this chronic mass disaster in South Texas, Operation Identification (OpID), a humanitarian project within the Forensic Anthropology Center at Texas State University (FACTS), was formed in 2013 to facilitate the recovery, identification, and repatriation of unidentified presumed migrants in collaboration with local jurisdictions, international governmental organizations, and other human rights groups (Spradley et al. 2019; Gocha, Spradley, and Strand 2018). OpID currently manages 330 active unidentified presumed migrant cases and has facilitated 63 identifications, with temporary custody for these cases obtained through Justice of the Peace permissions. In conjunction with the Forensic Border Coalition (FBC), and particularly the South Texas Human Rights Center (STHRC), OpID has conducted numerous forensic excavations and surveys in cemeteries throughout South Texas. Throughout years of fieldwork, OpID has repeatedly encountered challenges with the region's medicolegal system, including missing or deficient death certificates, case reports, and funeral home records, as well as missing case files in the NamUs database. Within the cemeteries, maps are either non-existent or inaccurate, and grave markers are temporary and flimsy, often being displaced by cemetery maintenance or missing all together (Gocha, Spradley, and Strand 2018; Spradley et al. 2016; Spradley et al. 2019). These insufficient burial and documentation practices have necessitated time and labor-intensive archaeological survey and excavation in order to locate remains for identification. Without these forensic exhumations, many individuals would have no chance of being found, and it is still unclear how many decedents have yet to be recovered.

The location, identification, and dignified handling of the dead are critical to safeguard the rights of migrant decedents and their families according to the international humanitarian and human rights standards previously discussed. Despite also being required by Texas state law to investigate all suspicious or unidentified deaths, local authorities simply lack the resources, training, and oversight to fulfill these legal and ethical obligations. Yet, the problem with this fragmented, overwhelmed system is complex. On the one hand, the perpetual neglect of the death crisis in South Texas by state and national actors is an intentional and biopolitical strategy that denies transnational migrants their identity, essentially allowing them to disappear. This neglect also impacts local Texas authorities as well as known community members, whose postmortem treatment can also suffer at the hands of the strapped system. On the other hand, the patterned mistreatment of certain groups in South Texas also reflects processes of othering within the medicolegal system itself in which financially poor citizens and migrants are handled in distinctly careless and disrespectful ways. These permeating, trickle-down impacts of Prevention through Deterrence on death investigation speak to the multi-tiered power structure governing life and death at the Texas southern border. It is within this structure that unidentified migrants are willfully forgotten, becoming *los nuevos desaparecidos*.

GOVERNING LIFE AND DEATH AT THE U.S.-MEXICO BORDER

To fully appreciate the concept of *los nuevos desaparecidos* and the mechanisms of disappearance affecting migrants in South Texas, it is important to review the theories that best speak to how structural forces and institutional actors can violently eradicate human beings. In terms of global migration, and particularly in South Texas, it is largely intentional and collective inaction that serves to further disappear individuals even after death.

Originally coined by Kjellén (1916) and re-conceptualized by Foucault (1997), biopolitics suggests that the sociopolitical structures of power and knowledge are used to order, restrain, and control human biological processes. For Foucault, these processes were contingent upon one another; political will and regulations were implicated in all aspects of biology and neither could be understood without the other. This is particularly important when considering mass migration across the U.S.-Mexico border in which the political dynamics of the migrant's country of origin create an unsustainable environment that not only forces individuals to find alternative means of survival and access to rights, but quite literally etches its effects on their bodies (Beatrice and Soler 2016; Soler and Beatrice 2018). Although the United States has also historically intervened in the sovereignty of Latin America, creating the conditions that force people to migrate to survive, it is U.S. legal frameworks and discourse on criminalizing migration that has most shaped the disposability—and hence disappearance—of migrants along the southern border.

While any person has the right to migrate under international law, their status as legal versus illegal is produced by the states that govern visa issuance and the provision of asylum and refugee status. A historic understanding of the current militarized stance on migration at the U.S.-Mexico border revolves around three key laws: the *Immigration and Nationality Act of 1965*, the *1986 Immigration Reform and Control Act (IRCA)*, and the *Illegal Immigration Reform and Immigrant Responsibility Act (IIRIRA)*. Together, these acts laid the groundwork for the othering of immigrants as illegal and not worthy of equitable treatment.

First, the *Immigration and Nationality Act of 1965* ended the quota system established by the *Immigration Act of 1924*, or the "National Origins Act", which established quotas for immigrants coming from different countries, effectively legitimizing "white" immigrants over "black" and "brown" immigrants (Hiemstra 2019). Although praised as progressive reform because of its elimination of the national-origins quotas, the *Immigration and Nationality Act of 1965* created restrictive limits on the number of annual immigrant visas that could be distributed to migrants coming from the Western Hemisphere (Hiemstra 2019).

The IRCA was later passed to decrease the large undocumented immigrant population branded as a "threat to national security" (Hiemstra 2019, 52). Marking a turning point in labeling certain persons as "illegal," IRCA allowed for criminal charges to be brought against people for violating immigration laws (Abrego et al. 2017). This act directly led to increased detention and the expansion of immigration enforcement to local governments, effectively criminalizing irregular migration throughout the country (Hiemstra 2019). Additionally, this policy coincides with the development of the "prison industrial complex" and the expansion of deterrence strategies at the southwest border, including increased surveillance and apprehension efforts (Slack and Martínez 2019) and the extension of the U.S.-Mexico border beyond territorial boundaries (Abrego et al. 2017). Directly in line with Foucault's concepts of governance through discipline, restraint, and surveillance (1997), the IRCA was a milestone for U.S. national control over migrant bodies and created the conceptual foundation for Prevention through Deterrence.

Finally, the IIRIRA passed in 1996 to further expand immigration officials' power to detain and deport immigrants. By broadening the list of criminal offenses associated with immigration, elevating the classification of minor offenses to aggravated felonies, and curtailing immigrants' rights to due process through the establishment of "expedited removal" in which immigration officials may order deportation rather than a judge, the IIRIRA solidified the criminalization and disposability of migrating persons considered "undesirable" and a threat to U.S. sovereignty (Abrego et al. 2017; Hiemstra 2019). Collectively, these policies of the last fifty years helped redefine *legal* versus *illegal* immigrant status in the United States, and their enactments follow historical events that contributed to heightened security fears produced by the state. Specifically, IRCA and IIRIRA helped to fill the post-Cold War vacuum, in which a new enemy of the state needed to be defined (Betts and Collier 2017; Hiemstra 2019). Overall, these policies contributed to tightening migration controls that broaden definitions of *illegal migration* while simultaneously reducing the opportunities for legal migration.

Yet, to fully understand the scope of the state's control over migration, it is also important to consider the systemic denial of refugee and asylum status as much as the expansion of detention and criminalization. While the idea of "refuge," defined as a place of shelter, protection, and safety, was developed through a common sense of humanity in the international arena, the status of *refugee* has become imbricated with the concept of the right to migrate (Betts and Collier 2017). Specifically, Betts and Collier (2017) suggest that nation-state fragility and feelings toward government legitimacy contribute to the mass violence that causes asylum seekers to have no choice but to flee their country of origin. However, as more people migrate because they are unable to obtain the basic needs that ensure their human dignity, often termed *survival migration*, migrants are stuck between legal definitions and their urgent experiences of harm. Considering the current U.S. stance on migration, the supposed definition that legitimizes refugee or asylee seeker claims is no longer applicable (Betts and Collier 2017). By denying asylum, conducting mass deportations, and prohibiting accessible avenues for legal migration, the government ubiquitously disregards the potential for individuals to experience extreme harm in their country of origin and thus denies the validity of survival migration claims. A possible solution to rectify the escalating disconnect between policy intention and reality lies in the notion of *force majeure*, in which those who migrate do so because they have no other option (Betts and Collier 2017). However, in the absence of this framework, restrictive U.S. policies currently cause individuals who feel they have no other option to seek out alternative, clandestine, and dangerous pathways to maintain their human rights. These individuals are then made to fight for survival on their journey when facing border enforcement policies that prioritize the perception of national security over life.

Finally, building upon the concept of biopolitics, Mbembe (2003) describes necropolitics, with regard to these concepts of life and death as coordinated through social and political power. According to Mbembe (2003), necropolitics explains how those who enact policies and operate within structures of power are afforded the right to dictate who should live and who should die. Through hegemonic strategies, the unspeakable can become rationalized, accepted, and expected. At the U.S.-Mexico border, necropolitical power is embedded in current Prevention through Deterrence policies, which were implemented to order and restrain the flow of migration by imposing tactics that would lead to sharp increases in death in the hopes that fear would deter other would-be migrants. By imbuing policymakers with ultimate power over the lives of immigrants, migrant deaths along the border came to be used as a metric for the success of the Prevention through Deterrence program (Kovic 2013; De León 2015). Beyond just deterrence by fear of death, however, these policies also serve to relegate even those who survive the journey to "less-than" spaces of illegality and statelessness, effectively controlling and denying their right to life once they are successfully in the country (Reineke 2019). Additionally, because clandestine migration is often only successful with the help of a coyote (i.e., a guide), migrants are further made vulnerable by the commodification of trafficking, as well as the extortion of families who lack knowledge about their loved one's whereabouts (Kovic 2013; Hiemstra 2019; Slack and Martínez 2019). For many individuals who succumb on the trail, biopolitical treatment then follows in death through the erasure of migrant bodies (Kovic 2013; Spradley et al. 2019).

These examples highlight how precariousness and vulnerability are produced and exploited by the state through the criminalization of immigration, denial of asylum, and development of policies that cause migrating individuals to be labeled as illegal, viewed as deportable, and consequently perceived as disposable. These processes of marginalization to constrain life are further made "natural" in death as efforts toward the identification of transnational migrants continue to be marred in systems of inaction.

SYSTEMS OF INACTION

Structural violence, broadly described as systemic inequity or oppression that hinders human beings from actualizing their potential, is embedded in many aspects of migration. While not always fully separated from interpersonal acts of violence, structural violence captures the institutionalized forces that both directly and indirectly deprive people of the equal opportunity for life (Galtung 1969). Often equated with social injustice, the theory of structural violence encompasses societal subjugation of various groups as well as large-scale unequal distributions of power and resources among nations (Galtung 1969).

In terms of migration, institutionalized systems of capitalist inequity such as the North American Free Trade Agreement (NAFTA) (Kovic 2013), corrupt governments, and cartel violence all serve as major violent forces driving irregular migration along the Central America-Mexico-U.S. migration corridor (Stephen 2008; Kovic 2018; Martínez et al. 2014; Vogt 2013). The high rates of migrant death at the U.S. southern border are also a product of the structural violence inherent to the "funnel effect" created by increased border militarization and prohibitive immigration policies described above (Rubio-Goldsmith et al. 2006; Martínez et al. 2014; Vogt 2013). Not only do these policies directly restrict movement, which in turn causes death, but they also serve to conceal and justify human suffering by placing responsibility on migrants themselves (Galtung 1969; Martínez et al. 2014).

Beyond the violence embedded in irregular migration routes, there has been an increasing awareness of the political and often violent nature of death investigation itself. Even within U.S. forensic casework, the management and handling of the dead can, intentionally or unintentionally, perpetuate systems of marginalization and exercise processes of erasure (Goad 2020; Reineke 2019; Davies, Isakjee, and Dhesi 2017; De León 2015; Mbembe 2003). For one, structural inequities for certain groups in life, such as a lack of access to resources or healthcare, can inhibit and delay identification by limiting the antemortem data available for reconciling cases (Goad 2020; Hughes et al. 2017). Additionally, investigative inaction or neglect, as well as the discriminatory treatment of remains can be considered both passive and active forms of necroviolence that deprive certain groups the equal opportunity to be identified (Reineke 2019; De León 2015). Specifically, the lack of federal or state support for death management in South Texas should be recognized as a primary dimension of necroviolence related to Prevention through Deterrence that functions cooperatively with the physical landscape to erase migrant bodies and conceal the vast scope of death in the region. Considering the difficulty of recovering visually identifiable remains from these harsh landscapes, ensuring optimal preservation of bodies and evidence is often the only way to obtain viable samples for DNA analysis, facilitate positive identifications, and provide answers to families (Anderson 2008; Fleischman et al. 2017; Spradley et al. 2019). To hinder or not guarantee that populations of unidentified decedents receive proper care, analysis, and curation is therefore in itself a political act of othering that classifies individuals with irregular migration status as people who can be "let" to die and left to be forgotten (Mbembe 2003).

Although the jurisdictional system in South Texas was already fragmented and under-resourced, the complete lack of governmental effort or political will to capacitate this system in the face of overwhelming migrant deaths both exploits and allows the perpetual overburdening of financially poor counties and represents a secondary tier of institutional violence. Many individual actors dedicate time and resources to ensure the decent treatment of unidentified remains, but are met with un-ending obstacles in communication, funding, transport, and services due to absent medicolegal infrastructure. Though racial discrimination, a tertiary dimension of violence, also contributes to poor case tracking and the undignified treatment of migrant remains, the regional inaction and careless treatment of dead bodies in South Texas is predominantly a product of willful negligence at the state and federal levels. Unfortunately, this willful negligence continues to have detrimental consequences for multiple living and deceased stakeholders in the Rio Grande Valley.

LOS NUEVOS DESAPARECIDOS: EXEMPLIFIED THROUGH THE TRES NORIAS CEMETERY

To explore the multi-tiered power structures and forms of (necro)violence occurring in South Texas, the chapter now turns to a case study of the Tres Norias Cemetery. It is here where forensic exhumations conducted by Operation Identification (OpID) revealed archaeological evidence of disappearance and undignified postmortem treatment of both unknown and known decedents. Characterized by dozens of unmarked burials of unidentified migrants intermixed with indigent local residents, Tres Norias exemplifies the nuanced, trickle-down effects of the systemic inaction and fragmentation of the South Texas medicolegal system.

Tres Norias is a small, privately owned cemetery located in Willacy County, approximately 35 miles north of the U.S.-Mexico border (figure 2.1). The cemetery was identified as an area of interest for recovering unidentified migrant decedents following an analysis of death certificate records by the Forensic Border Coalition (FBC), of which OpID is a founding member. The FBC, formed in 2013, is a collaborative team of forensic scientists, scholars, and human rights and non-governmental organizations working to support families in their search for missing loved ones and to address issues pertaining to the identification of human remains found near the U.S. southern border.

Death certificates filed with the state of Texas suggest that approximately seventeen unidentified individuals were buried at Tres Norias between 2007 and 2016. Prior to 2007, the southern section of Tres Norias Cemetery, where

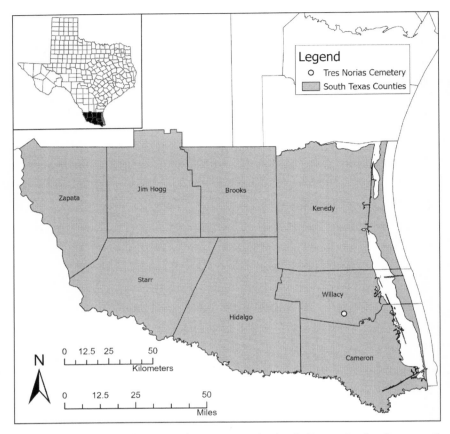

Figure 2.1 Location of Tres Norias Cemetery in South Texas. Credit: Courtney C. Siegert.

the majority of unidentified, presumed migrants were buried, was used as an agricultural field. Although Tres Norias is located in Willacy County, these cases originated from Cameron County to the south, according to a Cameron County death investigator and vital statistics records. Furthermore, records from NamUs suggested five burials of unidentified remains at Tres Norias, three of which correspond to filed death certificates.

The locations of these unidentified burials, however, were not available through any official record or map, but rather existed in memory, making pedestrian survey and further cemetery evaluation necessary. A county official who handled many of these cases pointed out thirty-one areas thought to contain an unidentified decedent, twenty-three of which were unmarked. These unmarked areas were clear, shallow depressions in the ground surface, most having marked differences in vegetation from the surrounding surface.

Thus, the areas pointed out to the FBC seemed credible as they exhibited textbook signatures of a burial. At this time, the county official also revealed that not all of the unidentified human remains buried at Tres Norias had DNA samples submitted to University of North Texas Center for Human Identification (UNTCHI), as had been required by law since 2005 (Texas Constitution and Statues 2020b).

Exhumation Findings

After this initial cemetery evaluation, it was clear to OpID and the FBC that exhumation would provide the only opportunity for identification for these individuals. However, once forensic excavations were under way, the team quickly realized that recovering unidentified presumed migrants would prove challenging. During exhumation efforts, OpID routinely conducts field intakes, similar to triage assessments to facilitate and expedite anthropological analysis and identification once cases are transferred back to the laboratory. During initial field intake procedures at Tres Norias, OpID encountered several individuals whose burial features suggested they were indigent or unclaimed community members rather than unidentified presumed migrants. This realization prompted the team to develop a contextual profile for burials that would be considered likely to represent unidentified migrants while conducting field exhumations.

Because indigent burials of known community members were also in unmarked graves and were interspersed among probable unknown migrant remains, every burial container that was encountered was opened and assessed to determine whether remains fit the scope of the OpID project. Several indicators were used to make these determinations including the positioning of the remains within the burial container (figure 2.2), placement of personal effects, associated documentation with names that did not match any migrant records, significant medical intervention suggestive of palliative care (e.g., central lines, catheters and feeding tubes), and indications of advanced age.

In total, seventy-eight individuals were uncovered during exhumations in January and June 2018 (figure 2.3). However, thirty-eight of these decedents were recognized as primarily elderly community members, many of whom had received medical intervention or died at hospitals and were subsequently interred in indigent or unclaimed burials by the county. These cases are hereafter referred to as *not forensically significant* since they do not meet the scope of the OpID project, which seeks to facilitate the identification and repatriation of unidentified, presumed migrants. In fact, thirteen of the decedents at Tres Norias Cemetery had names written on red tags or documents

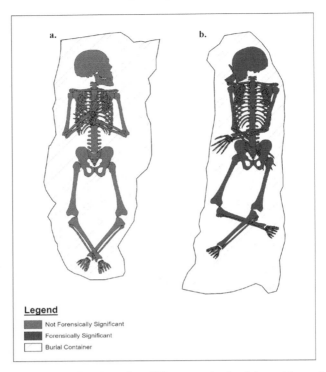

Figure 2.2 Schematic showing the differences in burial positions for a.) Not Forensically Significant and b.) Forensically Significant cases encountered at Tres Norias Cemetery. Credit: Courtney C. Siegert.

in the burials (16.9%), and yet only sixteen of the thirty-eight community member graves were marked (42.1%). Eleven such community member burials were also erroneously indicated by a county official as containing unidentified, presumed migrant remains; thus, demonstrating the fallibility of memory recall, particularly when used as the sole record of burial locations. Far from what international human rights accords and laws would recognize as dignified burials, eleven known individuals were also buried with medical intervention equipment, such as catheters, IVs, intubations, central lines, and electrode pads still present (28.9% of the thirty-eight known decedents). This unanticipated treatment of the indigent population in the region served as an identity erasure, relegating not only transnational migrants, but the community's financially poor to forgotten spaces—including them as another demographic of *los nuevos desaparecidos*. Furthermore, these burial practices necessitated more intensive and intrusive assessments to locate forensically relevant cases, thus increasing the risk that community member burials were potentially disturbed.

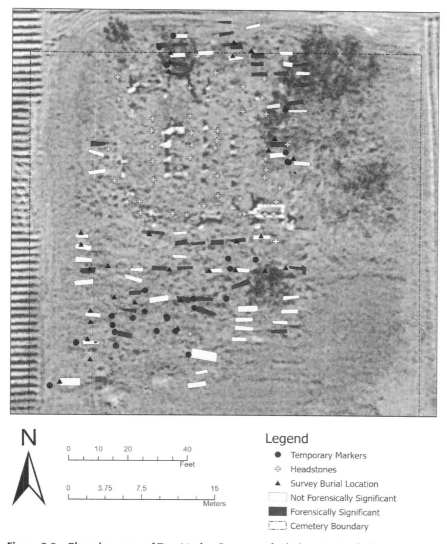

Figure 2.3 Plan view map of Tres Norias Cemetery depicting OpID's findings during a pedestrian survey and subsequent excavations. Credit: Courtney C. Siegert.

Despite this collective disregard for both indigent community members and unknown migrants, differences in the treatment between these two groups were also apparent. Most unidentified presumed migrants at Tres Norias Cemetery were buried in body bags (89.7%), while non-forensically significant burials were buried in more varied containers and wrappings, including plywood boxes. Although no migrant remains were located within plywood boxes, unconventional burial containers including biohazard and trash/plastic bags were utilized in four unidentified, presumed migrant interments (10.3%). One unknown decedent was recovered in a Styrofoam cooler intended for the medical transport of tissue.

While this distinction in burial containers assisted in determining which burials were forensically significant and in need of identification, it revealed additional processes of "othering" characterized by dehumanizing the migrant population. Although most burials were individual interments of similar depths, and organized in a somewhat linear pattern, the thirty-nine cases representing unidentified, presumed migrants differed significantly from other burials based on their body position (figure 2.2). Many indigent community members, or not forensically significant cases, were positioned with care, as suggested by their arms folded across the chest and feet neatly crossed at the ankles. Alternatively, unidentified presumed migrants, or forensically significant cases, were positioned without reverence as suggested by their encumbered arms and hyperflexion or hyperextension of their legs. Additionally, five forensically significant burials were placed face down or prone in the burial shaft (12.8%) and five burials were stacked with one individual on top of another in the same burial shaft (12.8%), including a bone bundle in a plastic bag that was placed on top of an indigent community member. Medical waste, including nitrile examination gloves, was found in twenty-two unidentified graves (56.4%), while additional, non-medical trash, such as food wrappings, was present in seven unknown persons' burials (17.9%).

Beyond the prominence of body positions, containers, and refuse that can only be classified as undignified, an overall lack of investigative attention was also apparent for the unidentified migrant decedents. Although twenty-two decedents exhibited skeletal evidence of autopsy (56.4%), including cranial or rib cuts, and the presence of an organ bag, seventeen cases exhibited no evidence of autopsy (43.6%) and lacked paperwork or records clarifying whether identification attempts had been carried out. Additionally, twenty-six cases lacked skeletal cuts consistent with DNA sampling (66.7%), while thirteen cases had clearly been sampled (33.3%). While this distribution of autopsied and DNA-sampled cases is more lawfully compliant than has been seen in other counties where OpID has conducted exhumations, autopsy and genetic sampling of remains serve no purpose if cases are not tracked and cannot be re-associated with missing persons. Because documentation linking unidentified remains to recovery reports or investigative files was not retained, any efforts toward identification are significantly hindered.

This hindrance is exacerbated when considering that only 20 percent of the unidentified, presumed migrant burials located at Tres Norias were marked on the ground surface and that only six of the eight total markers contained legible case information. Critically, the overwhelming lack of grave markers and dispositional records serves to physically disappear unidentified decedents underground so that most individuals cannot be re-located even if a DNA match to a missing person occurred. In addition to producing forgotten and ignored spaces, these irreverent burial practices and lack of case tracking contribute to the active removal of identity from human bodies. Of the thirty-eight individuals considered not forensically significant, and therefore thought to represent probable indigent community members, only thirteen retained identity records within their burial container. Although all thirty-eight individuals were likely buried as identified persons, the passively violent and ineffectual death management system acted to erase their names, relegating them to an intersectional existence as both the "unidentified" and "not forensically significant." Collectively, this evidence reinforces the notion that these groups' disappearance stems directly from the institutional breakdown of death investigation in South Texas, and indirectly from the biopolitical and necropolitical structures surrounding immigration at the U.S.-Mexico border. However, it must be recognized that the effects of these structures and institutions permeate beyond those politically deemed as dispensable—and, in turn, expand the category of dispensability to additional persons.

Challenges at Tres Norias

Aside from the difficulties locating unidentified burials due to a lack of record keeping or mapping, other issues concerning burial documentation were also soon discovered. During excavations at Tres Norias, several burials were encountered that had associated documentation containing names, including an individual with the name, Hugo Escobar Rodriguez (figure 2.4). To verify whether Hugo and others at the cemetery were in fact identified, a list of all the names encountered during excavations were sent the U.S. Border Patrol Missing Migrant Program (MMP) to ascertain whether missing persons cases remained open among any consulates or missing migrant advocacy groups.

The MMP reported that Hugo was detained and deported in December 2015 and found deceased in Brownsville, TX in January 2016. Based on previous work conducted by OpID and collaborators, it is known that identifications in other counties have been made when an individual is found with an identification card, with no additional forensic analyses to corroborate identity. This practice is problematic, as it is circumstantial and not based on scientific examination. Hugo, however, was identified through a fingerprint match to his detention record prior to deportation, and yet was still buried and lost in a cemetery because family members were not located at the time the identification was declared. OpID's collaboration with governmental

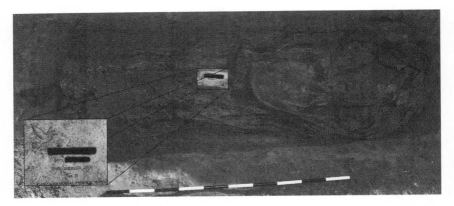

Figure 2.4 Hugo Escobar Rodriguez's burial showing the insert from a temporary marker found on top of his body bag. Credit: M. Kate Spradley.

and non-governmental organizations enabled the location of Hugo's family members in Brownsville, TX. In 2018, his daughter had been searching for him for two years, only to learn that he was buried thirty minutes away from her residence. On January 25, 2018, Hugo was released for repatriation, less than a month after being exhumed from an unmarked grave at Tres Norias. Although in this case Hugo had been identified, his family had originally not been notified, thus calling into question the meaning of a positive identification, especially when an individual is subsequently interred without a trace.

Other challenges at the cemetery centered more generally around red morgue tags. OpID personnel had been told that red tags were only used for identified individuals; yet, as exhumations progressed, the team encountered several illegible tags, which could neither confirm nor exclude an individual as being identified—and one clearly read, "Doe, John #9" (figure 2.5). Once again, this finding reiterates the imprecise and incomplete nature of memory recall as the only mechanism for case tracking in the context of death investigation. More urgently, it prompted re-evaluating the exhumation strategy and necessitated reinvestigation and *in situ* field assessment ("intake") of all burials found with an illegible morgue tag.

Another problem faced during excavations was the presence of multiple individuals within one burial. While most burials contained only one person, five had multiple individuals within one burial shaft. For example, Burial 58 had two stacked individuals. The bottom individual was in a black body bag in an extended, carefully placed position, while the top individual was bundled in a disintegrating white plastic bag that had skeletal elements exposed. During the excavation of this burial, a marker was found just below ground surface that read "John Doe" and listed a case number. Through further investigation, it was determined that the bottom individual was an indigent

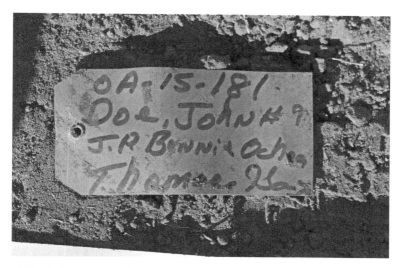

Figure 2.5   Red morgue tag for "Doe, John #9" which prompted reinvestigation of previously found illegible red morgue tags. Credit: M. Kate Spradley.

community member due to the positioning, presence of a hospital gown, and older age. The top individual was determined to be a presumed migrant due to the skeletonized bundle in the bag. While clearly undignified to have multiple individuals in one shaft without corresponding documentation, these multiple interments also exemplify the haphazard nature of burial practices occurring in South Texas as a result of the overwhelming numbers of death. This type of practice could be easily mitigated with minor additional oversight, training, or cemetery planning, which are sorely lacking.

The recovery of thirty-nine unidentified, presumed migrant decedents is a marked success of the Tres Norias exhumations; however, the challenges of locating these individuals among positively identified and unclaimed burials made OpID's field efforts particularly difficult and taxing. In the search for unidentified human remains at Tres Norias, OpID had to excavate much of the cemetery, increasing the likelihood of encountering community member burials to ascertain forensic significance and identification status. Designating separate areas in the cemetery to be reserved exclusively for unidentified remains, as distinct from known indigent or unclaimed burials, would greatly remedy this problem and assist in future recovery efforts should these individuals be positively identified post-deposition. Utilizing county cemeteries for the burial of unidentified remains, as opposed to land on private property, will also better ensure the county's ability to track unresolved cases. The fact that no policies or oversight exist to ensure the marking of graves and the prevention of intermixing of identified and known individuals in cemeteries is a systemic failing that constitutes violent inaction toward, and erasure of, these marginalized groups.

The overall lack of centralized and standardized documentation for individuals buried at Tres Norias Cemetery must also be addressed. The Texas Criminal Code of Procedures (TCCP) Article 49.09 mandates that burial records be maintained for all unidentified remains for a minimum of ten years, including documenting the final disposition of remains on death certificates filed with the state. The lack of any such records for Tres Norias and the reliance on memory recall from the sole death investigator for the county necessitated invasive, large-scale exhumation and the assessment of many burials that do not meet the purview of the OpID project. While the death investigator pointed out thirty-one burial locations during initial survey in 2016, more than two times that number of individuals were located by OpID in predominantly unmarked graves.

Although many unclaimed and indigent community members may have been interred in Tres Norias Cemetery as identified individuals, the lack of documentation and case tracking works as an erasure of many individuals' identities. If burials continue to be interred at Tres Norias, best practices to ameliorate this denial of identity and post-dispositional disappearance of individuals within the cemetery are essential.

CONCLUSIONS, RECOMMENDATIONS, AND THE SHIFTING ROLE OF FORENSIC ANTHROPOLOGISTS

South Texas is just one region along the U.S.-Mexico border, yet the area represents a microcosm of the systemic challenges inherent to migrant death investigation and serves as a critical case study for how anthropological research and humanitarian forensic action can be applied to mitigate mass fatalities from migration. U.S. border militarization and the current handling of unidentified migrant decedents in South Texas not only disregard basic human rights as outlined in international accords, such as the *Right to Know*, but serve to structurally and violently disappear individuals in such a way that deems them as not worthy of life nor dignity in death. As a political and philosophical approach to migration, Prevention through Deterrence knowingly perpetuates migrant death and justifies it using the narrative of border security, placing blame and agency on the dead themselves. Because these undocumented individuals in life are politically stigmatized as criminal and not deserving of equitable treatment, this leads to their negligent treatment in death, including a lack of political will or infrastructure to properly facilitate their identification and repatriation. Systemic under-resourcing of South

Texas counties and their efforts toward death investigation is another dimension of violence inherent to migrant death that leads to the overburdening of local jurisdictions and the haphazard interment and case tracking practices that are non-compliant with state law. Policy and practice reform at the federal, state, and local levels is therefore urgent, particularly within regions most impacted by clandestine migration.

Throughout the years of conducting forensic surveys and excavations in South Texas, OpID and the FBC have recognized several areas of improvement for migrant death investigation. Arguably the most urgent problem is a statewide lack of a regional medical examiner system and an overall shortage of pathologists. Currently, jurisdictions are largely unable to transport remains far distances across county lines to receive forensic analysis and DNA sampling, which results in the high numbers of unidentified remains interred without investigation. Yet, even when decedents are autopsied, as is the case with several of the unidentified individuals recovered from Tres Norias, few are sampled or entered into nationwide databases due to a lack of oversight, personnel, and the fragmentation of evidence that occurs when decedents are transferred across multiple agencies. Large caseloads for the few medical examiners and pathologists that do exist further create backlogs and increase the difficulty of hiring new positions, especially when they are contract-based (paid per autopsy) rather than salaried. Although the recent passing of the federal *Missing Persons and Unidentified Remains Act* (S.2174) marks a big step toward securing funding for local jurisdictions managing high numbers of unidentified decedents, the problems of DNA sampling and case fragmentation will continue in South Texas without access to centralized systems of forensic services.

The need for designated respectful burial sites for unidentified decedents in South Texas is as important as the need for a regional medical examiner system in the state. Considering that new deaths continue to occur at high rates and unidentified individuals are being further disappeared in unmarked graves, reforming burial practices throughout the region is critical. While, on a national level, policy reform supporting accessible, safe, and legal migration will ultimately be what prevents migrant death, these types of recommended changes to state and local investigative structures are where forensic professionals, and anthropologists in particular, have the most potential to have a profound impact. Not only do training and experience in decedent identification allow swift targeting of where reforms need to occur, but the collaborative relationships that anthropologists form with jurisdictional authorities, medical examiners, and non-governmental organizations can lead to advocacy that streamlines the flow of casework and enhances case resolution.

Over the past several years, the FBC has made great strides to improve medicolegal death investigation of migrant remains in South Texas. In 2013, for example, recognizing that a lack of funding largely contributed to the burial of unidentified decedents without autopsy or DNA sampling, the South Texas Human Rights Center partnered with the Brooks County Sheriff's Office to reach out to state senators and secure much-needed resources for the county to transport decedents to the medical examiner's office in Laredo, TX. Because of this advocacy, unidentified remains are no longer buried unmarked in Brooks County, but now receive an opportunity to have their identity known. Additionally, in 2018, the FBC, along with families of the missing, held a hearing with the Inter-American Commission on Human Rights to address ongoing challenges to transnational DNA comparison for unidentified migrant cases. This hearing has led to collaboration with the FBI and the development of a humanitarian DNA CODIS (Combined DNA Index System) database that should serve to expedite the comparison of unidentified remains with family reference samples and increase the number of positive identifications (Budowle et al. 2020).

Ensuring DNA collection and entry into CODIS therefore remains crucial, which is why a regional ME system in South Texas is of the utmost importance. Ongoing collaborative efforts with governmental and non-governmental agencies will continue to be essential both for resolving cases and for developing standards of practice that ensure unidentified decedents of all backgrounds receive equitable and dignified treatment. Although practitioners working in South Texas face unique challenges in which large numbers of migrant decedents are disappeared within the medicolegal system, forensic anthropologists and other professionals have the ability to spearhead structural reforms impacting casework in all medicolegal contexts. For some practitioners these changes might include applying humanitarian frameworks and broadened definitions of justice to medicolegal death investigation of recent and long-term cases. For others, it may be working to better integrate instruments and databases such as NamUs or CODIS into daily practice across institutions.

The role of forensic anthropologists has grown and shifted over the years and will continue to do so. Forensic anthropology today is much more than compiling the biological profile, assessing trauma and pathology, and assisting with death scene reconstruction. Rather, forensic anthropologists are actively contributing to the enhancement of death investigation and improving systems of our practice. This combination of forensic science and advocacy within varying medicolegal contexts brings visibility to the dead, facilitates identification and case resolution, and attempts to reform the systems that have led to individuals' disappearances through a collaborative approach centered on family rights.

NOTE

1. Acknowledgments: Thank you to the Forensic Border Coalition, the South Texas Human Rights Center, the Brooks County Sheriff's Office, and to all Texas State University students, faculty, and staff who have contributed to Operation Identification. This work would also not be possible without the International Committee of the Red Cross and the Office of the Governor of the State of Texas.

REFERENCES

Abrego, Leisy, Mat Coleman, Daniel E. Martínez, Cecilia Menjívar, and Jeremy Slack. 2017. "Making Immigrants into Criminals: Legal Processes of Criminalization in the Post-IIRIRA Era." *Journal on Migration and Human Security 5,* no. 3 (September): 694–715. https://doi.org/10.1177/233150241700500308.

Anderson, Bruce E. 2008. "Identifying the Dead: Methods Utilized by the Pima County (Arizona) Office of the Medical Examiner for Undocumented Border Crossers: 2001–2006." *Journal of Forensic Sciences 53*, no. 1: 8–15. https://doi.org/10.1111/j.1556-4029.2007.00609.x. https://www.ncbi.nlm.nih.gov/pubmed/18279232.

Beatrice, Jared S., and Angela Soler. 2016. "Skeletal Indicators of Stress: A Component of the Biocultural Profile of Undocumented Migrants in Southern Arizona." *Journal of Forensic Sciences 61*, no. 5: 1164–1172. https://doi.org/10.1111/1556-4029.13131.

Beck, Jess, Ian Ostericher, Gregory Sollish, and Jason De León. 2015. "Animal Scavenging and Scattering and the Implications for Documenting the Deaths of Undocumented Border Crossers in the Sonoran Desert." *Journal of Forensic Sciences 60* (s1): S11–S20. https://doi.org/10.1111/1556-4029.12597.

Betts, Alexander, and Paul Collier. 2017. *Refuge: Rethinking Refugee Policy in a Changing World.* New York: Oxford University Press.

Budowle, Bruce, Magdalena M. Bus, Melody A. Josserand, and Dixie L. Peters. 2020. "A Standalone Humanitarian DNA Identification Database System to Increase Identification of Human Remains of Foreign Nationals." *International Journal of Legal Medicine 134*, no. 6 (August): 2039–2044. https://doi.org/10.1007/s00414-020-02396-9.

Davies, Thom, Arshad Isakjee, and Surindar Dhesi. 2017. "Violent Inaction: The Necropolitical Experience of Refugees in Europe." *Antipode 49*, no. 5: 1263–1284. https://doi.org/10.1111/anti.12325.

De León, Jason. 2015. *The Land of Open Graves: Living and Dying on the Migrant Trail.* Berkeley: University of California Press. https://doi.org/10.1525/9780520958685.

Fleischman, Julie M., Ashley E. Kendell, Christen C. Eggers, and Laura C. Fulginiti. 2017. "Undocumented Border Crosser Deaths in Arizona: Expanding Intrastate Collaborative Efforts in Identification." *Journal of Forensic Sciences 62*, no. 4 (January): 840–9. https://doi.org/10.1111/1556-4029.13368.

Foucault, Michel. 1997. *The Politics of Truth.* Semiotext(e), accessed October 1, 2021. https://library.uoh.edu.iq/admin/ebooks/50893-foucault__the_politics_of _truth__semiotext_e__foreign_agents_series__compressed.pdf.

Frey, John Carlos. 2015. "Graves of Shame." *The Texas Observer*, July 6, 2015, accessed September 20, 2021. https://www.texasobserver.org/illegal-mass-graves -of-migrant-remains-found-in-south-texas/.

Gaggioli, Gloria. 2018. "International Humanitarian Law: The Legal Framework for Humanitarian Forensic Action." *Forensic Science International 282* (January): 184–94. https://doi.org/10.1016/j.forsciint.2017.10.035.

Galtung, Johan. 1969. "Violence, Peace, and Peace Research." *Journal of Peace Research 6*, no. 3: 167–91, accessed October 1, 2021. https://journals.sagepub.com /doi/pdf/10.1177/002234336900600301?casa_token=omAuBSplJrMAAAAA:Ry2 0egjIYyfYAHwCr1G7iQGev8XF2zTN_BwFg58iafR2H5R51t0TsHt9UESSRki9 6PAxdd1J6Iiy.

Goad, Gennifer. 2020. "Expanding Humanitarian Forensic Action: An Approach to U.S. Cold Cases." *Forensic Anthropology 3*, no. 1 (Winter): 50–8. https://doi.org /10.5744/fa.2020.1006.

Gocha, Timothy P., M. Katherine Spradley, and Ryan Strand. 2018. "Bodies in Limbo: Issues in Identification and Repatriation of Migrant Remains in South Texas." In *Sociopolitics of Migrant Death and Repatriation: Perspectives from Forensic Science*, edited by Krista E. Latham and Alyson J. O'Daniel, 143–56. Cham: Springer. https://doi.org/10.1007/978-3-319-61866-1_11.

Hanzlick, Randy. 2007. "The Conversion of Coroner Systems to Medical Examiner Systems in the United States: A Lull in Action." *The American Journal of Forensic Medicine and Pathology 28*, no. 4 (December): 279–83. https://doi.org/10.1097/ PAF.0b013e31815b4d5a.

Hiemstra, Nancy. 2019. *Detain and Deport: The Chaotic U.S. Immigration Enforcement Regime.* Athens: University of Georgia Press. https://doi.org/10.2307 /j.ctv5npj70.

Hughes, Cris E., Bridget F. B. Algee-Hewitt, Robin Reineke, Elizabeth Clausing, and Bruce E. Anderson. 2017. "Temporal Patterns of Mexican Migrant Genetic Ancestry: Implications for Identification." *American Anthropologist 119*, no. 2 (May): 193–208. https://doi.org/doi:10.1111/aman.12845.

International Committee of the Red Cross. 2003. *The Missing and Their Families: Conclusions Arising from Events Held Prior to the International Conference of Governmental and Non-governmental Experts (19–21 February 2003)*, accessed October 1, 2021. https://www.icrc.org/en/doc/resources/documents/report/5jahr8 .htm.

Interpol General Assembly. 1996. Disaster Victim Identification. In *Resolution No. AGN/65/RES/13.* ICPO - Interpol General Assembly, 65th session, accessed September 29, 2021. https://www.legal-tools.org/doc/d6aa95/pdf/.

Kjellén, Rudolf. 1916. Staten Som Lifsform. *Politiska Handböcker III.* Stockholm: Hugo Gebers Förlag. http://hdl.handle.net/2077/56383.

Kovic, Christine. 2013. "Searching for the Living, the Dead, and the New Disappeared on the Migrant Trail in Texas: Preliminary Report on Migrant Deaths in South

Texas." Texas Civil Rights Project. https://southtexashumanrights.files.wordpress
.com/2013/09/migrant-deaths-report-edited.pdf.

———. 2018. "Naming State Crimes, Naming the Dead: Immigration Policy, and
'The New Disappeared' in the United States and Mexico." In *Sociopolitics of
Migrant Death and Repatriation: Perspectives from Forensic Science*, edited by
Krista E. Latham and Alyson J. O'Daniel, 39–51. Cham: Springer. https://doi.org
/10.1007/978-3-319-61866-1_4.

Martínez, Daniel E., Robin C. Reineke, Raquel Rubio-Goldsmith, and Bruce O.
Parks. 2014. "Structural Violence and Migrant Deaths in Southern Arizona: Data
from the Pima County Office of the Medical Examiner, 1990–2013." *Journal
on Migration and Human Security 2*, no. 4: 257–86. https://doi.org/10.1177
/233150241400200401.

Mbembe, Achille. 2003. "Necropolitics." *Public Culture 15*, no. 1 (Winter): 11–40.
https://doi.org/10.1215/08992363-15-1-11.

Meyers, Deborah W. 2006. "From Horseback to High-Tech: U.S. Border Enforcement."
Migration Information Source, February 1, 2006, accessed October 1, 2021. https://
www.migrationpolicy.org/article/horseback-high-tech-us-border-enforcement.

Missing Persons and Unidentified Remains Act of 2019. 2020. Public Law 116–277.
U.S. Statutes at Large 166: 2174.

O'Connor, Allison, Jeanne Batalova, and Jessica Bolter. 2019. "Central American
Immigrants in the United States." *Migration Information Source*, August 15, 2019,
accessed October 1, 2021. https://www.migrationpolicy.org/article/central-ameri-
can-immigrants-united-states-2017.

Ortega. Bob. 2018. "Border Patrol Failed to Count Hundreds of Migrant Deaths on
US Soil." *CNN*, May 15, 2018, accessed October 1, 2021. https://www.cnn.com
/2018/05/14/us/border-patrol-migrant-death-count-invs/index.html.

Reineke, Robin. 2013. "Lost in the System: Unidentified Bodies on the Border."
NACLA Report on the Americas 46, no. 2: 50–3. https://doi.org/10.1080/10714839
.2013.11721998.

———. 2019. "Necroviolence and Postmortem Care along the U.S.-México Border."
In *The Border and its Bodies: The Embodiment of Risk along the U.S.-México
Line*, edited by Thomas E. Sheridan and Randall H. McGuire, 144–72. Tucson:
The University of Arizona Press. https://library.oapen.org/bitstream/handle/20.500
.12657/43879/external_content.pdf?sequence=1#page=153.

Rubio-Goldsmith, Raquel, Melissa McCormick, Daniel Martinez, and Inez Magdalena
Duarte. 2006. "The 'Funnel Effect' and Recovered Bodies of Unauthorized
Migrants Processed by the Pima County Office of the Medical Examiner, 1990–
2005." *Binational Migration Institute*. Tucson, AZ: University of Arizona. http://
dx/doi.org/10/2139/ssrn.3040107.

Slack, Jeremy. 2019. "5. Guarding the River: Migrant Recruitment into Organized
Crime." In *Deported to Death: How Drug Violence is Changing Migration on the
US-Mexico Border*, 107–30. Berkeley: University of California Press. https://doi
.org/10.1525/9780520969711-007.

Slack, Jeremy, and Daniel E. Martínez. 2019. "The Geography of Migrant Death:
Violence on the US-Mexico Border." In *Handbook on Critical Geographies*

of Migration, edited by Katharyne Mitchell, Reece Jones, and Jennifer L. Fluri, 142–52. Cheltenham: Edward Elgar Publishing. https://doi.org/10.4337/9781786436030.00020.

Soler, Angela, and Jared S. Beatrice. 2018. "Expanding the Role of Forensic Anthropology in a Humanitarian Crisis: An Example from the USA-Mexico Border." In *Sociopolitics of Migrant Death and Repatriation: Perspectives from Forensic Science*, edited by Krista E. Latham and Alyson J. O'Daniel, 115–28. Cham: Springer. https://doi.org/10.1007/978-3-319-61866-1_9.

Spradley, M. Katherine, Michelle D. Hamilton, and Alberto Giordano. 2012. "Spatial Patterning of Vulture Scavenged Human Remains." *Forensic Science International* 219, no. 1 (June): 57–63. https://doi.org/https://doi.org/10.1016/j.forsciint.2011.11.030.

Spradley, M. Katherine, Nicholas P. Herrmann, Courtney B. Siegert, and Chloe P. McDaneld. 2019. "Identifying Migrant Remains in South Texas: Policy and Practice." *Forensic Sciences Research* 4, no. 1 (October): 60–8. https://doi.org/10.1080/20961790.2018.1497437.

Spradley, M. Katherine, Robin Reineke, Mercedes C. Dorreti, and Bruce E. Anderson. 2016. "Death along the US Mexico Border: A Comparative View of Policy and Practice in Arizona and Texas." Las Vegas (NV): American Academy of Forensic Sciences.

Stephen, Lynn. 2008. "Los Nuevos Desaparecidos y Muertos Immigration, Militarization, Death, and Disappearance on Mexico's Borders." In *Security Disarmed: Critical Perspectives on Gender, Race, and Militarization*, edited by Barbara Sutton, Sandra Morgen, and Julie Novkov, 79–100. New Brunkswick: Rutgers University Press. http://www.jstor.org/stable/j.ctt5hj5b1.8.

Texas Constitution and Statutes. 2020a. Title 1. Code of Criminal Procedure. Chapter 63, Subchapter B: University of North Texas Health Science Center Fort Worth Missing Persons DNA Database.

———. 2020b. Title 1. Code of Criminal Procedure. Chapter 49: Inquests Upon Dead Bodies.

United Nations. 2018. Global Compact for Safe, Orderly and Regular Migration. Edited by Office of the United Nations High Commissioner for Human Rights, accessed September 29, 2021. https://refugeesmigrants.un.org/sites/default/files/180713_agreed_outcome_global_compact_for_migration.pdf.

United Nations General Assembly. 1948. United Nations Universal Declaration of Human Rights 1948.

United States Customs and Border Protection. 2020. "Southwest Border Deaths by Fiscal Year." U.S. Department of Homeland Security, accessed October 1, 2021. https://www.cbp.gov/sites/default/files/assets/documents/2020-Jan/U.S.%20Border%20Patrol%20Fiscal%20Year%20Southwest%20Border%20Sector%20Deaths%20%28FY%201998%20-%20FY%202019%29_0.pdf.

Vogt, Wendy A. 2013. "Crossing Mexico: Structural Violence and the Commodification of Undocumented Central American Migrants." *American Ethnologist* 40, no. 4 (November): 764–80. https://doi.org/10.1111/amet.12053.

Chapter 3

Qué pena con usted

The Struggle for Victim Identification in Colombia

Elizabeth A. DiGangi and Daniela Santamaria Vargas

INTRODUCTION

The country of Colombia is located at the northwestern corner of South America, and is organized as a republic with thirty-two departments, somewhat analogous to the states in the United States or Mexico.[1] Geographically, it is bordered by the Atlantic and Pacific Oceans to the north and west, part of the Amazon jungle occupies its southern borders with Brazil and Peru, and the northernmost part of the Andes Mountain range, divided into three major cordilleras, assist in separating the country into distinct ecological zones[2] (figure 3.1). This unique geography and its proximity to the equator are not mere footnotes to the Colombian story we will recount here: these factors have been starring characters that have served as buttresses to the country's longstanding internal conflict.

Despite its status as a longstanding democracy, Colombia has been beset by violence born out of sociopolitical conflict, which has increased in scope and severity since the mid-twentieth century; and according to Civico (2016), likely has its roots in the nineteenth-century animosity between the two founding generals, Simón Bolívar and Francisco de Paula Santander. This enmity evolved into longstanding fundamental disagreements especially pertaining to land rights (Tate 2007) which tend to juxtapose the land-holding elites vs. those of the working class and the rural poor, and strong allegiance to one of the two political parties, Conservative or Liberal. In the early twentieth century, increasing modernity in the cities led to a deepening divide with those in rural areas as well as with the working class (Rosa 2003).

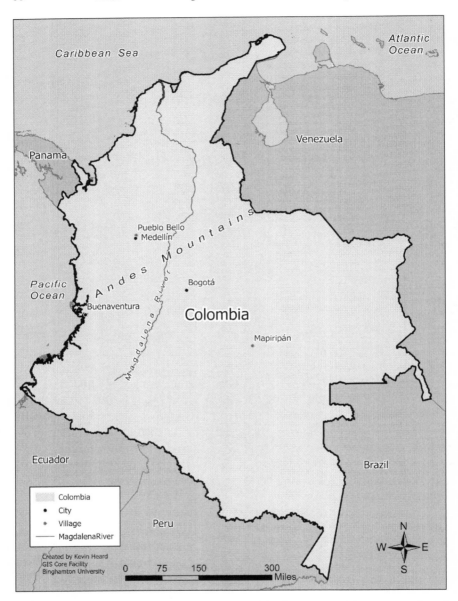

Figure 3.1   Map of Colombia depicting some of the locations and features mentioned in the chapter. Map created by Kevin Heard, GIS Core Facility, Binghamton University.

This division came to a head on April 9, 1948 with the public assassination of the leading Liberal candidate for President, Jorge Eliécer Gaitán, in the capital city of Bogotá. Radio broadcasts of the tragedy fanned the flames, and the subsequent riot and looting lasted for hours, resulting in near complete destruction of downtown Bogotá (Braun 1985; Pita Pico 2018; Tate 2007). More riots arose in other major cities, such as Medellín; reports as to the exact number of casualties vary but by the time the last fire burned out, thousands of people were dead and injured (Sánchez-Ángel 2008; Sharpless 1978). The severity of the events of *El Bogotazo* cannot be understated because they were the catalyst for a protracted period of violence, known as *La Violencia* (Ríos Sierra 2017) which included frequent homicides and massacres committed by hired assassins or armed gangs and the shocking shooting death of one politician against another on the floor of Congress (Tate 2007; Uribe 1990). This devastating period in Colombian history was only moderated in the 1950s with the commencement of Colombia's short-lived military dictatorship (1953–1957) and the subsequent agreement known as the National Front which dictated each political party would take turns holding Presidential and Congressional power (Tate 2007).

This power-sharing compromise was unable to solve the country's fundamental ideological and practical divisions between the elite, land-holding oligarchy and the rural and urban poor and working class. The power structure that was set up nationally therefore played out locally (Green 2004): the government's inability to satisfactorily address the needs and concerns of the poor and working class led to the rise of illegally armed leftist groups in the country's rural areas (Ríos Sierra 2017). In response, militias aligned with the right—both legal and illegal—arose to lethally combat the leftists. The subsequent violence in many rural and urban areas has led to the longest, ongoing internal conflict in the Western Hemisphere (Tate 2007) and for years Colombia had the highest number of internally displaced persons in the world, which by the end of 2019 was second only to Syria (Alsema 2018; Internal Displacement Monitoring Centre n.d.). The conflict has led to upward of 220,000 deceased persons[3] as of 2012, of which over 80 percent are civilians (Civico 2016; Guzmán and Sanabria Medina 2016), and many were disappeared or buried in clandestine or other non-official graves.

In this chapter, we bring the perspective of forensic anthropologists to the conflict, its causes, the identity of the victims, and the politics and complexity of identification. The first author is an American who lived and worked in Bogotá for several years, serving in an advisory and mentoring role with the country's forensic anthropologists; and the second author is a Colombian who has worked as a forensic anthropologist analyzing human remains for the Colombian national medical examiner's office. We bring our expertise and lived experience of the conflict and its aftermath to this discussion where we will briefly trace the origins of the major illegally armed groups combating each other and the government, will introduce the structures set in place to resolve or ameliorate the conflict, and finally, will discuss how victim identification—from the search for clandestine graves to the search for living family members willing to provide reference information—is affected by who the victims were during life: namely, largely marginalized, rural, and impoverished. We will contextualize this discussion using a structural violence framework enhanced by an understanding of the continuum of violence (Scheper-Hughes and Bourgois 2004) to appreciate the demands placed on rural citizenry to acquiesce to the power and authority (Arendt 1969) of various armed groups, and how victim suffering (Farmer 1997) is a multidimensional hallmark which has shaped modern Colombia.

The chapter title we have chosen—*qué pena con usted*—literally translates to "what a shame for you." Here, we use it to express an apology on our part as authors as a segue to discuss the difficulties surrounding conflict resolution and victim recovery and identification. While in practice *qué pena* is often used in lieu of expressing a contrite apology, and typically has a "too bad, how awful" undertone to it, we do not mean to suggest that the attitude surrounding the conflict is exclusively one of complacency—to the contrary, there are many victims' rights groups, human rights defenders, and government officials who work tirelessly on the behalf of victims and families. However, from a structural perspective, not all lives are seen as equal (Sanford 2003), least of all those killed because of suspicion of guerrilla sympathizing or because of having identities deemed by others to be undesirable. The story of the conflict, its beginnings and trajectory, is one that demonstrates how this attitude is supported, condoned, and perpetuated by the Colombian state and its sociopolitics.

ES COMPLICADO: COLOMBIAN GEOGRAPHY AND THE SITUATING OF THE GUERRILLA, PARAMILITARIES, NARCOTRAFFICKERS, AND THE GOVERNMENT

Es complicado—in English, "it's complicated"—is an apt phrase often uttered by Colombians when discussing the conflict, its causes, and possible solutions. While the period known as *La Violencia* may have dissipated by the early 1960s, violence as a backdrop to Colombian life, especially for people in rural and poverty-stricken urban areas, has continued as the *status quo*. Tate (2007) discusses the unique nature of Colombian violence, as it occurs in multiple categories that are not always mutually exclusive: *political* (members of one political party against the other or against those deemed by the party as targets), *common* (crimes ostensibly having nothing to do with politics), *domestic* (committed against and by members within a single household), and *organized* (under the auspices of or for illegal drug/activity syndicates). Understanding the broader conflict requires teasing out entanglements between the categories and their actors, disentanglements made more challenging with the necessary consideration of the physical setting of Colombian geography where the violence takes place, as well as how structural factors contribute to its manifestation and persistence.

The latter can be conceptualized as structural violence, where sociopolitical and economic factors can and do lead to human suffering essentially because of lack of access to clean water and nutritious food and/or adequate healthcare, education, employment, and housing (Farmer 2003). Such suffering is inherently violent, because violence cannot be defined solely as physical force—it also involves an onslaught against fundamental human rights, to include dignity (Scheper-Hughes and Bourgois 2004). Further, structural as well as other types of violence occur along a continuum (Scheper-Hughes and Bourgois 2004) where violence cannot be conceptualized as having distinct start and end points. This is particularly true in Colombia, where despite the complexity of the situation, a bird's-eye view of the violence since *El Bogotazo* reveals the non-stop loop on which it is playing: the players may come and go, but entrenchment of ideological differences coupled with thirst for revenge, aspiration, lack of opportunity, greed, and/or corruption maintain the pattern.

As noted, Colombia boasts a diversity of ecological zones, from oceanside beaches to dense tropical jungle to high-altitude mountain passes; lakes that dot the countryside and rivers that cascade across the landscape add to its diversity (figure 3.2). Two major factors inherent to this geography have contributed to the conflict for decades. First, the three cordilleras of the Andes Mountains as well as major rivers such as the Magdalena physically divide the country, making travel between distinct areas time consuming if not close to impossible; extensive dense rainforest also serves as a physical barrier to ingress and egress. Second, the country's proximity to the equator coupled with a variety of elevations means that the climate varies from cold to tropical with minor seasonal variation; the temperate and tropical areas in particular are especially conducive to agriculture and animal husbandry.

Farmers—from poor *campesinos* (peasants) to multinational agricultural firms—have taken advantage of the land's fertility to grow major crops for export such as coffee and bananas; cattle ranching is widespread, and coca, native to the Andes, grows almost without effort. It is the dovetailing of the existence of valuable, productive farmland and the geographical physical barriers in place that while not causes of the conflict, have been among the obstacles to resolution. Control for land and the subsequent wealth, or simply,

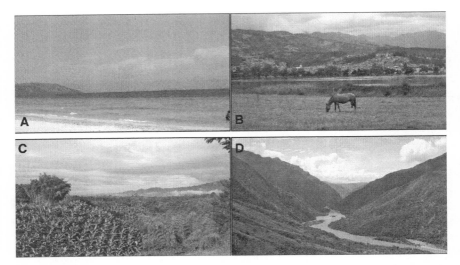

Figure 3.2 The diverse Colombian countryside: lakes, rivers, beaches, and mountain ranges are all typical. A: Beach of the Lago de Tota, the largest natural lake in Colombia, department of Boyacá, central Colombia. B: Countryside outside of Paipa, department of Boyacá, central Colombia. C: Banana trees growing outside of Pereira, department of Risaralda, west-central Colombia. D: Mountains and a river that are part of the Cordillera Oriental of the Andes near Bucaramanga, department of Santander, eastern Colombia. Credit for all photographs: Elizabeth A. DiGangi.

subsistence, it can bring have been defining factors in the persistence of political and other types of violence (Tate 2007). Running parallel to this are the geographical barriers such as mountains, rainforest, and rivers that dually dissuade government authorities from readily enforcing order while preventing some citizens who desire to be law-abiding from growing anything but illegal crops because of limited infrastructure to get perishable goods to market.[4]

The FARC

The existence of rural areas isolated by geography, relatively devoid of any state officials charged with law enforcement, and populated with *campesinos* working for a pauper's wage on vast tracts of land owned by large corporations or wealthy individuals led to the birth in 1964 of the country's major guerrilla group, the *Fuerzas Armadas Revolucionarias de Colombia-Ejército del Pueblo* (FARC-EP) (Revolutionary Armed Forces of Colombia—People's Army). Initially, the FARC and other guerrilla groups saw themselves as champions of *campesinos* and their original goals included political organization of peasants (Civico 2016). In fact, a popular slogan, as seen on the t-shirt of a slain FARC guerrillero goes as follows:

Against imperialism
for the motherland...
Against oligarchy
for the people...
We are FARC, Army of the people.[5]

As the FARC expanded its reach to include more rural areas, its tactics scaled up as well to include land seizures, imposition of protection taxes, and kidnappings—especially of government officials such as police officers or Army soldiers (Civico 2016). Over the decades, the organization grew to have a formalized military structure, with several different *bloques* (essentially, garrisons) in different parts of the country and a hierarchical leadership structure (Molano 2000). The existence of various social problems led to the formation of several other guerrilla groups, each with its own tactics and ideology (Rosa 2003).

Peace talks have been attempted at various points, and Porch and Rasmussen (2008) characterize their being stalled as a Colombian political tradition. However, a landmark moment occurred in 2016 when a four-year peace talk process resulted in an accord with the FARC. Sadly, and perhaps predictably, implementation of the agreement has not gone well. Several guerrilleros, including some former FARC leaders, reinitiated aggressions shortly thereafter (Binningsbø et al. 2019; Human Rights Watch 2020); and as of late 2020, over 200 former FARC members had been killed upon their reintegration into society (*La Semana* 2020).

The Paramilitaries and Narcotrafficking

Overt public displays of terrorism by the various guerrilla groups such as placing land mines in the countryside, forceful possession of rural property, and kidnappings led to public disapproval of the insurgency, and a narrative that supported the rise of paramilitary groups expressly for public protection partially because the state was too impotent to intervene (Civico 2016). Since the guerrillas were decidedly leftist, the paramilitaries, or "counter terrorists" as they referred to themselves, were expressly extreme right (Huhle 2001). Their mission was to rid the towns of what they saw as human waste—not only the guerrillas, but people involved with social movements, such as union organizers or human rights defenders, and anyone not fitting a particular mold and deemed by them to be hazardous to society, including those addicted to drugs or alcohol, people who were lesbian or gay, and sex workers (Civico 2016).

Fears about Communism that were widespread following WWII coupled with the increase in violence by guerrilla groups led to a governmental decree in 1965 giving citizens the right to organize against leftist ideology; made into law in 1968, it essentially legalized private self-defense groups (García-Godos and Lid 2010). The law was only struck down in 1989 when the violence had become pervasive and almost intractable (Tate 2007), but by then, the damage from official government approval of such groups had already been done. The illegality of such groups was not to last: legal rural defense forces known as the *Convivir* were established in 1995 and were involved in numerous human rights abuses.

Tate (2007) divides the history of Colombian paramilitaries into three periods. The first, contemporary with the FARC's founding, were the roving death squads in the 1970s and 1980s, formed primarily to rout out the guerrilla who had taken near-full control of many rural areas.

The state's impotency to exert control was commonly understood and the paramilitaries acted with impunity; in addition to rape and murder, they regularly increased the amount of protection taxes imposed on landowners and businesses (Civico 2016). By the late 1980s, the second phase of paramilitaries had begun with the organization of private armies funded by narcotraffickers (Tate 2007). The guerrilla had also discovered that the illegal drug trade was an ideal way to help finance their operations, and so the lines between the guerrilla and the paramilitaries became blurred: control of illegal coca, marijuana, and poppy fields as well as the related routes to market gave them another thing to fight about, and the influx of drug cartels complicated the picture even further.

The third phase of paramilitary evolution in Colombia was with their unification in 1997 into the group known as *Autodefensas Unidas de Colombia* (AUC), (United Self-defense Forces of Colombia) (Tate 2007). Following unification, a major calling card of the AUC was massacres in rural areas, with another popular tactic being limb dismemberment with machetes, knives, or chainsaws, often while the victim was still alive[6] (Campos Varela and Morcillo 2011). Massacres in Colombia were not novel when the AUC was founded; incidentally, *Rutas del Conflicto*, a journalistic project to archive, document, and investigate reports of conflict violence, has information on 1,982 massacres committed between 1982 and 2012, of which 730 are fully documented. The paramilitaries relied on massacres in particular to exert control; of the nearly 2,000 massacres over the thirty-year documented period, paramilitaries were responsible for almost 60 percent (Castro 2014). As noted below, such excesses fit into the quest for authority, even when considering the individual paramilitary rank-and-file who was just carrying out orders (Civico 2016).

Such terror techniques were expressly part of the modus operandi of the AUC so that they could legitimize their power and authority; to follow Hannah Arendt's (1969) definitions of *power* as being bestowed to a group by others, and *authority* being an end in and of itself where its recognition compels others to obey. It was in the pursuit of such power and authority that massacres occurred. A cursory review of the documented massacres by *Rutas del Conflicto* (n.d.) reveals a trend of assassins arriving suddenly, oftentimes having lists of targeted people, other times with the seeming goal of random murder, sometimes killing children, pregnant women, or other vulnerable people.

Witnesses were often present who could hear the wailing or gunshots, and not infrequently, they were made to watch their loved ones being mutilated, raped, or murdered (Sánchez-Moreno 2018); to bestow such suffering on bystanders illustrates the scope of violence as beyond physical pain (Scheper-Hughes and Bourgois 2004). For the armed groups, we argue that the more important element is the inflicted psychic and emotional pain on the family members and community. This psychic pain confers power to the offending group and authority to the individual assassin. Unfortunately, many rural townspeople were placed in an impossible position with knowing whose authority to respect; as Sanford (2003, 65) has described it, civilians were "everywhere in between" the locations of guerrilla, Army, and paramilitaries, leaving many *campesinos* no option but to flee.

Paramilitary killing statistics and modus operandi are especially chilling when you consider that their existence was largely supported by the urban middle and upper classes, seen as a necessary evil to combat the guerrilla and leftist ideology (Civico 2016). Many of the elite had been subjected to kidnapping or extortion by the guerrilla (Civico 2016); however, their daily lives did not necessarily include exposure to the reality of rural violence: blood, screaming, terror, fear, and pain. The disconnect between those living amidst the horror of the violence and those who were not as directly affected is characterized by Feldman (1994, 404) as "cultural anesthesia," and in Colombia is perhaps best highlighted by the 2016 popular referendum on acceptance of the peace accords with the FARC. While the measure failed nationally by less than a percentage point, only about 40 percent of eligible voters turned out, and there was a substantial divide between areas, with many of the worst affected, such as Guaviare and the Caribbean and Pacific coasts, overwhelmingly voting to accept the accord (Barragan 2017; *El Tiempo* 2016; Eventon 2016). The overwhelming support in many of the hardest hit areas indicates the desire of many citizens most directly affected by the conflict for the violence to cease (García-Godos and Lid 2010), despite the existence of significant controversies over parts of the agreement, such as mechanisms for reintegration of ex-guerrilleros into society and mandating their involvement as legitimate political actors (Eventon 2016).

In 2005, a specific legal structure was set in place to demobilize and reincorporate former paramilitaries into society while providing for victim reparation that included the stipulation that ex-combatants must refrain from future criminal activity (see upcoming discussion). However, the violence continued with ex-paramilitaries and ex-guerrilleros forming criminal gangs (*Bandas Criminales*), and in 2008, with the founding of the spin-off group known as the *Autodefensas Gaitanistas de Colombia* (AGC) (Gaitanista Self-Defense Forces of Colombia), who as of this writing continue to engage in similar activities to that of the demobilized AUC (Colombia Reports 2019; Human Rights Watch 2020). The Gaitanistas are not alone in their endeavors as Paramilitaries 2.0; several other new paramilitary groups have arisen to fill the vacuum left by the AUC, and a major departure with pre-demobilization paramilitaries is collaboration with the guerrilla when it symbiotically benefits their mutual interests in the drug trade (Civico 2016).

The government's relationship through time with the paramilitaries has been a reciprocal, yet uneven, one. Because the guerrilla were anti-government, with the pre-demobilization paramilitaries' founding objective being anti-guerrilla, the Colombian state had a vested interest in whether paramilitaries were successful at eradicating guerrilla and guerrilla sympathizers. The resulting support, either overtly or covertly, has led at least one observer to declare the paramilitaries as being another branch of the Colombian military (Molano 2000). Simultaneously however, the government's active involvement with fighting the drug trade (in which the paramilitaries were intimately involved) has led to killings of hundreds of judges and other law enforcement officers at the hands of paramilitary assassins (Tate 2007). Figure 3.3 illustrates the overlapping relationship between the government, paramilitaries, narcotraffickers, and the guerrilla.

Human Rights Violations

This fractured nature of the Colombian state's response to the violence is especially apparent when considering the human rights abuses committed by the military. On any given day that peace negotiations on the behalf of the

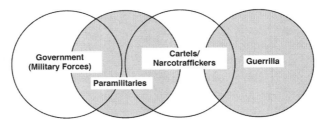

Figure 3.3 Approximate relationship between the Colombian Armed Forces, paramilitary groups, narcotraffickers, and the guerrilla, circa early 1990s. Note the larger share of complicity with the drug trade ascribed to paramilitaries as opposed to the guerrilla (Sanford 2003). Credit: Elizabeth A. DiGangi.

government were underway with the guerrilla, the Army would be actively trying to kill guerrilleros (Richani 2000). Part of this strategy included collusion with the paramilitaries, a model created in 1982 when the fallout from a guerrilla kidnapping of a prominent cartel member included the creation of a self-defense group to kill kidnappers, and the Army's provision of that group with intelligence, training, and other resources (Carrigan 1995).

One especially poignant example of military overt and covert support of paramilitary violence is evident with the massacre at Mapiripán, Meta (central Colombia) in July 1997. One hundred AUC combatants landed at the local Army-guarded airstrip and systematically began killing people on predetermined lists (Chernick 1998). The town's judge called local Army leadership multiple times over the next several days begging for help (Vargas Meza 1998); the Army finally arrived on the sixth and last day of the massacre. At that point, anywhere between thirty and forty-nine people[7] were dead and dozens more had fled (Chernick 1998). Shamefully, this is but one of many examples of the Army's complicity during violent attacks on civilians perpetrated by paramilitaries. Carlos Castaño, the architect of the Mapiripán massacre, was adamant that the victims were not "innocent peasants," rather, they were "despicable . . . guerrillas in peasant clothing" (Chernick 1998). Such a statement betrays the rationalization behind his killing initiatives, which were ultimately about social cleansing, power, and control.

In addition to this hear-nor-see-no-evil approach, the military has also been implicated in purposeful killings of civilians to increase their reported body counts[8] of guerrilleros. The common scenario could involve civilians being lured away with the promise of money for a day's labor, or arbitrary arrest on false charges; victims would then be shot and dressed in military fatigues to pass them off as guerrilleros[9] (Lindsay-Poland 2014). Known as "false positives" (*falsos positivos*), victims included people the Army likely reasoned would not be missed, such as those addicted to drugs, but students and young professionals were targeted as well (Lindsay-Poland 2014). Military cover-ups of such abuses were rampant (Carrigan 1995) and the problem was substantial—in 2021, the Special Jurisdiction for Peace put the number of *falsos positivos* at just over 6,400 victims during the period 2002–2008 (Emblin 2021). Further, many were only subjected to an abbreviated medicolegal death exam, hindering the ability to ultimately identify them as well as comprehensively document the cause and manner of death (Guzmán and Sanabria Medina 2016).

FORENSIC ANTHROPOLOGY IN LATIN AMERICA

In general, forensic anthropology in Latin America more broadly was initiated in the 1980s and 1990s on a country-by-country basis. Several Latin

American countries share a similar origin story with regard to the discipline of forensic anthropology, to include Argentina, Guatemala, Chile, and Peru; namely, that anthropologists formed NGOs to respond to exhumation and victim identification needs following gross human rights violations. The common threads these teams faced of method standardization and the regional context under which forensic anthropology was necessary led to the creation of the Latin American Association of Forensic Anthropology (*Asociación Latinoamericana de Antropología Forense*—ALAF). Instituted in 2003, it was created as a professional organization to connect forensic anthropology professionals, establish scientific and ethical practices, and promote the use of forensic anthropology and archaeology in medicolegal death investigations, from mass disasters to human rights violations. In 2012, ALAF became the third organization worldwide[10] to institute a board certification process for individual forensic anthropologists.

GOVERNMENTAL RESPONSE TO THE CONFLICT: THE POLITICS OF IDENTIFICATION

Forensic Anthropology in Colombia

Colombia's development of forensic anthropology is somewhat distinct from the aforementioned countries in Latin America, with its beginnings not unlike that of the discipline in the United States, where anatomists or physical anthropologists began providing consults for law enforcement when human skeletal remains were discovered (DiGangi and Bethard 2021). In Colombia in the 1980s, Dr. José Vicente Rodríguez, a physical anthropologist from the *Universidad Naciónal* in Bogotá, began providing his expertise for governmental agencies, to include consultation on high-profile cases (Guzmán and Sanabria Medina 2016). However, unlike the earlier development of the discipline in the United States, Dr. Rodríguez was the primary physical anthropologist doing such work and most anthropology programs in Colombia were focused on sociocultural anthropology, which to this day has limited the academic development of skeletal biology in biological anthropology more broadly.

Even though the conflict was well entrenched by the late 1980s with presumably a substantial number of bodies in advanced stages of decomposition to be autopsied, there was no lasting development of a non-governmental Colombian forensic anthropology team as established in other South American countries such as Argentina and Peru. Instead, the catalyst for the discipline were two mass disasters within a month of each other in late 1989—a bomb on a domestic flight that killed 107 people and a detonated car bomb in front of the Security Police's headquarters that added 110 to the body count (Guzmán and Sanabria Medina 2016).

Shortly after these events, the director of the National Institute for Legal Medicine and Forensic Sciences, the country's national medical examiner system, established the first forensic anthropology laboratory. Within four years, the law enforcement branch (*Cuerpo Técnico de Investigación*-CTI) of the National Prosecutor's Office had also established its first laboratory. By 2005, CTI had six laboratories around the country (Guzmán and Sanabria Medina 2016), and Legal Medicine had at least one. The Security Police (disbanded later in 2008) and the National Police had also established at least one lab each in the early 2000s. During the first decade of the twenty-first century, all nationwide labs employed a total of about thirty forensic anthropologists. At the time of this writing, this number has approximately doubled, and they are divided unequally between three government agencies of CTI, Legal Medicine, and the National Police, as well as the nascent Search Unit for Disappeared Persons (*Unidad de Búsqueda de Personas Dadas por Desaparecidas*—UBPD) (discussed below).

Practically, the diversity of state organizations having forensic anthropology labs meant that there were several different ways of practicing forensic anthropology, and unfortunately the agencies did not necessarily meet to discuss best practices or how to streamline efforts. In fact, when the first author began work in Colombia in 2008, it was in her training courses that some of the anthropologists from the different agencies met each other for the first time. This is a unique situation distinct from that in other parts of South America where a single organization conducts all forensic anthropology casework associated with the conflict, such as with the Argentinean Forensic Anthropology Team (EAAF).

In general, there is a non-unified strategy to best practices, case resolution, and continuing education which we attribute to the fractured nature of the collective approach to forensic anthropology and each agency's specific charge with whether it exhumes or analyzes bodies or both, which experts are involved in those endeavors, what protocols and methods will be followed, what the hiring qualifications are, and what the onboarding training process will entail. This is in part illustrated by the six Colombians as of 2020 certified as Diplomates of ALAF. Diplomate status is conferred after an extensive review of qualifications followed by a rigorous, comprehensive written and practical exam. Each of the Colombians who are Diplomates as of this writing were at some point in their careers affiliated with Legal Medicine rather than the other government institutions. This illustrates the distinctive emphasis this institution places on continuing education and certification for its personnel.

As evidence of the increasing internationalization of the conflict (Tate 2000; Vargas Meza 1998), the Colombian government has not been alone in its endeavors to improve the forensic sciences. Foreign governments and NGOs have provided their assistance through the years in the form of equipment donations, mentorship of forensic professionals, provision of continuing education, and sponsorship to attend forensic conferences. For example, the United States has been continuously involved for several decades with funding provided by the State Department and Department of Justice, through its ICITAP program (International Criminal Investigative Training Assistance Program). Major NGOs such as the International Committee of the Red Cross have also been involved with mentorship of forensic professionals. Internal NGOs have been active as well, with a notable one being the *Equipo Colombiano Interdisciplinario de Trabajo Forense y Asistencia Psicosocial* (EQUITAS) (Colombian Interdisciplinary Forensic and Psychosocial Assistance Team), formed in 2003 with its focus being an extra-governmental check on forensic analyses for families as well as scientific research into improving grave location techniques (Camacho Cortés, Adriana Pérez, Arango Gómez 2020; Guzmán and Sanabria Medina 2016).

Relevant Legislation

Regardless of the agency forensic anthropologists work for, the job has become more complex, especially as new laws surrounding evidence admissibility, transitional justice, and victims' rights have been instituted, introducing new procedures with which to comply. Complicating matters is that there are two distinct criminal procedure codes (Law 600 of 2000 and Law 906 of 2004); the former is inquisitorial, and the latter adversarial including rules of evidence admissibility similar to those clarified by the *Daubert* trilogy rulings in the United States.[11] The application of one code or the other depends on when the crime was thought to be committed, with crimes after 2004 being under Law 906/2004.

One of the first major pieces of legislation dealing with the conflict was Law 589 of 2000. It formally outlawed forced disappearance, displacement, and torture among other crimes against humanity while establishing the National Search Commission for Missing Persons (*Comisión de Búsqueda de Personas Desaparecidas*—CBPD), designed to search for victims of forced disappearance. It also established the National Registry of Missing Persons, meant to include all the victims from the conflict (Semma Tamayo 2020; Vivas Díaz and Vega Urueña 2020). Conflict victims include more than just those people who were forcibly disappeared (i.e., displaced persons); therefore, years later the peace accord (discussed below) included a special mechanism to also account for other categories of victims.

In 2005, the law of *Justicia y Paz* (Justice & Peace) was instituted (Law 975/2005) which was Colombia's first example of legislated transitional justice, and among other things, provided a means for demobilization for paramilitaries and their reintegration into society while calling for victim identification and restitution for affected families (Vivas Díaz and Vega Urueña 2020). Also in 2005, the *Acta Urgente* law (Mechanism of Urgent Search, Law 971/2005) was enacted to alleviate some of the red tape surrounding searches and recoveries when there is a report of a missing person believed to have been forcibly disappeared (Vivas Díaz and Vega Urueña 2020) or upon unexpected discoveries of graves or human remains. The law establishing databases specific to disappearances was instituted in 2010 (Law 1408/2010) (Semma Tamayo 2020), and in 2011, the Victims' and Land Restitution Law created the Victims' Unit, charged with documenting victims for the purpose of reparations.

Finally, the 2016 Peace Accord established five separate mechanisms for restorative justice, to include the creation of the UBPD for those missing because of the conflict (Vivas Díaz and Vega Urueña 2020). The UBPD is independent from the aforementioned government institutions and also employs forensic anthropologists who conduct exhumations in support of Legal Medicine. It is set apart from the other initiatives because it was created by the peace accord process to search for all victims missed by the other agencies and laws, such as children recruited by the various armed groups and people who have been forcibly displaced. Further, it includes a National Search Plan (*Plan Nacional de Búsqueda*) which was uniquely constructed not only by government experts, but with input from NGOs, victims, civil society, academics, and artists; taking into account that an interdisciplinary approach incorporating historical context will be more likely to succeed (*Plan Nacional* 2020).

Practical Impact of Legislation

Each piece of legislation impacts the practicing forensic anthropologists because confusingly, they govern slightly different aspects of the conflict, in addition to establishing new units to oversee or coordinate certain areas. For example, Law 975/2005 requires that the prosecutor in charge of the case accompany the anthropologist and their exhumation team in the field; other laws do not and practically this can result in logistical problems during fieldwork because the prosecutor is able to facilitate necessities such as the guarantee of team security. Further, the Justice & Peace law applies to those victims of paramilitaries or guerrilleros who have demobilized; while investigations prior to exhumations may uncover some information about presumptive perpetrators, this is obviously not universal and many bodies are completely divorced from any such interpretive context. Finally, starting in 2010 with the increasing suspected *falsos positivos* case count, the prosecutor or judge in charge of each case began requesting second autopsies which involves exhumation, analysis, and full documentation to include comparison with any previous autopsy report (Guzmán and Sanabria Medina 2016); this process is more involved than those skeletal analyses under Justice & Peace or other laws.

Justice & Peace ushered in a new era for Colombian forensic anthropology, as part of the law required *postulados* (ex-combatants) to confess all their crimes, including where they had buried or disposed of all the bodies of their victims. Within the first few years of the law, thousands of graves had been discovered and exhumed (García-Godos and Lid 2010; Guzmán and Sanabria Medina 2016). *Postulado* confessions were not the sole mechanism by which graves were discovered; family and community members often had direct knowledge of grave location, in some cases because they had buried their loved ones themselves.[12]

Many graves are of a clandestine nature remotely located and/or under active conflict, and it is not uncommon for exhumation teams to have an hours-long hike through the jungle or farmland to get to the scene. Given this ongoing, inherent safety concern, exhumation teams must include escorts from the police or Army (figure 3.4), which is supposed to be organized by the prosecutor in charge of the case. Unfortunately, it has not been unheard of for teams to arrive at the rendezvous point to discover that security had not been arranged or was delayed, or for teams to be fired upon in the field. As a result, the general exhumation strategy has been to get in and out on the same day. This time constraint obviously means that corners must be frequently cut with doing the most scientific excavation possible.

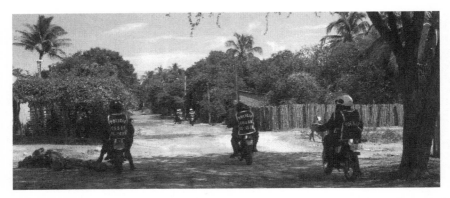

Figure 3.4   Police escort to an exhumation site in a small village located near the city of Valledupar in the Cesar department, northeastern Colombia. Photograph credit: Elizabeth A. DiGangi.

With the influx of human remains to the various laboratories comes associated problems. One is that of scale in terms of having a limited number of people to do the analyses—Guzmán and Sanabria Medina (2016) estimate that each anthropologist at Legal Medicine analyzes approximately sixty skeletons a year (that's more than one individual a week).[13] Another is the dearth of antemortem information or family reference samples with which to compare the biological profile or generated DNA profile, respectively. This is compounded by many of the analyzed skeletons sharing a biological profile of being male (c. 88%) and being between 17 and 35 years of age (Segura and Ramírez 2013). Antemortem information may not exist for those victims who have been reported missing, or family members may not have made a report out of fear or are not willing to provide DNA reference samples; inability for next-of-kin to travel may also impact this important collection of reference data. Some families have been decimated by the conflict, with several siblings dead or displaced in different parts of the country, and multiple missing siblings from one family also complicates DNA identifications when reference samples are available (Guzmán and Sanabria Medina 2016). Finally, as will be discussed in more depth below, a sizable proportion of victims have been buried as John or Jane Does (in Spanish, *ningún nombre*, "no name") in cemeteries which have later removed the bones and placed them in a common ossuary (Guzmán and Sanabria Medina 2016), making identification at that point close to impossible barring extraordinary measures.

STRUCTURAL VIOLENCE AND VICTIMOLOGY

As introduced at the beginning of this chapter, structural violence is the imposition of suffering on people because of the systems—social, political, and economic—that are designed to benefit the few at the expense of the many. Practically, this results in lack of access to necessities such as clean water, adequate housing, education, and legal employment opportunities. In Colombia, where many of the conflict victims are impoverished (Rettberg 2015), it is not only the conflict itself which has created the structure within which their victimization occurs, but the macro-economic and political structure of capitalism which has placed them in a position which restricts their agency (see Farmer 1997). For *campesinos* joining the guerrilla or paramilitaries, or working to grow illegal drug crops, their choices often revolve around a viable yet illegal economic opportunity with higher wages (Holmes et al. 2007), destitution, or death—not much of a choice at all. This also lends many *guerrilleros* and paramilitary combatants a unique intersectional identity (Crenshaw 1997): they are simultaneously victim and perpetrator.

Further, as noted, many living victims are placed in impossible situations—with the conflict continuing and the murderers of their loved ones or perpetrators of their own displacement at large, there is no reconciliation, only the perpetuation of fear and terror. Green (1998) characterized such terror as being *diffused* into all aspects of life, and Farmer (1997, 2003) as being *embodied*; both have irreparably shaped what it means to be Colombian in the twentieth and twenty-first centuries.

As an example, of the estimated six million living victims, only 7 percent are registered with some victim organization, and such organizations number in the thousands (Rettberg 2015). This general culture of victim non-involvement can perhaps best be understood in the context of the diffused terror. Victims have seen what happens when people are involved in any kind of social movement, or when they are even suspected or accused of being involved: their lives are taken for it. In this way, the power of the guerrilla, paramilitaries, and Army units involved in human rights violations is not exclusively in the violence that they perpetrate, but in the silencing of the victims left alive.

Green (1998) discussed how remaining silent was a "survival strategy" for victims in Guatemala, and the same is true for Colombia. While silence does not necessarily guarantee survival, it certainly facilitates it. Further, Farmer (1997) discussed how the suffering itself of the impoverished is silenced—without agency, without a unified political voice, their experience is left largely unspoken, a mere footnote to the history of the country and the conflict. Only recently have the National Center for Historical Memory, created in 2011 by the Law of Victims and Land Restitution (Law 1448/2011), in concert with the extra-judicial Commission for the Clarification of Truth, Coexistence, and Non-Repetition resulting from the 2016 peace accord, actively acted to combat this silence by documenting the diversity of victims' experiences (Tate 2016).

Who Are the Victims?

In this chapter, we have spent a large part of the preceding discussion on the actors rather than the victims. It is our position that you cannot begin to understand who the victims are and exactly how they have been victimized until you have contextualized who the perpetrators are and their motives. As noted, it is a complex contextualization, one which we have barely begun to summarize here. However, as Chernick (1998) aptly noted, in the end the story is ultimately about the victims. It is their suffering and pain born from the violence—direct and structural—which has shaped the cultural landscape of Colombia over the past several decades.

The conflict has been so protracted and has influenced essentially every aspect of Colombian society that devising an encompassing description of who the victims are is not possible. Some are wealthy and are to various extents complicit in the conflict, as in a kidnapped cartel member or assassinated high-ranking politician; many are impoverished, as in a *campesino* forced off her land or a squatter killed when an assassin arrives in the *barrio*; many are children, recruited from a young age or as teenage sisters disappeared by paramilitaries who rape, torture, and murder them; some are young men with insecure employment lured by the military on the promise of a day's wage who are killed to increase the body count and earn the killers an extra weekend of leave; some are combatants forced or compelled to join one side or the other for lack of other viable employment opportunities or to avenge a murdered loved one; some have no choice but to grow coca because of limited infrastructure or restrictive market forces preventing cultivation of other crops; some are trapped when the armed groups invade their land to fight; some are mothers, forcibly displaced from their homes in the countryside who wind up nursing their babies while selling trinkets by the side of the road in Bogotá; some are community leaders bravely risking their lives to advocate for social change or union rights; some are simply in the wrong place at the wrong time when a bomb goes off in a mall or in front of a building; most are civilians; they span all ages from elderly to unborn; all are human.

Despite this disparate picture of who the victims are, here we focus on those victims who are from impoverished rural or urban backgrounds. A survey of all victims revealed that half have less than a high school education and most fall into the lowest *estratos* (socioeconomic status level) (Rettberg 2015). Such impoverishment is abject and the city of Buenaventura, located in the department of Valle de Cauca on the Pacific Coast and having a population of over 300,000, is one example. Within the past decade, 65 percent of households did not have indoor plumbing for sewage and 45 percent did not have potable water (Nicholls and Sánchez-Garzoli 2011).

Structural violence obviously disproportionally affects people who have scant access to resources that would help them live healthier and safer lives, and the conflict only serves to exacerbate this, because it is their very lack of access that primes them for victimization. Ironically, even the wealthy victims, such as kidnapped politicians or cartel members, are also undergirded by structural violence because of their participation in and benefit from the system that has served to disenfranchise a large segment of Colombians. It is the structures that have created the poverty typifying the majority of victims which have been the primary driver behind their susceptibility to victimization. The 1990 massacre in the town of Pueblo Bello as well as the pervasive misplacing of bodies by cemeteries are two examples that serve to highlight how structural violence plays out with victim identification, as well as how victimization itself does not necessarily have an end (Taussig 2004).

Pueblo Bello Massacre

In January 1990, paramilitaries led by Carlos Castaño's elder brother, Fidel, entered the village of Pueblo Bello in Antioquia, and disappeared forty-three civilians because the guerrilla had stolen forty-three of Fidel's cattle. After a few months of decomposition, twenty-four bodies were exhumed without regard for evidence preservation; unthinkably, state agents asked families to identify their decomposing loved ones without providing any psychosocial support (Guzmán and Sanabria Medina 2016; Miric 2016). Family members identified six people based on clothing and other personal effects, and the remaining unidentified bodies were placed into an unmarked mass grave at the local cemetery. Recall that these events were at the infancy of the establishment of forensic anthropology as a part of state forensic services, and despite subsequent attempts to rectify the situation, thirty-seven people remain disappeared (Guzmán and Sanabria Medina 2016). In 2021 after substantial effort, the state located a presumptive mass grave site for the unidentified individuals who were interred in 1990. As of the time of this writing in early 2022, the analysis of these recovered remains continues (Francis Paola Niño Ruíz, personal communication, February 7, 2022). In this instance, the families were victimized three times: during the massacre itself, when the state asked them to inspect the decomposing bodies of those murdered, and when the state lost the rest of the recovered bodies through cemetery mismanagement and incompetence. With the 2021 discovery, the chance exists now for resolution to finally occur.

Cemetery Burials of N.N.s (Ningún Nombre, No Name)

In 2010, an inter-institutional agreement was established between the National Civil Registry, the Ministry of the Interior, and Legal Medicine to identify 35,000 people buried as unknowns (*ningún nombre*, N.N.) between 1970 and 2010 (Vivas Díaz and Vega Urueña 2020). The agreement was to cross-check available records such as autopsy fingerprint cards with national identity cards for these individuals to determine if some of them could at last be identified (Vivas Díaz and Vega Urueña 2020). By 2016, over 28,000 people had been identified through such record checking alone (Semma Tamayo 2020). However, similar to the situation following the Pueblo Bello massacre, many of these people were buried at cemeteries in mass or single graves that were later subjected to exhumation and placement in a common ossuary by cemetery officials.[14] Further, many of the cemeteries have poor or non-existent record-keeping practices (Guzmán and Sanabria Medina 2016; Vivas Díaz and Vega Urueña 2020), meaning that (1) locating the grave(s) on the grounds of the cemetery is difficult, (2) if an unmarked grave is located, it is unclear as to who might be in it, (3) cross-referencing who is still in the grave(s) with who had been placed in the ossuary is impossible, and (4) resolving the commingling in the ossuary with people who had been identified and perhaps were not even conflict victims with those who had been buried as N.N.s is almost insurmountable.

Both examples demonstrate how Colombian victimization has no end, à la Taussig (2004): the question of where the bodies may be remains perpetually open, an eternal question mark. Living victims are not allowed to move through stages of grief—they are kept in limbo, stuck waiting on the state for answers—the same state which either victimized them outright or indirectly via its dereliction of duty to keep its citizens safe in their own communities, what Sanford (2003, 64) calls "state violence by proxy." Further, the structures in place that have led to rural and urban poverty are also those that have contributed to revictimization via cemetery loss of remains where the people at the bottom are seen as disposable, "waste" in the parlance of the paramilitaries. The structural violence thus continues, even in death.

How to Define Suffering—The Meaning of a Loved One's Death

How does one define human suffering? The late Paul Farmer, a physician and anthropologist, posed this question as he pondered the suffering he had seen his patients in Haiti experience (1997). It seems clear that the most extreme suffering is easy to identify, but what of the other types—the insidious suffering of living in fear, of not knowing the fate of a loved one, of not having enough to make ends meet? A related question is how to ascribe meaning to the suffering—of the living survivors as well as that experienced by the dead in their last moments. Tate (2007) discusses how the statistics of the victim count—absolute deaths attributed to each actor, numbers of community members displaced, numbers of mourning family and community members— are problematic because they aid in concealing the enduring meaning behind each death. This meaning is unmeasurable in terms of the suffering for those left behind and the impact this continues to have on Colombian society and culture, for those mourning the identified and unidentified alike.

The first author once attended a repatriation ceremony in Medellín for a number of victims where each set of bones was in its own miniature plain wooden coffin accompanied by a cross and photograph of the deceased. While this was a large ceremony and many families were present, one family member in particular was notable. Based on her age and how young the victim appeared in his photo, she was presumably his grandmother, and she was distraught. Standing near her grandson's coffin, this elderly woman wept openly, yet silently, while photographers from the media converged on her until ceremony officials made them stop. That moment—a grandmother's enduring love and silent grief made tangible—encapsulates the story of

Colombian suffering. We do not know her name; but naming her is not necessary to understand that the combined suffering experienced by every grandparent, parent, pibling, child, sibling, cousin, nibling, spouse, neighbor, and friend is incomprehensible.

NOTES

1. Acknowledgments: Many of our friends and colleagues in Colombia have dedicated their professional careers to conflict resolution and victim identification; we thank them for their friendship, collegiality, and commitment in the face of enormous obstacles. We thank Dr. Nancy Applebaum for her insightful comments which substantially assisted us with improving this chapter within the space allotted; and we are grateful to Dr. César Sanabria for providing information about the UBPD. A special thanks to Francis Paola Niño Ruíz and the entire team of experts who have been diligently working on the Pueblo Bello case. Finally, we acknowledge the two anonymous reviewers. EAD would like to thank former and current ICITAP-Colombia leadership, especially the late Dr. Dan Garner, for the opportunities to contribute her expertise to capacity building in Colombia; as well as her Colombian friends who have helped teach her much about the tension of joy and pain that characterizes Colombian life. DSV would like to thank her sisters and everyone who has listened to her non-stop talk about the conflict in Colombia, and to her mentor who has solidified her passion for forensic anthropology. We are grateful to the editors of this volume for their invitation and especially thank them for spearheading this conversation about forensic anthropology's role in social justice. Finally, we humbly acknowledge the millions of victims, living and deceased, and we hope we have approached an adequate account for them here.

2. This unique geography has also contributed to the country's rich biodiversity, counting it second worldwide to Brazil (World Wildlife Fund 2017).

3. The estimates of deceased persons vary widely, depending on the consulted database or reporting organization. Regardless of the absolute number, it is clear that the problem is of enormous magnitude.

4. In fact, concerns about infrastructure for farmers to grow legal crops are so great that a commitment to building new roads in rural areas was part of the 2016 peace accord with the FARC (*Presidencia de la República* 2016).

5. The authors' English translation of:
Contra el imperialismo
por la patria...
Contra la oligarquia
por el pueblo...
Somos FARC, Ejercito del pueblo.

6. The dismemberments served a practical function in addition to terror and inflicting of maximum physical pain: the problem of body disposal is simplified when only parts rather than a whole remain; smaller graves can be dug making their

discovery less likely while reducing the effort needed for digging, and transportation for disposal in waterways is similarly facilitated.

7. Reports as to the number of victims vary; many were thrown into the Guaviare River and their remains were never recovered.

8. This body count mentality sprung from the emphasis military leaders put on the absolute numbers of guerrillas killed as a metric to demonstrate the armed forces were successfully waging the war. The individual perpetrators directly benefited when their commanding officers granted privileges such as extra leaves when dead guerrilla quotas were met (Guzmán and Sanabria Medina 2016; Winograd 2017). Unfortunately, this body count mentality, the underlying principle of which is that the absolute numbers are more important than conflict resolution itself and that they symbolize the legitimacy of the state's efforts, is ubiquitous. Prosecutors have been known to rejoice when site exhumations turn up more bodies than the investigation indicated there would be, because it allows them to increase their recovered body counts in their reports. Such a mentality misses the forest for the trees.

9. One of the ways this was discovered was at autopsy by medical examiners or anthropologists who astutely noted the lack of any bullet holes in the fatigues, an impossibility for someone shot in a part of the body presumably covered by clothes (Olarte-Sierra and Castro Bermúdez 2019).

10. After the American Board of Forensic Anthropology (ABFA) and the Forensic Anthropology Society of Europe (FASE).

11. The *Daubert* trilogy refers to a series of Supreme Court rulings that allowed the Court to clarify the admission of expert testimony in federal judicial proceedings (Bethard and DiGangi 2019).

12. Unfortunately, the government has been inefficient at solicitation of such witness information (López Cerquera 2018).

13. The average numbers for CTI are likely lower because those anthropologists also participate in field exhumations, sometimes for weeks at a time.

14. The removal of burials after a given amount of time (a few years) is typical in Colombia and many other places worldwide because of the limited amount of space for multiple single long-term burials.

REFERENCES

Alsema, Adriaan. 2018. "Colombia has highest number of internally displaced people." *Colombia Reports*, June 19, 2018. https://colombiareports.com/colombia -has-highest-number-of-internally-displaced-people/

Arendt, Hannah. 1969. *On Violence*. New York: Harcourt, Brace, and Company.

Barragan, Yesenia. 2017. "To end 500 years of great terror. For Afro-Colombian communities, the struggle for peace and justice is centuries long—and remains far from over." *NACLA Report on the Americas* 49, no. 1: 56–63.

Bethard, Jonathan D. and Elizabeth A. DiGangi. 2019. "From the laboratory to the witness stand: research trends and method validation in forensic anthropology." In

Forensic Anthropology and the United States Judicial System, edited by Laura C. Fulginiti, Kristen Hartnett-McCann, and Alison Galloway, 41–52. Wiley & Sons Ltd.

Binningsbø, Helga Malmin, Dahl Marianne, Mokleiv Nygård Håvard, Abbey Steele, and Michael Weintraub. 2019. "Colombia's historic peace agreement with the FARC is fraying. We talked to 1,700 Colombians to understand why." *The Washington Post*, 7 August 2019. https://www.washingtonpost.com/politics/2019/08/06/colombias-historic-peace-agreement-with-farc-is-fraying-we-talked-colombians-understand-why/

Braun, Herbert. 1985. *The Assassination of Gaitán: Public Life and Urban Violence in Colombia*. Madison: University of Wisconsin Press.

Camacho Cortés, Ginna P., Luz Adriana Pérez, and Diana Arango Gómez. 2020. "Complex scenarios and technological innovation: Brief case report from Colombia." In *Forensic Science and Humanitarian Action: Interacting with the Dead and the Living*, edited by Roberto C. Parra, Sara C. Zapico, and Douglas H. Ubelaker, 257–71. John Wiley & Sons.

Campos Varela, Isla Y., and Maria Morcillo. 2011. "Dismemberment: Cause of death in the Colombian armed conflict." *Proceedings of the 63rd Annual Meeting of the American Academy of Forensic Sciences* 17, 356.

Carrigan, Ana. 1995. "A chronicle of a death foretold: State-sponsored violence in Colombia." *NACLA Report on the Americas* 28, no. 5: 6–10. https://doi.org/10.1080/10714839.1995.11722937

Castro, Daniela. 2014. "The trail of death: 30 years of massacres in Colombia." *Insight Crime*, May 8, 2014. https://insightcrime.org/news/analysis/the-trail-of-death-30-years-of-massacres-in-colombia/

Chernick, Marc W. 1998. "The paramilitarization of the war in Colombia." *NACLA Report on the Americas* 31, no. 5: 28–33. https://doi.org/10.1080/10714839.1998.11722772

Civico, Aldo. 2016. *The Para-State: An Ethnography of Colombia's Death Squads*. Oakland, CA: University of California Press.

Colombia Reports. 2019. "*Gaitanista Self-Defense Forces of Colombia (AGC) / Gulf Clan*". October 22, 2019. https://colombiareports.com/agc-gulf-clan/

Crenshaw, Kimberlé W. 1997. *On Intersectionality: Essential Writings*. New York: The New Press.

DiGangi, Elizabeth A. and Jonathan D. Bethard. 2021. "Uncloaking a lost cause: Decolonizing ancestry estimation in the United States." *American Journal of Physical Anthropology* 175, no. 2: 422–36. https://doi .org /10 .1002 /ajpa .24212

El Tiempo. 2016. "Polarización del país, reflejada en resultados del escrutinio." *Polarization of the Country, Reflected in Poll Results*. October 2, 2016. https://www.eltiempo.com/archivo/documento/CMS-16716558

Emblin, Richard. 2021. "Colombia's war atrocities emerge with JEP's revised 'false positives'." *The City Paper*, February 19, 2021. http://thecitypaperbogota.com/news/scale-of-colombias-war-atrocities-emerge-with-6400-false-positives/26822

?fbclid=IwAR3IsgKOT8CE6viQ1w-pxsh3cFm-Pbq7ypOHhymWKgYe2hhKDO
_PFoNPNzo

Eventon, Ross. 2016. "War and democracy in Colombia. Guerrilla demobilization or otherwise, Colombia will remain a country with deep social conflicts and a far cry from a functioning democracy." *NACLA Report on the Americas* 48, no. 4: 303–6. https://doi.org/10.1080/10714839.2016.1258270

Farmer, Paul. 1997. "On suffering and structural violence: A view from below." In *Social Suffering*, edited by A. Kleinman, V. Das, and M. Lock, 261–83. Berkeley: University of California Press.

———. 2003. *Pathologies of Power: Health, Human Rights, and the New War on the Poor*. Berkeley and Los Angeles: University of California Press.

Feldman, Allen. 1994. "On cultural anesthesia: From Desert Storm to Rodney King." *American Ethnologist* 21, no. 2: 404–18.

García-Godos, Jemima, and Knut Andreas O. Lid. 2010. "Transitional justice and victims' rights before the end of a conflict: The unusual case of Colombia." *Journal of Latin American Studies* 42, no. 3: 487–516. http://www.jstor.org/stable /40984893

Green, Linda. 1998. *Fear as a Way of Life: Mayan Widows in Rural Guatemala*. New York: Columbia University Press.

———. 2004. "Response to an anthropology of structural violence." *Current Anthropology* 45, no. 3: 319–20.

Guzmán, Angélica and César Sanabria Medina. 2016. "The origin and development of forensic anthropology and archaeology in Colombia." In *Handbook of Forensic Anthropology and Archaeology*, edited by Soren Blau and Douglas Ubelaker, 2nd edition, 75–93. New York: Routledge.

Holmes, Jennifer S., Gutiérrez de Piñeres, Sheila Amin, and Kevin M. Curtin. 2007. "A subnational study of insurgency: FARC violence in the 1990s." *Studies in Conflict & Terrorism* 30: 249–65. https://doi.org/10.1080/10576100601148456

Huhle, Rainer. 2001. "La violencia paramilitar en Colombia: Historia, estructuras, políticas del Estado e impacto politico." *"Paramilitary violence in Colombia: history, structures, state politics, and the political impact."* *Revista Del CESLA* 2: 63–81.

Human Rights Watch. 2020. *"Colombia Events of 2020"*. Date of last access February 23, 2021. https://www.hrw.org/world-report/2021/country-chapters/colombia# 2020.

Internal Displacement Monitoring Centre. Date of last access February 23, 2021. Retrieved from https://www.internal-displacement.org/ n.d.

La Semana. "La matanza de los excombatientes de las Farc: un lunar del acuerdo de paz." "The killing of ex-FARC combatants: a stain on the peace agreement." Date of last access May 19, 2021. https://www.semana.com/nacion/articulo/la-matanza -de-los-excombatientes-de-las-farc-una-gran-deuda-del-acuerdo-paz/202002/ 24 November 2020.

Lindsay-Poland, John. 2014. "Guerrillas killed in combat" and the Colombian military's persistent impunity." *NACLA Report on the Americas* 47, no. 2: 6–10. https://doi.org/10.1080/10714839.2014.11721842

López Cerquera, Maria Alexandra. 2018. "The Law of Justice and Peace and the Disappeared: A Critical Evaluation of Forensic Intervention as a Tool of Transitional Justice in Colombia." PhD Diss., The University of Tennessee.

Miric, Milja. 2016. "Pueblo Bello Massacre v. Colombia." *Loyola of Los Angeles International and Comparative Law Review* 38: 1294–326.

Molano, Alfredo. 2000. "The evolution of the FARC: A Guerrilla group's long history." *NACLA Report on the Americas* 34, no. 2: 23–31. https://doi.org/10.1080 /10714839.2000.11722627

Nicholls, Kelly and Gimena Sánchez-Garzoli. 2011. "Buenaventura Colombia: Where Free Trade Meets Mass Graves." *NACLA Report on the Americas* 44, no. 4: 4–7. https://doi.org/10.1080/10714839.2011.11722142

Olarte-Sierra, María Fernanda, and Jaime Enrique Castro Bermúdez. 2019. "Notas forenses: conocimiento que materializa a los cuerpos del enemigo en fosas paramilitares y falsos positivos." "Forensic Notes: knowledge that reveals the bodies of the enemy in paramilitary graves and false positives." *Antipoda. Revista de Antropología y Arqueología* 34: 119–40. https://doi.org/10.7440/antipoda34.2019.06

Pita Pico, Roger. 2018. "Violence, censorship and media in Colombia: Effects of the "Bogotazo" and the collapse in radio broadcasts". *Anagramas Rumbos y Sentidos de la Comunicación* 37, no. 33: 153–73. https://dx.doi.org/10.22395/angr .v17n33a7

Plan Nacional de Búsqueda de la Unidad de Búsqueda de Personas Dadas por Desaparecidas en el Contexto y en Razón del Conflicto Armado. National Search Plan of the Search Unit of Persons Reported as Disappeared in the Context and Due to the Armed Conflict. 2020. Bogotá D. C., Colombia.

Porch, Douglas and María José Rasmussen. 2008. "Demobilization of paramilitaries in Colombia: Transformation or transition?" *Studies in Conflict & Terrorism* 31: 520–40. https://dx.doi.org/10.1080/10576100802064841

Presidencia de la República. 2016. *Acuerdo Final para la Terminación del Conflicto y la Construcción de una Paz Estable y Duradera. Final Agreement for the End of the Conflict and the Construction for a Stable and Lasting Peace.* Oficina del Alto Comisionado para la Paz, Bogotá, Colombia. Accessed on 23 February 2021. https://www.jep.gov.co/Documents/Acuerdo%20Final/Acuerdo%20Final %20Firmado.pdf

Segura, Jaime Andrés and Ramírez, Diana. 2013. "Comportamiento del fenómeno de desaparición, Colombia". "Behavior of the disappearance phenomenon, Colombia." *Forensis 13.* Instituto Nacional de Medicina Legal y Ciencias Forenses. Bogotá, Colombia: Imprenta Nacional.

Rettberg, Angelika. 2015. "Victims of the Colombian Armed Conflict: The Birth of a Political Actor." In *Colombia's Political Economy at the Outset of the Twenty-First Century: From Uribe to Santos and Beyond*, edited by B. M. Bagley and J. D. Rosen, 111–39. Lanham, MD: Lexington Books.

Richani, Nazih. 2000. "The Paramilitary Connection." *NACLA Report on the Americas* 34, no. 2: 38–48. https://doi.org/10.1080/10714839.2000.11722632

Ríos Sierra, Jeronimo. 2017. *Breve historia del conflicto armado en Colombia. Brief history of the armed conflict in Colombia.* Madrid: Los Libros de la Catarata.

Rosa, Fidel. 2003. "Los grupos paramilitares en Colombia". "Paramilitary groups in Colombia." *Boletín de Información* 279: 15–50.

Rutas del Conflicto. n.d. www.rutasdelconflicto.com Routes of Conflict. Date of last access February 23, 2021.

Sánchez-Ángel, Ricardo. 2008. "Gaitanismo y nueve de abril." Gaitanism and the 9th of April. *Papel Politico* 13, no. 1: 13–52.

Sánchez-Moreno, Maria McFarland. 2018. *There Are No Dead Here: A Story of Murder and Denial in Colombia*. New York: Nation Books.

Sanford, Victoria. 2003. "Learning to Kill by Proxy: Colombian Paramilitaries and the Legacy of Central American Death Squads, Contras, and Civil Patrols." *Social Justice* 30, no. 3 (93): 63–81. http://www.jstor.org/stable/29768209

Scheper-Hughes, Nancy and Philippe Bourgois. 2004. "Introduction: Making sense of violence". In *Violence in War and Peace, An Anthology*, edited by Nancy Scheper-Hughes and Philippe Bourgois, 1–27. Oxford: Blackwell.

Semma Tamayo, Alexandra. 2020. "Missing Persons and Unidentified Human Remains: The Perspective from Armed Conflict Victims Exhumed in Granada, Colombia." *Forensic Science International* 317: 110529. https://doi.org/10.1016/j.forsciint.2020.110529

Sharpless, Richard E. 1978. *Gaitán of Colombia: A Political Biography*. Pittsburgh, PA: University of Pittsburgh Press.

Tate, Winifred. 2000. "Repeating past mistakes: Aiding counterinsurgency in Colombia." *NACLA Report on the Americas* 34, no. 2: 16–9. https://doi.org/10 .1080/10714839.2000.11722625

———. 2007. *Counting the Dead: The Culture and Politics of Human Rights Activism in Colombia*. Berkeley and Los Angeles: University of California Press.

———. 2016. "Chronicle of a Peace Foretold." *NACLA Report on the Americas* 48 no. 1: 18–21. https://doi.org/10.1080/10714839.2016.1170292

Taussig, Michael. 2004. "Talking terror." In *Violence in War and Peace: An Anthology*, edited by Nancy Scheper-Hughes and Philippe Bourgois, 171–4. Malden, MA: Blackwell Publishing.

Uribe, María Victoria. 1990. "*Matar, rematar, y contramatar: Las masacres de la violencia en el Tolima, 1948–1964*". "Killing, rekilling, and counterkilling: The massacres of the violence in Tolima, 1948–1964." Vol. 159–160. Bogotá: CINEP.

Vargas Meza, Ricardo. 1998. "A military-paramilitary alliance besieges Colombia." *NACLA Report on the Americas* 32, no. 3: 25–43. https://doi.org/10.1080 /10714839.1998.11722737

Vivas Díaz, Jairo and Claudia Vega Urueña. 2020. "The Colombian experience in forensic human identification." In *Forensic Science and Humanitarian Action: Interacting with the Dead and the Living,* edited by Roberto C. Parra, Sara C. Zapico, and Douglas H. Ubelaker, 693–702. John Wiley & Sons.

Winograd, Miguel. 2017. "In search of peace amidst a history of violence in Colombia's Jardines de Sucumbíos, years of violence and state neglect generate both hope and skepticism about peace." *NACLA Report on the Americas* 49, no. 1: 95–101. https://doi.org/10.1080/10714839.2017.1298255

World Wildlife Fund. 2017. "A look at the natural world of Colombia." *World Wildlife Magazine*, Winter. https://www.worldwildlife.org/magazine/issues/winter -2017/articles/a-look-at-the-natural-world-of-colombia

Chapter 4

Devaluing the Dead

The Role of Stigma in Medicolegal Death Investigations of Long-Term Missing and Unidentified Persons in the United States

Cate E. Bird and Jason D. P. Bird

INTRODUCTION

In the United States, the problem of long-term missing and unidentified persons has been described as a "Silent Mass Disaster" (Ritter 2007)[1]. Each year in the United States, over 600,000 individuals go missing and over 4,400 unidentified bodies are recovered; while many of these cases are resolved, tens of thousands of people remain missing or unidentified for more than a year (NamUs n.d.). As time progresses and active cases become cold, the likelihood of resolving them diminishes. Establishing the identity of unknown decedents may serve several overlapping and related purposes, such as fulfilling legal obligations outlined in medicolegal statutes, tracking vital statistics, addressing issues related to wills/inheritance, and ensuring public health/safety. Identification also serves *humanitarian functions* in both international (Cordner and Tidball-Binz 2017) and domestic contexts (Goad 2020), by protecting the dignity of the dead and clarifying the fate of the missing for their families.

Investigation of missing and unidentified persons can be problematic for any number of reasons related to systemic hindrances, such as lack of capacity (e.g., resources, trained personnel, analyses, expertise, time), lack of will, and/or fragmentation of databases. The differential treatment of missing and unidentified person cases can disproportionately affect socially disadvantaged populations and lead to inequitable rates of personal identification, a phenomenon we refer to as *identification disparities*. One issue that has been understudied is the role that *stigma* can play during the investigation process.

Donald Black (1976) posited in *The Behavior of Law* that there is considerable variation in how the criminal justice system operates across time, location, and population, arguing that what is defined as a crime, which investigations are undertaken, and who is surveilled or protected is influenced by deeply embedded structural biases that disenfranchise vulnerable groups in society. He contends that this variation is related to discretion afforded to law enforcement agents during investigations, where decisions, interpretations, and conclusions may be influenced by the social characteristics of victims/perpetrators and location of crimes. Today, this framework remains robust and may help shed light on medicolegal death investigations in the United States, where vulnerable groups (e.g., chronically homeless, migrants, sex workers, among others) are disproportionately represented among long-term missing and unidentified person cases (Goad 2020; Kimmerle, Falsetti, and Ross 2010). In death, these individuals may continue to experience identification disparities in the medicolegal system due, in part, to lower socioeconomic/societal/legal statuses and lack of cohesive group mobilization for advocacy.

This chapter evaluates the process of stigmatization, which includes devaluing and dehumanizing non-normative individuals or groups, in the context of long-term missing and unidentified persons. We illustrate various examples of pejorative language in written descriptions from medicolegal cold case reports used to describe decedents from particular groups. Focusing on language surrounding immigration in the United States, we consider how *stigma* affects the construction of migrants in death as "deviant" and contributes to the process of marginalization in death. We propose an equity-based approach for missing and unidentified persons to address identification disparities, which includes acknowledging biases, advocating for a better understanding of forensic casework, developing community-based partnerships, practicing empathy, and prioritizing humanitarianism.

THE PROCESS OF STIGMA

Social stigma describes a process by which certain individuals, groups, or communities are devalued in society, which can potentially lead to dehumanization and/or marginalization (figure 4.1). *Stigma* is defined as discrediting attributes, characteristics, or behaviors that are viewed as incongruent with those considered to be "normative." Goffman's (1963) groundbreaking research argued that stigma manifests as three primary types: 1) abominations of the body, such as those related to disability and disease; 2) blemishes of individual character related to the engagement in specific types of non-normative activities (e.g., homosexuality, prostitution, unemployment,

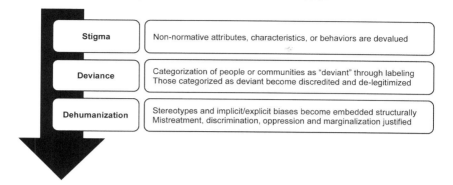

Figure 4.1   Process of stigma, deviance, and dehumanization. Credit: Cate and Jason Bird.

addiction); and 3) stigmas associated with group affiliations, such as those that deviate from normative ethnicity, race, nationality, or religion. During this process, attributes or characteristics perceived as normative are assigned positive value while non-normative attributes are marked as stigmas and constructed as negative (Bos et al. 2013).

Affiliation with a stigmatized attribute, characteristic, or behavior de-legitimizes the individual or community, signifying them as a threat to society or desired social norms (Goffman 1963; Elliott et al. 1982). In other words, those individuals associated with stigmatizing attributes are at risk of being labeled as "deviant." Therefore, the public management or control over the individual's stigma is critical to the overall impact that stigma has on their relationships and access to societal resources and opportunities.

DEVIANCE

The concept of *deviance* refers to a violation of an accepted and valued norm, belief, and/or behavior (Goffman 1963; Becker 1963). More specifically, deviance can be conceptualized as a process by which a stigmatized attribute, characteristic, or behavior (i.e., one that has been identified as non-normal, illegitimate, and discrediting) becomes labeled as problematic (i.e., deviant), which can result in social sanctioning. This social sanctioning can be informal (i.e., being denied access to social resources and/or opportunities) or formal (i.e., fines, legal restrictions, and incarceration) for violations constructed as illegal (Anderson, Chiricos, and Waldo 1977). It is important to note that in this conceptualization, not all violations of a social norm are considered "deviant"—a violation might be seen as eccentric, unusual, unconventional, or "different" but not "bad" or negative (Becker

1963; Jensen 2011; Best 2011). Stebbins (2011) refers to this as *tolerable* or *acceptable deviance*.

Constructions of deviance are dynamic and may change over time and vary across cultures, communities, and generations, allowing a "deviant" and previously socially sanctioned attribute or behavior to become more accepted as positive or neutral over time. Conversely, previously perceived excepted norms (e.g., racial segregation) may also become constructed as deviant (Bryant 2011; Best 2011). Constructions of deviance are *subjective* and embedded in the public sphere as a part of a shared social and cultural understanding of the world. Furthermore, constructions of deviance are entrenched in structural stigma, whereby shared meanings of "non-normative" attributes, characteristics, or behaviors are replicated, perpetuated, and/or amplified through social institutions such as in families, schools, and media (Best 2011; Bryant 2011; Jensen 2011; Bos et al. 2013). These meanings become embedded in individuals' ideological frameworks or understandings about how the world is organized (Day 2008). In this way, constructions of deviance reflect underlying societal values and fractures in the consensus on these values, exposing competing perceptions of right versus wrong (Best 2011).

Deviance works as a mechanism of social control at multiple levels. On one hand, categorizations of deviance have been justified as reinforcing *social solidarity* by creating predictable social expectations that help smooth and facilitate social interactions and relationships (Best 2011; Jensen 2011). On the other hand, however, constructions of deviance can be used to maintain the *status quo*, keeping power and position consolidated among societal elites and protecting elitist interests (Best 2011; Conyers 2011). For example, Black Codes, which were developed in southern states after the Civil War and the passage of the Thirteenth Amendment, included vagrancy laws that specifically targeted Black men, ensuring their re-enslavement (i.e., through imprisonment) as a labor force for White, southern landowners (Alexander 2012). More contemporarily, the resistance of companies to raise the minimum wage and the fact that raises to the federal minimum wage must occur through congressional action as opposed to regular, automatic increases tied to inflation, denies low-wage laborers economic self-sufficiency or accessible pathways out of poverty and maintains a dependent and cheap workforce (Ruan 2017).

Finally, constructions of deviance serve as mechanisms for maintaining social, cultural, and structural privilege, which influence how groups compete for status, resources, and opportunities. These mechanisms, therefore, benefit and maintain the interests of dominant groups (e.g., White, male, heterosexual, Christian, U.S. citizens) and decrease perceived challenges to the privileges and resources controlled by these groups. In this sense, constructions of deviance maintain social stratification (e.g., racial, class, gender, sexuality, ability, age) that requires members of society to conform to the expected norms, if they can, and makes examples of those who will not, or cannot, conform through social and legal sanction and marginalization (see Merton's Strain Theory) (Best 2011; Heitzeg 2011; Jensen 2011). In other words, the threat of being categorized as deviant serves as a *deterrent* to keep people from engaging in stigmatized behaviors or exhibiting stigmatized attributes/ characteristics while *constraining* and *isolating* those people or groups who will not, or cannot, assimilate to normative expectations (Best 2011; Jensen 2011). These sanctions become levied at multiple levels, from family abandonment to exclusion from social resources to imprisonment.

The process by which an individual becomes categorized as deviant is multi-faceted (Becker 1963). Those who wield societal control and power (i.e., the privileged) construct both the normative expectations and the categories of deviance as they relate to those expectations. According to Merton's Strain Theory, those normative expectations, as a part of our social structure, put strain on individuals to conform (Merton 1938). Individuals who cannot conform to the expectations, and/or whose stigmatized attributes are public, are thereby labeled as deviant and categorized with others who share that label (see Labeling Theory) (Becker 1963; Best 2011; Heitzeg 2011; Goffman 1963; Merton 1938). In other words, the engagement in a non-normative or deviant behavior (e.g., drug use) can result in the association of the individual with a deviant identity (e.g., drug user). In this way, deviant behaviors are separate yet interconnected to deviant identities or labels.

In the eyes of the observer, the label then associates the individual or group with a cognitive representation of the stigmatized attribute or characteristic, which in turn can trigger negative reactions or actions toward that individual and/or group (Bos et al. 2013). Both the construction of categories of deviance and the process of labeling is stratified and hierarchical: vulnerable groups nearly always fit into a category of *difference* as opposed to "normal," while the privileged almost never do because they control the construction of what constitutes "normal" (Becker 1963; Best 2011; Heitzeg 2011; Goffman 1963).

An intersectional lens, which examines social positionality across multiple social dimensions (e.g., gender, race, ethnicity, sexuality, socioeconomic class, ability, nationality), helps to conceptualize how this process of categorization and labeling play out differently across and within groups and why the process results in differential, unequal and/or discriminatory treatment (Best 2011; Crenshaw 1991; Heitzeg 2011). Individuals possess attributes and characteristics (i.e., identities) across these multiple dimensions. For example, an individual embodies a gender, race and/or ethnicity, a socioeconomic class, and sexuality. Some of these identities are more privileged in society; others are more devalued. An intersectional lens illuminates how these different identities intersect at the micro-level (i.e., within an individual or small group) to create interconnected systems of oppression or privilege depending on one's positionality experienced by an individual at the macro-level. For example, an individual may face privilege because of their wealth; however, this privilege may be decreased or nullified because of racial, gender, or sexual discrimination (Crenshaw 1991).

This social positionality then shapes whether and how an individual or group becomes labeled and classified as deviant. For example, "drug user" is a category of deviance; however, race and socioeconomic privilege shapes the labeling process so that more vulnerable members of society (i.e., people of color, poorer people) are disproportionately labeled as "deviant" (i.e., fitting into the category of deviance) than more privileged members of society. These are primary reasons why racial minorities and the poor are disproportionately engaged in the criminal justice system (i.e., more often labeled as criminal) while White and wealthier individuals are more likely to engage in mental health or substance use treatment programs and thereby become labeled as "ill" (Heitzeg 2011). This process has played out differently in responses to drug-use "epidemics" in the United States. The crack-cocaine "epidemic" in the 1980s, which was constructed as a primarily inner-city, Black phenomenon, resulted in the War on Drugs that emphasized the moral failings of the user and strict prison sentences for even minor possession. This response stands in stark contrast with the opioid "epidemic," which has been constructed as a primarily White, middle-class phenomenon, with an emphasis on empathy, the victimhood of the user, and the de-stigmatization of treatment. In both of these cases, race and socioeconomic conditions shaped public perceptions of the epidemics that supported the different political responses to the health crises (Netherland and Hansen 2017).

Language is key to the process of categorization and labeling. Language represents an important mechanism through which social relationships are maintained and underlie the development of ideological frameworks, which are value-based assumptions regarding how the world works. These frameworks include commonly held beliefs about what constitutes right or wrong behavior and help shape our biases and stereotypes (Day 2008). Through language we create meaning and build consensus toward shared conceptions or frameworks for interpreting the world around us (Best 2011).

Language is both social and political and thus it exists as contested space. The perception of language as merely reflecting and responding to a natural, neutral reality helps hide the ways in which mechanisms of power and privilege operate through language to codify particular social values, norms, and expectations. This process of legitimizing meaning through language helps to naturalize certain biases as truth. It also hides the influences of power and privilege on the process of meaning-making and the ways in which the process is used to preserve the consolidation of power in particular groups in society (Ehrlich and King 1994).

A raciolinguistic perspective is useful for further examining these social and political underpinnings. Flores and Rosa (2015) argue that dominant (e.g., White, male, heterosexual) norms, expectations, and perspectives are privileged in the process of standardizing language (i.e., establishing "appropriate" usage and meaning), which is then used as a measure of legitimacy (i.e., those who adhere to the standards are seen as worthy, those who do not or cannot as unworthy). What constitutes legitimate language is not only influenced by historical bias that is used to consistently marginalize members of non-dominant groups, but also by the use of socially acceptable language, based on dominant language and grammatical conventions, that becomes associated with legitimacy. Therefore, by controlling what constitutes "appropriate" language, certain populations become constructed as more worthy and deserving of societal resources and opportunities while others are labeled as problematic and unworthy of societal investment (Rosa and Flores 2017; Flores and Rosa 2015). This construction shifts responsibility for hardship, emphasizing an individual's poor fit with normative expectations while obscuring the structural constraints and bias that serve to marginalize and disconnect the de-legitimized groups (Merton 1938).

While this process of legitimization requires a degree of agreement, both on the meaning and usage of language (Best 2011), unanimous consensus is neither required nor often achieved, especially when concerning contested constructions of deviance. However, agreement must be broad enough that its common meaning is largely understood, and its usage is accepted as appropriate, or at the very least tolerated. The acceptance or tolerance serves to legitimize language's meaning, including any bias, assumptions, or stereotypes the language implies. It also helps to justify actions taken based on how the language categorizes an individual (i.e., referring to people as criminals justifies imprisoning them). For example, the classification of *homosexuality* as a mental disorder in the first *Diagnostic and Statistical Manual of Mental Disorders* (*DSM*) in 1952 justified the use of involuntary institutionalization as a means of protecting the public from corruption and re-alignment therapy (APA n.d.). These constructions can have long-term negative effects. For example, while the American Psychiatric Association (APA) removed *homosexuality* from the DSM in 1973 (APA n.d.), homosexuality remained a *criminal offense* throughout much of the United States during the twentieth century and was used to justify arrests and imprisonment. Sodomy laws, which have been disproportionately imposed against gay men, were only ruled unconstitutional by the U.S. Supreme Court in 2003 through the *Lawrence et al. v. Texas* ruling (Kennedy and the U.S. Supreme Court 2003).

Language is key not only for describing categories of difference and deviance, but also for *how* "deviants" become labeled (Best 2011). Labels allow us to engage cognitive shortcuts when making determinations about which categories an individual person fits (Markowitz and Slovic 2020). In other words, labels provide a way to circumvent cognitively intensive processes of interpersonal engagement and allow for rapid determinations about another person's position in society, status, and worth. Unfortunately, the shortened cognitive process triggered by a label relies on the positive and negative values embedded in the label, and relies on both conscious and unconscious stereotypes, assumptions, and biases embedded in the constructed meaning of the label and its association with a particular category.

DEHUMANIZATION

In many ways, this process of devaluation is, ultimately, a process of *dehumanization*, which has serious consequences on the treatment of, and suffering experienced by, stigmatized individuals and groups. Dehumanization manifests within both interpersonal and intergroup contexts and goes beyond violence or direct conflict; it is reflected in the relationships people have with each other and in the ways people engage gatekeeping mechanisms to deny the devalued access to resources in society (Bandura, Underwood, and Fromson 1975; Haslam 2006; Esmeir 2006; Markowitz and Slovic 2020).

Underlying the construction of dehumanization is the belief supported by dominant values and norms, that a person and/or group is less worthy, that there is a hierarchy of worth and a line under which an individual or group becomes not only unworthy but worthless. In other words, they become constructed as having no worth to society, and as such, a danger to that society. In this sense, the constructions of worthlessness generate hostility toward the group. Marginalization and a disinvestment of societal resources are seen as justified and a legitimate consequence for being worthless (Haslam 2006).

Language and labeling are critical to this process of dehumanization. The language used helps to shape perceptions, stimulate hostility, and propagate negative beliefs about the group. Language can be used to explicitly *deny membership amongst humans* by comparing individuals to other species (e.g., referring to people as apes, monkeys, dogs, pigs, parasites, cockroaches, or vermin). Language can be used to *infantilize* individuals, constructing a person or group as naïve, childlike or childish, and/or bereft of mature cognitive capacities and therefore incapable of agency, freedom of choice, or equal treatment, such as when adult women are referred to as "girls." Language can also be used to *objectify* members of a group. This process of objectification constructs people as existing merely for, or against, the interests of others. In other words, the person or group becomes abstracted as a representation of a category, as opposed to being seen as fully autonomous, in such a way as to bring their behavior under control of another group and/or into alignment with expected norms (Haslam 2006). This has often been observed in the ways that women in positions of power are referred to as being "bossy," "aggressive," or "cold" for exhibiting behavior that is unremarkable, or positive, when exhibited by men.

Ultimately, an objective of dehumanization and dehumanizing language is to deny members of the group "moral consideration" to the extent that members are seen as unworthy of equal treatment or equal consideration, which can then be used to justify or legitimize that unequal treatment (Haslam 2006). Assumptions regarding the "deservingness" of medical care have shown to have negative health outcomes for certain marginalized populations, such as migrants (Holmes et al. 2021). This process of dehumanization decreases feelings of empathy by dominant members of society toward the dehumanized groups and undermines calls for justice, equality, and equity (e.g., referring to sex workers as "whores" or substance users as "junkies"). For example, the label "bum" to describe someone who is homeless and/or unemployed is a value-based term that elicits a construction of someone as lazy, irresponsible, and/or unmotivated. The term reflects negative societal beliefs about the homeless or unemployed and shapes the negative emotional response of both the user and the audience. In essence, the term "bum" denotes someone who is unworthy of resource allocation because they have not earned their access to those resources in society and its use in conversation justifies the negative beliefs an individual might feel toward homeless or unemployed persons, thus short-circuiting any attempt at understanding or empathy.

Therefore, this process by which social stigmas are used to construct and define categories of deviance facilitates and justifies the dehumanization of deviants as unworthy and worthless to society and creates both micro- and macro-level consequences. At the micro-level (i.e., individual or small-group level), this process can be used to justify criticism, rejection, and separation of individuals and groups from the resources and protections afforded to mainstream society (Haslam 2006). At the macro-level (i.e., structural or societal levels) the process justifies, replicates, and exacerbates oppressive and marginalizing laws and policies (Owusu-Bempah 2017).

LANGUAGE IN MEDICOLEGAL DEATH INVESTIGATIONS

Language used in the medicolegal and/or criminal justice systems can also play an integral role in reinforcing stigma and constructing deviance.

Recognition of pejorative language used to describe or label missing or unidentified persons can illuminate obvious biases. For instance, even the distinguished forensic anthropologist and human rights advocate, Clyde Snow openly used stigmatizing language to describe decedents, noting that, "each year in this county, police harvest the skeletons of a pitiful army of aging derelicts-skid-row alcoholics, bag-ladies, and the like—who live on the fringes of society and die alone of neglect and disease in out of the way places. Usually they are edentulous and are dressed in a manner suggesting that someone has fired them from a cannon through a Salvation Army Thrift Shop" (Snow 1982, 126). While there is an air of jest in this passage, the language used describes unknown persons based on perceived (i.e., stigmatized) attributes (i.e., chronically homeless, poor, substance users). Examples of similar types of pejorative language used to describe or haphazardly categorize unknown persons can be found in other sources from medicolegal death investigations.

Stigma toward missing and unidentified persons is highly visible in written texts from medicolegal reports (i.e., autopsy, investigator, anthropology, law enforcement). In these documents, investigators, broadly defined here as anyone in the medicolegal or criminal justice community who works missing or unknown person cases, may haphazardly categorize or label unknown persons according to perceived group affiliation. Numerous examples of pejorative language written in medicolegal reports have been observed during cold case reviews (1960s-2000s) of unidentified persons from several medicolegal jurisdictions in the United States (figure 4.2). While a systematic evaluation of these reports is beyond the scope of this chapter, undertaking this type of review would be an essential next step.

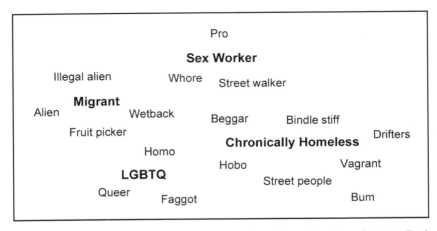

Figure 4.2   Examples of pejorative language used to refer to decedents from medicolegal reports in the United States. Credit: Cate and Jason Bird.

In case reports where unidentified persons have been negatively labeled according to perceived group affiliation, it is often included casually and with explicit bias and prejudice. Dysphemisms, particularly those that are pejorative in nature (e.g., "bum," "addict," "wetback"), reflect and continue to construct certain groups as "deviant" or less valued in society. For example, by labeling a decedent as a "wetback," investigators are devaluing that person. "Wetback" is a value-based term that elicits a construction of someone as dangerous, deceptive, interloping, intrusive, criminal, uncivilized, and even threatening to personal or national security. The use of that specific term reflects how the investigator views a decedent. At the same time, it shapes the perception of a decedent for others. In essence, the term "wetback" denotes someone who is unworthy of resource allocation because they have not earned their access to those resources in society.

In fact, immigration and the construction of immigrants represents a critical area in which stigma, constructions of deviance, and dehumanization through language play out in law, policy, and practice. Immigration is intricately entwined in the nation-building history of the United States and reflected in language used to describe the *other* in relation to the State and "citizens." Popular characterizations of non-citizens in U.S. history ebb and flow between the extremes of "victim" and "criminal" largely in response to labor supply and demand, and distinct political conditions. Further complicating the issue is that immigration and those viewed as legitimate versus illegitimate immigrants is often intertwined with race, ethnicity, religion, language, and class (Chavez 2008; Thomas 2020).

Terms used to label immigrants have a long and controversial history in the American lexicon. Analyzing immigration discourse illuminates how words and their meanings have changed over time. As some linguists have pointed out, the "euphemism treadmill" or changing of acceptable lexicon represents a framing of political discourse (Nowrasteh 2017). For example, the meaning and connotation of the term "alien" has shifted considerably during the last 200 years (Florido 2015). Codified in the *Naturalization Act of 1790*, this law defined eligibility for U.S. citizenship for "aliens" who were "free white persons" of "good character" (U.S. Congress, House 1790). While citizenship later changed to include non-Whites, criminality and questions of legality became entangled with the definition of "alien." The *Immigration and Nationality Act of 1965* re-defined "alien" as "any person not a citizen or national of the United States," but differentiated between asylum seeker, refugee, resident and non-resident, immigrant and non-immigrant, and documented and undocumented persons (U.S. Congress, House 1965).

Despite the increased nuance of this definition, there remained a hierarchy of narrative construction that categorized immigrants, based on dominant norms, into those believed to be "worthy" versus "unworthy." In 1970, the phrase "illegal alien" was viewed as a way of combating racism in the United States, as highlighted by an appeal from UCLA law students following the publication of an editorial in the Los Angeles Times in which the word "wetback" was used to describe Mexicans living and working in the United States (Hawkins 2017). The terms "alien" and "illegal alien" which were reinforced in U.S. laws, such as the *Immigration Reform and Control Act of 1986*, were perceived as improving the problematic labeling of immigration policies, such as "Operation Wetback" (U.S. Congress, Senate 1986; Hawkins 2017).

Over time, however, the word "alien" took on more negative value, becoming more pejorative. In 2015, the State of California removed the word "alien" from its labor code, as the word was viewed as disparaging to immigrants (McGreevy 2015). No doubt, in the twenty-first century, the debate over the use of the terms "alien" and "illegal" has been highly politicized and has played out contentiously in legal-political spaces, as well as in media outlets. In 2013, the Associated Press modified its stylebook to exclude phrases such as "illegal alien" or "illegal immigrant," as the term "illegal" should only be used to describe actions, not people (Colford 2013). They also rejected the term "undocumented," as people may have many documents, but not the legally required ones. Entering, residing, or working in a U.S. territory without authorization by the State (whether one agrees or disagrees with the laws) does constitute a prohibited act under federal law. But at the center of this debate is the issue of labeling people, rather than behavior: "illegal immigrant" vs. "illegal immigration." This framework largely stems from a concept advanced by political activist, Nobel Laureate, and Holocaust survivor, Elie Wiesel, who famously stated, "You who are so-called illegal aliens must know that no human being is illegal" (Gambino 2015, 6). The Associated Press is not alone in taking up the issue, and other popular news outlets have since followed suit (Hiltner 2017). Acceptable use of language related to migrants in government agencies is still in contention. According to an agency-wide email obtained and published by CNN in 2018, the U.S. Department of Justice explicitly instructed U.S. attorney offices to continue using the phrase "illegal alien" rather than "undocumented" immigrant (Kopan 2018) in response to an increase in heated rhetoric around immigration that began with the 2016 presidential election. However, under the Biden administration, new guidance was issued instructing U.S. immigration enforcement agencies to replace the phrases "illegal alien" and "assimilation" with "undocumented noncitizens" and "integration" (Rose 2021).

Today, the use of the terms "illegal" vs. "irregular" vs. "undocumented" vs. "unauthorized" in reference to immigrants frequently denotes one's political leanings or views on U.S. immigration (Demby 2013; Nelson and Davis-Wiley 2018). Still, research has demonstrated how dehumanizing language toward migrants can lead to negative emotional responses and attitudes (Utych 2018). Partly because of the value-laden ambiguity embedded in political discourse, many researchers and organizations attempt to use terminology that is currently viewed as more neutral, such as "immigrant" or "migrant" to label individuals who have engaged in the act of crossing international borders, without reference to their known or perceived legal status. Consensus-based glossaries have also been developed, such as the International Organization for Migration's (IOM) Glossary on Migration (2019), which attempt to harmonize terminology across the global stakeholder landscape and avoid dehumanizing language while recognizing that terminology is fluid and needs to be regularly updated.

Words, alone, are not the problem. Linguistic trends move in and out of fashion, and researchers exploring certain issues using acceptable terminology at one point in time, are at risk of being framed as bigots by future generations as new terms become acceptable in the American lexicon. Nonetheless, words express ideas or explicit framings. Outwardly derogatory depictions or descriptions of decedents are problematic. The use of pejorative terms or phrases accomplishes multiple tasks. They project negative stereotypes on decedents. They construct decedents as deviant and "non-normal." And they relegate decedents as "outsiders" and potentially less human. A decedent is no longer a person, but a "wetback" or a "bum" or a "whore." Language used to describe decedents reifies an investigator's, and society's, general sentiments toward them (Bandura, Underwood, and Fromson 1975).

Haphazard labeling can be problematic in medicolegal death investigations if decedents are categorized in negative terms. But purposeful, tactful, and considerate labeling may in fact help the identification of unknown persons. One unique model for assessing group affiliation of decedents was pioneered by forensic anthropologists at the Pima County Office of the Medical Examiner (PCOME). Applying a biocultural approach, the PCOME assesses several lines of data, including those related to scene context, material culture, and biological indicators to categorize decedents as "undocumented border crossers" or UBCs; this label is used to denote suspected or known migrants who share a common attribute of dying while crossing into southern Arizona (Anderson 2008; Anderson and Parks 2008; Birkby et al. 2008; Reineke and Anderson 2010; Soler et al. 2014). In this context, migrants frequently enter the southern Arizona border through irregular means along migration corridors running through Central America and Mexico. As travel is typically performed on foot through remote desert areas to avoid border enforcement, the scenes (i.e., locations) where bodies are discovered represent an important indicator in the biocultural assessment. Furthermore, migrants who die in southern Arizona are frequently discovered in possession of, or in close proximity to, material culture (i.e., personal effects) used for concealment (e.g., carpeted shoe cover, camouflage clothing) or survival (e.g., water jugs). Other culturally significant personal effects may include jewelry, religious items, foreign currency, and personal documents. Finally, biological indicators represent a meaningful indicator of group affiliation, including dental modifications, tattoos with distinct cultural significance, demographic profiles, signs of medical intervention, and non-specific indicators of physiological stress (Reineke and Soler 2013; Beatrice and Soler 2016).

This biocultural approach for assessing group affiliation for unknown persons has proven advantageous in various contexts and for several reasons. First, this approach allows investigators to account for patterns of death in at-risk or vulnerable communities which may be overlooked or undercounted if deaths are neglected at an aggregate level. Accounting for migrants who go missing or die during transit is key to understanding the scale, scope, and ubiquity of public health concerns (e.g., migrants dying of exposure) and for developing preventive mechanisms. Currently, comprehensive accounting of migrant deaths around the globe is incomplete (IOM 2014). However, because the PCOME categorizes decedents as suspected migrants, they can account for and report migrants dying within their jurisdiction even when bodies are unidentified (Humane Borders 2021; PCOME 2019).

Second, the categorization of suspected migrants also helps the PCOME cater their investigative route for identification by informing them of the relevant community partners or stakeholders, such as NGOs, consulates, and international organizations (Bird and Maiers 2017). Similar biocultural strategies may be useful for developing hypotheses of group affiliation for unidentified persons in other contexts (e.g., LGBTQ community). However, the question arises of how to strike a balance between not further marginalizing vulnerable or at-risk communities in death through the labeling process and managing their bodies in a dignified manner.

DISCUSSION

Although those in the medicolegal community strive for pure objectivity, they are never separate from the social, historical, and political forces of the structures in which they operate. A report recently published by the Independent Civilian Review on shortcomings in missing person investigations in Toronto illustrates how stigma can translate into marginalization, bias, and missed opportunities in the investigation of missing person cases (Epstein 2021). Instead of striving for pure objectivity, an approach of "mitigated objectivity," which actively recognizes that bias exists while attempting to limit it, is more realistic and practical (Clemmons and Winburn 2021; Winburn 2018). One of the commonly accepted tenets of the Western justice system is that there is equal justice before the law. But society values certain groups of people more than others; without conscious and regular reflection on the management of missing and unidentified person cases at micro- and macro-levels, implicit bias can quietly affect important decision-making processes, such as resource prioritization.

Resource Scarcity and Prioritization

Despite ranking one of the highest in the world in terms of economic prosperity (e.g., gross domestic product), resource scarcity for medicolegal death investigations in the United States remains problematic. The United States has a decentralized medicolegal system which contributes, in part, to fragmentation and inconsistent practices within the medicolegal community. A report produced by the National Academy of Sciences (NAS) illuminated variations and deficits in medical examiner and coroner (ME/C) offices related to facilities, equipment, staff, education, and training. As a consequence, the report noted "the depth, reliability, and overall quality of substantive information arising from the forensic examination of evidence available to the legal system vary substantially across the country" (2009, 6). A subsequent report by the National Science and Technology Council (NSTC) on strengthening the medicolegal death system through improvement of data systems noted similar findings, as well as noting that death investigators were "overworked and overburdened with casework" (2016, 5). Finally, a recent report by the National Institute of Justice (NIJ) regarding needs assessment of forensic laboratories and ME/C offices found that variability in resources, capabilities, and services can "result in the inequitable application of death investigations, which may have deleterious effects on the fair administration of justice" (2019, 77).

If medicolegal resources are variable across the United States, with some ME/C offices and law enforcement agencies lacking necessary resources, it is no surprise that those on the margins of society would be the first casualty in this system. From a cost-benefit perspective, ME/C offices and law enforcement agencies with limited resources must weigh expending resources on investigating missing and unidentified person cases against other competing priorities (e.g., opioid overdoses, untested sexual assault kits, homicides, handling infectious disease cases, among others).

This economic dilemma in medicolegal death investigation is not unique to missing and unidentified person cases. Speaker (2019) developed a return of investment (ROI) metric which measured the societal benefit of testing backlogged sexual assault kits when medicolegal or forensic resources were scarce at a jurisdictional level. His research found that net benefits to survivors and the public, through prevention of repeated assaults, were high in relation to resource expenditure. While future research could assess similar

ROIs for the investigation of long-term missing and unidentified person cases in the United States, any cost-benefit analyses should incorporate humanitarian-based, not just economic-driven, metrics as affected persons frequently arise from vulnerable communities who may not be viewed as "worthy" or providing a high return on investment.

The *Missing Persons and Unidentified Remains Act* of 2019 which was signed into federal law at the end of December 2020 is promising for potentially providing additional funding for long-term missing and unidentified person cases. Of course, increased funding alone cannot modify systems of inequities, but perhaps one of the greatest strengths of this new legislation is the requirement for government agencies to account for missing migrants dying along the border. However, to be effective, these developments at a federal policy level should be implemented in tandem with the willful, collaborative effort of the medicolegal community to recognize and address identification disparities.

An Equity-Based Approach

Discussions of equality versus equity have been raised in numerous fields, such as education (Cramer, Little, and Alvarez McHatton 2018) and healthcare (NAS 2017). While the definition of *equality* has developed over time, today it refers to an equal distribution of resources or treatment of people as a means to achieving fairness, promoting impartiality, providing accountability, and combating bias (Takeuchi et al. 2018). *Equity* also stresses fairness but recognizes that not all people or communities begin in the same place, so providing the same resources to all people maintains hierarchies and perpetuates privilege. An equitable approach focuses on supporting communities in achieving the same goal and understanding that different communities will likely need different resources or strategies to achieve the same goal.

An approach in forensics which values *equality* treats every missing or unidentified persons case in the exact same manner, expending the same number or type of resources/strategies for investigation. However, this approach ignores that identification inequities exist in the United States, whereby 1) certain communities are disproportionately affected by missing and unidentified person cases, 2) communities face different challenges for reporting their missing and identifying their dead, and 3) the same process of stigma that leads to the devaluing of communities in life can persist into death through the medicolegal investigation.

We contend that an equity-based approach in forensics is required to adequately address the missing and unidentified person problem in the United States. An approach which values *equity* in forensics recognizes that different communities may have different needs and that current mechanisms to resolve missing and unidentified persons may not be adequate or effective in all cases. An equity-based approach focuses on the end goal (i.e., personal identification, dignity in death, clarifying the fate of the missing for families) and caters the investigative or identification strategy according to the *needs of that community*. The first step toward pursuing an equity-based approach is *accounting* for those who are subject to identification disparities. This entails that investigators perform in-depth assessments of their casework and understand from which communities unidentified persons arise. Applying biocultural strategies, such as conscientious, non-value-laden labeling of group affiliation may be warranted and contribute to the identification process. However, it is important to recognize that any strategy that promotes labeling or categorization of the dead, particularly unidentified persons, is inherently an etic approach. Forensic investigators who hypothesize group affiliation should do so cautiously, as identities projected onto the dead 1) may not be embraced by their surviving families or communities, and 2) could potentially exacerbate disengagement of families or communities in the investigatory process due to fears of associative (or courtesy) stigma. In this way, the hypothesized group affiliation could potentially perpetuate stigma and dehumanization, and thus must be approached cautiously, taking into account the context in which categorization will be perceived (see Haug, this volume).

Embracing equity-based casework necessitates empathetic engagement, as opposed to emotional disengagement. *Empathy* refers to the ability to understand the emotional state and feelings of another person. This engagement can help to individualize and humanize a person, recognizing them as a whole and complete individual as opposed to merely an extension of their group or community. The process, therefore, can help to interrupt the use of stereotypes and cognitive shortcuts in making determinations about an individual's worthiness or importance. Through these mechanisms, we believe the medicolegal community can continue to explore the root social, political, economic, environmental, and/or structural causes that contribute to identification inequities and pursue policies that help ameliorate these inequities. Research focusing on structural vulnerabilities and harm reduction in forensic casework represents promising developments in this regard (Michael et al. 2021; Joseph 2021; Soler et al. 2020).

An equitable approach in forensics will require those in the forensic community to move out of their comfort zones and interact with affected communities in order to understand specific challenges to identification, build trust, and develop joint, community-based solutions (e.g., partnerships, prevention/protection plans, and so on). Communication and transparency are integral in this process. Forensic experts often play primary roles during investigations but do not come from the disenfranchised communities of the missing or deceased for whom they are responsible for identifying. Given this power differential, families and communities must be considered primary stakeholders and afforded agency in the investigation of missing and unidentified persons and there must be a commitment to the collective responsibility to address inequities, many of which follow marginalized communities from life into death.

CONCLUSION

Today, there is a discernible will to recognize and address structural causes of persistent inequities embedded within the sociopolitical framework of the United States, evidenced by increased discourse around racial injustice, sexual harassment, homophobia/transphobia, ableism, among others. This moment of re-evaluating how systemic inequality is woven into the fabric of institutions presents an opportunity for the medicolegal community in the United States to reflect on its own explicit, and implicit, biases. Forensic experts should not claim to be above the systems in which they are embedded (i.e., merely passive "observers of fact") but rather acknowledge their roles as active participants in perpetuating constructions of the world. Indeed, reproducibility is at the heart of scientific objectivism, and nothing seems more "scientific" than measuring bones or evaluating the number of impacts associated with blunt force trauma. However, our disciplines are situated in a society and medicolegal system that is biased; this bias is structural, replicated through our shared values, beliefs, stereotypes, relationships, and actions. No matter how dedicated the medicolegal community is to performing objective scientific analyses or investigations, we are never truly removed from the social, historical, racial, gendered, and political forces of the biased structures in which we operate. As such, every person embedded in this system is influenced by this bias. Recognizing this bias does not create it—it already exists —but it can help to mitigate its unconscious impact on our decisions, interpretations, framings, and actions.

This is not to say that we should shy away from recognizing differences as a means of identification. Indeed, the application of a biocultural approach for unidentified persons has proven beneficial in accounting for certain groups who are vulnerable to going missing, and for catering unique investigative strategies for their identification. However, it must be applied considerately and with the recognition of the implied social and political outcomes for the dead, their families, and broader communities. This chapter provides examples of how stigma and labeling reflect devaluing of certain people in death. It does not represent a systematic content analysis to evaluate its frequency in medicolegal reports. While this is a logical next step, an important consideration for any future work is that stigma may be difficult to quantify as written texts represent only one source for evaluating constructions of deviance and dehumanization. The oral or spoken components of investigations are, regrettably, lost to time.

Better scientific methodologies or more funding alone will not resolve the problem of long-term missing and unidentified persons in the United States. We need to engage communities, embrace the role of empathy, and commit to the value of equity. This shift in our ideological frameworks will ultimately help us understand how poverty, class, racism, and other structural inequalities affect identification in medicolegal settings and lead to productive changes in policy and effective practice, perhaps helping us better address this "Silent Mass Disaster."

NOTE

1. Disclaimer: The views and opinions expressed in this paper do not necessarily represent those of the authors' employers or committees on which they serve.

REFERENCES

Alexander, Michelle. 2012. *The New Jim Crow: Mass Incarceration in the Age of Colorblindness*. New York: The New Press. https://doi.org/10.4324/9781912282586.

American Psychiatric Association (APA). 2021. "DSM: History of the manual." Accessed April 13, 2021. https://www.psychiatry.org/psychiatrists/practice/dsm/history-of-the-dsm.

Anderson, Bruce E. 2008. "Identifying the dead: Methods utilized by the Pima County (Arizona) Office of the Medical Examiner for undocumented border crossers: 2001–2006." *Journal of Forensic Sciences* 53, no. 1: 8–15. https://doi.org/10.1111/j.1556-4029.2007.00609.x.

Anderson, Bruce E., and Bruce O. Parks. 2008. "Symposium on border crossing deaths: Introduction." *Journal of Forensic Sciences* 53, no. 1: 6–7. https://doi.org/10.1111/j.1556-4029.2007.00608.x.

Anderson, Linda S., Theodore G. Chiricos, and Gordon P. Waldo. 1977. "Formal and informal sanctions: A comparison of deterrent effects." *Social problems* 25, no. 1: 103–114. https://doi.org/10.2307/800471.

Bandura, Albert, Bill Underwood, and Michael E. Fromson. 1975. "Disinhibition of aggression through diffusion of responsibility and dehumanization of victims." *Journal of Research in Personality* 9, no. 4: 253–269. https://doi.org/10.1016/0092-6566(75)90001-X.

Beatrice, Jared S., and Angela Soler. 2016. "Skeletal indicators of stress: A component of the biocultural profile of undocumented migrants in southern Arizona."

Journal of Forensic Sciences 61, no. 5: 1164–1172. https://doi.org/10.1111/1556 -4029.13131.

Becker, Howard. 1963. *Outsiders: Studies in the Sociology of Deviance.* New York: The Free Press. https://doi.org/10.1093/sf/42.3.389.

Best, Joel. 2011. "Constructing deviance." In *Routledge Handbook of Deviant Behavior*, edited by Clifton D. Bryant, 17–23. New York: Routledge. https://doi .org/10.4324/9780203880548.

Bird, Cate E., and Justin Maiers. 2017. "Dialog across border states: Juggling ethical concerns of forensic scientists at the border." In *Sociopolitics of Migrant Death and Repatriation: Perspective from Forensic Science*, edited by Krista Latham and Alison O'Daniel, 157–168. New York: Springer International Publishing. https:// doi.org/10.1007/978-3-319-61866-1.

Birkby, Walter H., Todd W. Fenton, and Bruce E. Anderson. 2008. "Identifying Southwest Hispanics using nonmetric traits and the cultural profile." *Journal of Forensic Sciences* 53, no. 1: 29–33. https://doi.org/10.1111/j.1556-4029.2007 .00611.x.

Black, Donald. 1976. *The Behavior of Law.* New York: Academic Press. https://doi .org/10.2174/1874945301406010001.

Bos, Arjan E. R., John B. Pryor, Glenn D. Reeder, and Sarah E. Stutterheim. 2013. "Stigma: Advances in theory and research." *Basic and Applied Social Psychology* 35, no. 1: 1–9. https://doi.org/10.1080/01973533.2012.746147.

Bryant, Clifton. 2011. "Part I: Conceptualizing deviance." In *Routledge Handbook of Deviant Behavior*, edited by Clifton D. Bryant, 1–10. New York: Routledge. https://doi.org/10.4324/9780203880548.

Chavez, Leo. 2008. *The Latino Threat: Constructing Immigrants, Citizens, and the Nation.* California: Stanford University Press. https://doi.org/10.1080/1369183X .2010.523226.

Clemmons, Chaunesey, and Allysha P. Winburn. 2021. "The Forensic Sciences' Toxic Entanglement with the Myth of Objectivity." *Forensic Magazine.* Accessed February 22, 2021. https://www.forensicmag.com/573476-The-Forensic-Sciences -Toxic-Entanglement-with-the-Myth-of-Objectivity/.

Colford, Paul. 2013. "'Illegal immigrant' no more." *Associated Press Blog.* Accessed April 15, 2021. https://blog.ap.org/announcements/illegal-immigrant-no-more.

Conyers, Addrain. 2011. "Conflict theory." In *Routledge Handbook of Deviant Behavior*, edited by Clifton D. Bryant, 135–142. New York: Routledge. https://doi .org/10.4324/9780203880548.

Cordner, Stephen, and Morris Tidball-Binz. 2017. "Humanitarian forensic action—Its origins and future." *Forensic Science International* 279: 65–71. https://doi.org/10 .1016/j.forsciint.2017.08.011.

Cramer, Elizabeth, Mary E. Little, and Patricia Alvarez McHatton. 2018. "Equity, equality, and standardization: Expanding the conversations." *Education and Urban Society* 50, no. 5: 483–501. https://doi.org/10.1177%2F0013124517713249.

Crenshaw, Kimberlé. 1991. "Mapping the margins: Intersectionality, identity politics, and violence against women of color." *Stanford Law Review* 43, no. 6: 1241–1299. https://doi.org/10.2307/1229039.

Day, Phyllis J. 2008. *A new history of social welfare.* Boston: Pearson Education.

Demby, Gene. 2013. "Immigration debate, 'undocumented' Vs. 'illegal' is more than just semantics." *NPR.* Accessed April 15, 2021. https://www.npr.org/sections/itsallpolitics/2013/01/30/170677880/in-immigration-debate-undocumented-vs-illegal-is-more-than-just-semantics.

Ehrlich, Susan, and Ruth King. 1994. "Feminist meanings and the (de) politicization of the lexicon." *Language in Society* 23, no. 1: 59–76. https://doi.org/10.1017/S004740450001767X.

Elliott, Gregory C., Herbert L. Ziegler, Barbara M. Altman, and Deborah R. Scott. 1982. "Understanding stigma: Dimensions of deviance and coping." *Deviant Behavior* 3, no. 3: 275–300. https://doi.org/10.1080/01639625.1982.9967590.

Epstein, Gloria J. 2021. "Missing and missed: Report of the independent civilian review into missing persons investigations." Toronto Police Services Board. Accessed April 15, 2021. https://www.missingpersonsreview.ca/report-missing-and-missed.

Esmeir, Samera. 2006. "On making dehumanization possible." *PMLA/Publications of the Modern Language Association of America* 121, no. 5: 1544–1551. https://doi.org/10.1632/S0030812900099843.

Flores, Nelson, and Jonathan Rosa. 2015. "Undoing appropriateness: Raciolinguistic ideologies and language diversity in education." *Harvard Educational Review* 85, no. 2: 149–171. https://doi.org/10.17763/0017-8055.85.2.149.

Florido, Adrian. 2015. "Tracing the shifting meaning of 'alien'." *NPR.* Accessed April 15, 2021. https://www.npr.org/sections/codeswitch/2015/08/22/432774244/tracing-the-shifting-meaning-of-alien.

Gambino, Lauren. 2015. "'No human being is illegal': Linguists Argue Against Mislabeling of Immigrants." *The Guardian.* Accessed April 15, 2021. https://www.theguardian.com/us-news/2015/dec/06/illegal-immigrant-label-offensive-wrong-activists-say.

Goad, Gennifer. 2020. "Expanding humanitarian forensic action: An approach to US cold cases." *Forensic Anthropology* 3, no. 1: 50–59. https://doi.org/10.5744/fa.2020.1006.

Goffman, Erving. 1963. *Stigma: Notes on the Management of Spoiled Identity.* New York: Simon & Schuster.

Haslam, Nick. 2006. "Dehumanization: An integrative review." *Personality and Social Psychology Review* 10, no. 3: 252–264. https://doi.org/10.1207%2Fs15327957pspr1003_4.

Hawkins, Derek. 2017. "The long struggle over what to call 'undocumented immigrants' or, as Trump said in his order, 'illegal aliens'." *The Washington Post.* Accessed April 15, 2021. https://www.washingtonpost.com/news/morning-mix/wp/2017/02/09/when-trump-says-illegals-immigrant-advocates-recoil-he-would-have-been-all-right-in-1970/.

Heitzeg, Nancy. 2011. "Differentials in deviance: Race, class, gender, and age." In *Routledge Handbook of Deviant Behavior*, edited by Clifton D. Bryant, 53–60. New York: Routledge. https://doi.org/10.4324/9780203880548.

Hiltner, Stephen. 2017. "Illegal, undocumented, unauthorized: The terms of immigration reporting." *The New York Times.* Accessed April 15, 2021. https://www

.nytimes.com/2017/03/10/insider/illegal-undocumented-unauthorized-the-terms-of
-immigration-reporting.html.

Holmes, Seth M., Ernesto Castañeda, Jeremy Geeraert, Heide Castaneda, Ursula
Probst, Nina Zeldes, Sarah S. Willen, et al. 2021. "Deservingness: Migration and
health in social context." *BMJ Global Health* 6, no. Suppl 1: e005107. http://dx.doi
.org/10.1136/bmjgh-2021-005107.

Humane Borders. 2021. Arizona OpenGIS initiative for deceased migrants. Accessed
April 4, 2021. https://humaneborders.info/.

International Organization for Migration (IOM). 2014. *Fatal Journeys: Tracking
Lives Lost During Migration.* Volume I. Geneva, Switzerland: International
Organization for Migration. https://publications.iom.int/system/files/pdf/fataljour-
neys_countingtheuncounted.pdf.

———. 2019. *Glossary for migration.* Geneva, Switzerland: International
Organization for Migration. https://publications.iom.int/system/files/pdf/iml_34
_glossary.pdf.

Jensen, Gary. 2011. "Constructing deviance." In *Routledge Handbook of Deviant
Behavior,* edited by Clifton D. Bryant, 11–16. New York: Routledge. https://doi
.org/10.4324/9780203880548.

Joseph, A. Skylar. 2021. "A modern trail of tears: The missing and murdered
Indigenous women (MMIW) crisis in the US." *Journal of Forensic and Legal
Medicine* 79: 102136. https://doi.org/10.1016/j.jflm.2021.102136.

Kennedy, A. M. and Supreme Court of The United States. 2003. U.S. Reports:
Lawrence et al. v. Texas, 539 U.S. 558. https://supreme.justia.com/cases/federal
/us/539/558/.

Kimmerle, Erin H., Anthony Falsetti, and Ann H. Ross. 2010. "Immigrants, undocumented workers, runaways, transients and the homeless: Towards contextual identification among unidentified decedents." *Forensic Science Policy and Management*
1, no. 4: 178–186. https://doi.org/10.1080/19409041003636991.

Kopan, Tal. 2018. "Justice department: Use 'illegal aliens,' not 'undocumented'."
CNN. Accessed April 15, 2021. https://edition.cnn.com/2018/07/24/politics/justice
-department-illegal-aliens-undocumented.

Markowitz, D. M., and P. Slovic. 2020. Social, psychological, and demographic
characteristics of dehumanization toward immigrants. *Proceedings of the National
Academy of Sciences of the United States of America* 117, no. 17: 9260–9269.
https://doi.org/10.1073/pnas.1921790117.

McGreevy, Patrick. 2015. "Gov. Brown doesn't want California to use this word
for immigrants." *Los Angeles Times.* Accessed April 15, 2021. https://www.lat-
imes.com/local/political/la-me-pc-gov-jerry-brown-signs-bills-to-help-immigrants
-20150810-story.html.

Merton, Robert K. 1938. "Social structure and anomie." *American Sociological
Review* 3, no. 5: 672–682. https://doi.org/10.2307/2084686.

Michael, Amy, Mariyam I. Isa, Lee Redgrave, and Anthony Redgrave. 2021.
"Structural vulnerability in transgender and non-binary decedent populations:
Analytical considerations and harm-reduction strategies." *Proceedings of the 73rd
Annual Scientific Meeting of the American Academy of Forensic Sciences,* virtual.

Missing Persons and Unidentified Remains Act of 2019. 2020. Public Law 116-277. *U.S. Statutes at Large* 166: 2174.

NamUs. 2021. "The Nation's Silent Mass Disaster." Accessed April 13, 2021. https://www.namus.gov/About.

National Academy of Sciences (NAS). 2009. *Strengthening forensic science in the United States: A path forward.* Washington, DC: The National Academies Press. Accessed April 15, 2021. https://www.ojp.gov/pdffiles1/nij/grants/228091.pdf.

National Academy of Sciences (NAS). 2017. *Communities in action: Pathways to health equity.* Washington, DC: The National Academies Press. https://doi.org/10.17226/24624.

National Institute of Justice (NIJ). 2019. *Report to congress: Needs assessment of forensic laboratories and medical examiner/coroner offices.* US Department of Justice Office of Justice Programs, Washington, DC. Accessed April 15, 2021. https://nij.ojp.gov/library/publications/report-congress-needs-assessment-forensic-laboratories-and-medical.

National Science and Technology Council (NSTC). 2016. Strengthening the Medicolegal Death Investigation System: Improving Data Systems. Accessed April 15, 2021. https://www.ojp.gov/pdffiles1/NIJ/251423.pdf.

Naturalization Act of 1790. 1790. Public Law 1-3. *U.S. Statutes at Large* 3: 103–4.

Nelson, Robin Lee, and Patricia Davis-Wiley. 2018. "Illegal or undocumented: An analysis of immigrant terminology in contemporary American media." *International Journal of Social Science Studies* 6: 8–15. https://doi.org/10.11114/ijsss.v6i6.3254.

Netherland, Julie, and Helena Hansen. 2017. "White opioids: Pharmaceutical race and the war on drugs that wasn't." *BioSocieties* 12, no. 2: 217–38. https://doi.org/10.1057/biosoc.2015.46.

Nowrasteh, Alex. 2017. "You say 'illegal alien.' I say 'undocumented immigrant.' who's right?" *Newsweek.* Accessed April 15, 2021. https://www.newsweek.com/you-say-illegal-alien-i-say-undocumented-immigrant-whos-right-750644.

Owusu-Bempah, Akwasi. 2017. "Race and policing in historical context: Dehumanization and the policing of Black people in the 21st century." *Theoretical Criminology* 21, no. 1: 23–34. https://doi.org/10.1177%2F1362480616677493.

Pima County Office of the Medical Examiner (PCOME). 2019. Annual Report. Tucson, Arizona: PCOME. https://webcms.pima.gov/UserFiles/Servers/Server_6/File/Government/Medical%20Examiner/Resources/Annual-Report-2019.pdf.

Reineke, Robin C., and Bruce E. Anderson. 2010. "Sociocultural factors in the identification of undocumented migrants." *Proceedings of the 62nd Annual Scientific Meeting of the American Academy of Forensic Sciences*, Seattle, WA.

Reineke, Robin C., and Angela Soler. 2013. "Dental Ornamentation among Southwest Hispanic Border Crossers at the Pima County Office of the Medical Examiner." *Proceedings of the 65th Annual Scientific Meeting of the American Academy of Forensic Sciences*, Washington, DC.

Ritter, Nancy. 2007. "Missing persons and unidentified remains: The nation's silent mass disaster." National Institute of Justice (NIJ) Office of Justice Programs.

Accessed April 15, 2021. https://nij.ojp.gov/topics/articles/missing-persons-and-unidentified-remains-nations-silent-mass-disaster.

Rosa, Jonathan, and Nelson Flores. 2017. "Unsettling race and language: Toward a raciolinguistic perspective." *Language in Society* 46, no. 5: 621–47. https://doi.org/10.1017/S0047404517000562.

Rose, Joel. 2021. "Immigration agencies ordered not to use term 'illegal alien' under new Biden policy." *NPR*. Accessed April 15, 2021. https://www.npr.org/2021/04/19/988789487/immigration-agencies-ordered-not-to-use-term-illegal-alien-under-new-biden-polic?t=1643153622250.

Ruan, Nantiya. 2017. "Corporate masters & low-wage servants: The social control of workers in poverty." *Wash. & Lee J. Civ. Rts. & Soc. Just.* 24: 103–68. https://scholarlycommons.law.wlu.edu/crsj/vol24/iss1/6.

Snow, Clyde C. 1982. "Forensic anthropology." *Annual Review of Anthropology* 11: 97–131. https://doi.org/10.1146/annurev.an.11.100182.000525.

Soler, Angela, Robin C. Reineke, Jared S. Beatrice, and Bruce E. Anderson. 2014. "An integrated approach to the identification of human remains: The biocultural profile of undocumented migrants." *Proceedings of the 66th Annual Scientific Meeting of the American Academy of Forensic Sciences*, Seattle, WA.

Soler, Angela, Jared S. Beatrice, Robin C. Reineke, and Daniel L. Martínez. 2020. "Beyond identification: Structural vulnerability and the investigation of migrant deaths." *Proceedings of the 72nd Annual Scientific Meeting of the American Academy of Forensic Sciences,* Anaheim, CA.

Speaker, Paul J. 2019. "The jurisdictional return on investment from processing the backlog of untested sexual assault kits." *Forensic Science International: Synergy* 1: 18–23. https://doi.org/10.1016/j.fsisyn.2019.02.055.

Stebbins, Robert. 2011. "Tolerable, acceptable, and positive deviance." In *Routledge Handbook of Deviant Behavior*, edited by Clifton D. Bryant, 24–30. New York: Routledge. https://doi.org/10.4324/9780203880548.

Takeuchi, David T., Tiziana C. Dearing, Melissa W. Bartholomew, and Ruth G. McRoy. 2018. "Equality and equity: Expanding opportunities to remedy disadvantage." *Generations* 42, no. 2: 13–9. https://www.jstor.org/stable/26556355.

Thomas, Nina. 2020. "Immigration: The "illegal alien" problem." *International Journal of Group Psychotherapy* 70, no. 2: 270–92. https://doi.org/10.1080/00207284.2020.1718504.

U.S. Congress, House. 1790. A bill to establish an uniform rule of naturalization, and enable aliens to hold lands under certain conditions (Naturalization Act). 1st Congress, Pub. Law. 1-3. Accessed April 15, 2021. https://govtrackus.s3.amazonaws.com/legislink/pdf/stat/1/STATUTE-1-Pg27.pdf.

U.S. Congress, House. 1965. Immigration and Nationality Act of 1965. 89th Congress, H.R. 2580; Pub.L. 89–236, 79 Stat. 911. Accessed April 15, 2021. https://www.govtrack.us/congress/bills/89/hr2580/text.

U.S. Congress, Senate. 1986. Immigration Reform and Control Act (IRCA). 99th Congress, S. 1200; Pub.L. 99–603, 100 Stat. 3445. Accessed April 15, 2021. https://www.govtrack.us/congress/bills/99/s1200/summary.

Utych, Stephen M. 2018. "How dehumanization influences attitudes toward immigrants." *Political Research Quarterly* 71, no. 2: 440–52. https://doi.org/10.1177%2F1065912917744897.

Winburn, Allysha Powanda. 2018. "Subjective with a capital S? Issues of objectivity in forensic anthropology." In *Forensic Anthropology: Theoretical Framework and Scientific Basis*, edited by C. Clifford Boyd, Jr. and Donna Boyd, 19–37. New Jersey: John Wiley & Sons, Ltd.

Part II

AT THE INTERSECTION

SOCIAL IDENTITIES AND
FORENSIC ANTHROPOLOGY

Chapter 5

Theorizing Social Marginalization for Forensic Anthropology

Insights from Medical Anthropology and Social Epidemiology

Allysha P. Winburn, Meredith G. Marten,
Taylor Walkup, Enrique Plasencia,
and Allison Hutson

The forensic anthropologist has just received a new case, this one originating from Flint, Michigan. They break the evidence seal on the 4-mil-plastic evidence bags holding the skeletal remains of a young child. As they position the cranium within its cushioning cork ring, inferior aspect up, the child's poor dental health becomes immediately apparent. The forensic anthropologist begins to annotate their odontogram with depictions of the many carious lesions, making note that a carbohydrate-rich diet and/or lack of access to dental care may be possible causes. Weeks later, when the case goes to peer review, the reviewer points out the cariogenic effects of some environmental toxins, and the analyst decides to send an enamel sample for isotopic testing. Results show that lead levels of the child's enamel are dangerously elevated.

The forensic anthropologist is speaking with a medicolegal death investigator. Intending to submit anonymized case data to a database, they are preparing a list of their agency's identified cases. Cross-checking the list with their case files, the forensic anthropologist realizes that many of their trauma cases are not on it. Specifically, few of the female or women homicide victims found in contexts suggestive of sex work are on the list. The anthropologist looks up from the list, "Seriously, none of our sex workers have been identified?" The death investigator frowns. "I know. Sad, right? But you know how it is...."

The forensic anthropologist is suspended on a plank of wood over a mass grave in Guatemala, pedestaling the intertwined remains of several desaparecidos. *While comprehensive analyses must wait until the remains have been mapped, photographed, bagged, labeled, transported, transferred, and cleaned, the anthropologist cannot help but notice the evidence of gunshot trauma to the decedents' occipital bones. Much of the biological and material evidence surrounding the decades-old skeletal remains has decomposed, but it appears to the excavator that the extant textiles are consistent with Indigenous clothing.*

Scenarios resembling these hypothetical vignettes characterize much of forensic anthropological casework. Each scenario is directly relevant to the contents of this chapter, which strives to unite forensic anthropological methods with broader anthropological theories to better serve decedents of marginalized social identities. Each vignette will be discussed throughout the chapter to illustrate the potential value of the theoretical approaches described herein.

We begin by acknowledging the fact that most of this chapter's authors identify as White, cisgender women. We are making knowledge claims about individual and group experiences that are outside of our own lived experiences, and we do so from positions of privilege. As such, we acknowledge that ours may not be the most appropriately situated voices to discuss issues of social marginalization. It is our hope, however, that our voices contribute in productive ways to conversations that are vital to ensuring that the problematically WEIRD (Clancy and Davis 2019) and whitewashed (Tallman and Bird 2022) discipline of forensic anthropology includes a plurality of voices in the future.

INTRODUCTION

Forensic anthropological casework more frequently involves the remains of individuals from socially marginalized than privileged groups (Bethard and DiGangi 2020; Goad 2020; Kimmerle, Falsetti, and Ross 2010; Winburn et al. 2022). Decades of research from medical anthropology and public health indicate that living with the acute and chronic stressors of social marginalization can be physically incorporated into human bodies, with detrimental *in vivo* effects in body systems including adrenal, cardiovascular, immune, neurological, and reproductive (Calvin et al. 2003; Gravlee, Dressler, and Bernard 2005; McDade 2002; MacDorman et al. 2016; Sapolsky 2004). Yet, the myriad ways in which social marginalization might impact the hard tissues of the body are incompletely understood, in terms of both their embodiment over the life course and their postmortem manifestations.

The field of forensic anthropology has recently begun to examine the potential for structural violence to be skeletally and dentally embodied (Beatrice and Soler 2016; Moore and Kim this volume; Soler and Beatrice 2018; Soler, Beatrice, and Martínez this volume). In the allied sub-discipline of medical anthropology, however, theoretical frameworks have already been developed that may contextualize a forensic anthropological understanding of social processes impacting skeletal biology. Chief among these is the *violence continuum*, which captures the "multisided character of violence" and the tangled ways in which types of violence—in both war and peacetime contexts—are experienced, enacted, and normalized (Bourgois 2004, 425). Coined by Scheper-Hughes and Bourgois (2004), the *violence continuum* analyzes how structural, everyday, symbolic, and direct political violence impact physical and mental health and well-being. Similarly, social epidemiologists often use ecosocial theory to address how population patterns of health, well-being, and disease are reflected in socially based health inequalities. The core constructs of ecosocial theory— embodiment in particular (Krieger 2001)—illuminate the mechanisms by which various forms of violence can become physiologically embodied (e.g., via the *weathering hypothesis*; Geronimus 1992) and potentially tempered by the effects of resilience and resistance (Berkman and Kawachi 2014; Krieger 2001).

In this chapter, we first provide a brief introduction to the theoretical constructs that medical anthropologists and social epidemiologists frequently use to describe these phenomena and illustrate how they may inform forensic anthropological interpretations of marginalization. We then consider specific ways in which the various forms of violence may be discernible in the hard-tissue remains of people of marginalized social identities, potentially with consequences for forensic anthropological analysis and ultimately medicolegal identification. We conclude by translating these theoretical contributions into methodological recommendations.

MEDICAL ANTHROPOLOGY AND SOCIAL EPIDEMIOLOGY: A BRIEF OVERVIEW

Medical anthropology is an expansive subfield of anthropology that studies disease, healing, and the social and cultural factors that interact with and impact health. Two primary orientations within medical anthropology—critical medical anthropology and biocultural anthropology—bring specific attention to the role of social marginalization in health, disease, and well-being. Critical medical anthropologists emphasize the political economy of health and social inequality (Singer and Baer 2018), while biocultural anthropologists generally focus their work on how sociocultural factors including racism (see Gravlee 2009) impact human biology (Hoke and Schell 2020).

Social epidemiology is a rapidly growing subdiscipline of epidemiology that examines patterns in the distribution of disease and health in relation to the broad range of "socioenvironmental exposures" individuals encounter over the course of their lives (Berkman and Kawachi 2014, 5). Similar to many biocultural medical anthropologists, social epidemiologists focus on the social determinants of health and the mechanisms through which social forces impact human biology and shape disease and suffering. Nancy Krieger is one of the most prolific theorists in this field, and as we describe below, developed ecosocial theory to frame health and disease, focusing on the process of embodiment, or "how we literally incorporate, biologically, the material and social world in which we live, from conception to death" (2001, 672).

Shared Goals and History of Medical Anthropology and Social Epidemiology

Medical anthropology and social epidemiology are both rooted in efforts to foreground the social, economic, and political forces that conspire to create disproportionately poorer health outcomes and higher mortality among marginalized peoples. These analyses reorient attention to the contributions of society for health inequities among populations, rather than frameworks that overemphasize personal responsibility and individual behavior change, dominant in the United States (Holmes 2013). For example, what forces are ultimately responsible for the premature death of the child in Flint, Michigan, referenced in our opening vignette? A faithful accounting of this child's death requires biosocial analysis, incorporating the consequences of injurious policy decisions enacted upon a majority-Black city into the official records of death investigation (see also Farmer et al. 2013).

The tension between individual and social contributions to health and disease is an outgrowth of the culturally and historically constructed analytic dualisms—mind/body and individual/society, for example—that emerged from work of seventeenth-century French philosopher René Descartes (Scheper-Hughes and Lock 1987). The broad theoretical orientation of Cartesian dualism changed medicine in dramatically effective ways, giving rise to germ theory and the exclusion of the magical and divine in understandings of sickness and health. Its legacy simultaneously contributed to the diminishment of social factors in our understanding of health. Instead, overly individualistic perceptions of health gained prominence, which Krieger and Davey Smith (2004, 94) describe as being determined by an "individual lifestyle plus faulty genes" perspective.

Before that epistemological shift, skeletal evidence formed the basis of much of the earliest work in epidemiology and anthropology. For example, in the 1820s, French physician and pioneer of social epidemiology Louis René Villermé found striking skeletal differences between economic classes, with poor populations being of shorter stature and having more skeletal deformities, as well as higher mortality (Krieger and Davey Smith 2004). Similarly, anthropologist Franz Boas noted the effects of environmental changes on the cranial forms of descendants of migrants to the United States, illustrating the biological plasticity that can occur within a single generation (Boas 1912, 1940; Gravlee, Bernard, and Leonard 2003). His findings called into question the accepted scientific ideas of race, which at the time were largely determined by head shape (Goodman, Moses, and Jones 2020).

The development of germ theory in the mid-1800s to early 1900s drove social variables to the background, as an emphasis on pathogens, rather than the broader social environment, became the focus of biomedical inquiry (Krieger and Davey Smith 2004; Packard 2016). Theories such as Social Darwinism and eugenics also gained traction, which framed poor health as a consequence of innate racial inferiority rather than social inequities. These ideas contributed to a scientific consensus at the time that naturalized social hierarchy, with White, male Westerners as the pinnacle of civilization (Blakey 2021; Dennis 1995; Watkins 2018).

Scholarly attention to the social contributions of poor health outcomes tends to ebb and flow over time, generally in accordance with large-scale socioeconomic trends and particularly amid periods of widespread immiseration. The depression of the 1930s, the social movements of the 1960s, and recent global recessions have all increased the urgency to examine how society "gets under the skin" (Krieger and Davey Smith 2004). As we describe in more detail below, medical anthropologists and social epidemiologists have been building theories for decades that address this. These conceptual approaches first required a fundamental epistemological shift that rejected the various dualisms that proliferated in the West since Descartes's day. These efforts are well underway in epidemiology and constitute much of medical anthropological work today.

RELEVANT THEORIES FROM MEDICAL ANTHROPOLOGY AND SOCIAL EPIDEMIOLOGY

The specific causes and mechanisms of human injury and death are well known to forensic anthropologists, but the larger-scale, contextual factors that undergird those causes remain less frequently examined. In the following section, we outline some of the primary theories and hypotheses framing health-related work in medical anthropology and social epidemiology today: the violence continuum, embodiment, and weathering. We begin by theorizing the violence continuum, which includes structural, everyday, symbolic, and direct political violence, all of which disproportionately affect individuals with marginalized social identities. We then describe the mechanisms by which these different forms of violence are biologically embodied.

Experiencing Marginalization: The Violence Continuum

Structural Violence

Structural violence is exerted systemically, indirectly, and often invisibly; it is, as Farmer notes, "the social machinery of oppression" (2004, 307). The concept of structural violence is rooted in 1960s liberation theology and characterized by *social inequality*, *racism*, and *sexism* (Galtung 1969; see also Farmer 2004). The concept foregrounds the political, economic, and other social structures that inhibit individuals' opportunities and potential—particularly those from marginalized groups (Galtung 1969). Structural violence highlights that these structural inequities are *violent* much in the same way a physical attack may be; a society's policies, laws, norms, and practices cause injury to bodies and premature death.

One of our opening vignettes illustrates the structural violence of policy decisions on Flint, Michigan citizens—particularly children. The state-appointed emergency manager's decision to switch the city's water source from Lake Huron to the more innately corrosive Flint River, without necessary corrosion control, eroded Flint's pipes and leached lead into the city's water supply (Hanna-Attisha et al. 2016). The consequences of this decision had dramatic health effects, with significant increases to blood lead levels of children, particularly those living in the most socioeconomically disadvantaged neighborhoods (Hanna-Attisha et al. 2016). There is no "safe" lead level for children, and when this neurotoxin is absorbed in high levels during childhood development, its detrimental impacts on neurological processes can have life-long repercussions in terms of cognition and behavior (Bellinger 2016). In our vignette, the forensic anthropologist initially posited that poor diet was a factor in the severity of the Flint child's dental disease. The subsequent isotopic analysis revealed the likely role of lead poisoning. Even if diet also played a role in the child's dental disease, their lack of access to safe drinking water proved a particularly powerful force. Applying a structural violence perspective to this case would enable the acknowledgment that societal-level, systemic factors might be more influential than individual-level parental decisions.

Some theorists have criticized the widespread use of the concept of structural violence, noting its limitations as "one catchall category liable to generate more moral heat than analytical light" (Wacquant 2004, 322). Chief among these critiques is its failure to illuminate the number of complex ways in which violence is perpetuated, normalized, and experienced. To better do so, Scheper-Hughes and Bourgois (2004) proposed a *violence continuum* including everyday violence (Scheper-Hughes 1993), symbolic violence (Bourdieu 2001), and political violence (Bourgois 2004), and structural violence. These forms of violence have synergistic qualities as they work together to fuel and perpetuate each other.

Everyday Violence

Everyday violence was initially outlined by Scheper-Hughes (1993) to illuminate the daily, routinized, and legitimated ways in which violence becomes commonplace and overlooked—a "social production of indifference" (Scheper-Hughes 1993, 268; Bourgois 2004). Through constant repetition and sheer banality, powerful systems of violence can operate in society unchecked and unchallenged. They are routine, "just the way it is." Scheper-Hughes (1993) first developed this concept to make sense of the violence exerted against women and their infants and children in a shantytown in northern Brazil. Here, infant mortality was exceedingly high—mothers in Scheper-Hughes's sample each averaged 3.5 infant deaths—and infant and child death was completely normalized (Scheper-Hughes 2013). In one example, she asked a mother in the town why the church bells ring so often. "It's nothing," the mother responded, "just another little angel gone to heaven" (268). Rather than working to address the excessive child mortality, local authorities made promises to increase the supply of free infant coffins.

Disproportionate, everyday violence against marginalized women and children can be seen in the medicolegal context in backlogs of cold cases, as illustrated in our vignette about the cases of unidentified sex workers. Women and children are much more likely than men to be victims of homicidal domestic violence (Cooper and Smith 2011), which, because it takes place in private, is often invisible to society at large (Mendenhall 2012). Victims of domestic homicide may also be less likely to be reported as missing, given that the perpetrator is a member of the family (Kimmerle, Falsetti, and Ross 2010). Our vignette highlights that women sex workers are particularly vulnerable to assault and are disproportionately the victims of homicidal violence compared with other women (Cunningham et al. 2018). Using an intersectional lens to analyze risk (Crenshaw 1991), transgender women, Black and Indigenous women, and other women of color are disproportionately victims of homicide and more likely to become cold cases (Dinno 2017;

Human Rights Campaign Foundation 2018; Lucchesi and Echo-Hawk 2018; Winburn et al. 2022).

Symbolic Violence

Symbolic violence describes the powerful processes through which inequality and oppression are made invisible, and therefore unchallenged, by members of a society. Importantly, it diminishes the blame placed on larger-scale, more powerful forces of violence and oppression (Bourgois 2004) and instead incorporates the contribution of marginalized peoples to their own oppression—the "unwitting consent of the dominated" (Bourdieu 2001, 8). For example, survivors of traumatic military repression may experience "survivor's guilt" that is characterized by either self-blaming or blaming the family or community members, rather than the perpetrators of terror (Bourgois 2004).

This type of violence somewhat builds on everyday violence in that the complicity among dominant and marginalized peoples requires the widespread normalization and internalization of social hierarchies, and the misrecognition of inequality as natural and common sense (Holmes 2013). The naturalization of hierarchy is the product of the constant reproduction, over time, of various mechanisms that reinforce these beliefs. In this case, symbolic violence is *symbolic* because it depends on a constellation of culturally relevant symbols in which perceptions of value and prestige come to be established and inhere in certain groups of people, and over time become unconscious (Bourdieu 1984).

Direct Political Violence

Structural, everyday, and symbolic violence are all more indirect forms of violence that occur to produce poor health and early death, but more direct violence and the social, political, and economic factors that underpin them are also important components to Scheper-Hughes and Bourgois's (2004) violence continuum. Direct political violence describes the targeted violence enacted by official authorities (and oppositional political forces) and includes police brutality and torture, military repression, and armed resistance (Bourgois 2004). This type of violence is often overt, but because of its entanglements with other forms of violence may also be made invisible. For example, in the United States, the historical failure to disaggregate citizen deaths by police based on race—a form of structural violence—has specifically obscured the political violence against Black Americans (Lett et al. 2020). Conversely, as critiqued by Bourgois (2003), the multiple, simultaneous forms of violence experienced *within* the ranks of the oppressed, such as the sexual assault of women by marginalized men, may be "sanitized" and minimized by anthropologists concerned with protecting informants suffering from political violence—an ultimately dehumanizing perspective that ignores the complicated lives, hierarchies, and power structures that operate within families and communities.

In one of our opening vignettes, an anthropologist excavated a mass grave containing the remains of *desaparecidos* executed by agents of the Guatemalan government during its decades-long civil conflict in the second half of the twentieth century. The excavator's observation that the decomposing textiles in the grave resemble Indigenous garments is consistent with the fact that most of the Guatemalan *desaparecidos* from rural contexts were of Indigenous descent (Snow et al. 2008). This targeting of socially marginalized individuals by government forces is an example of direct political violence (see also Bourgois 2004).

Embodying Marginalization: Embodiment Theory and the Weathering Hypothesis

The experience of living as a member of a marginalized group in a segregated or otherwise unequal society can detrimentally impact an individual's physical health and well-being (Krieger et al. 1993; Krieger 2003; Mulligan 2016; Rej et al. 2020). To use an example from our current pandemic, disproportionate numbers of Black, Indigenous, and People of Color (BIPOC) have been impacted by COVID-19, resulting from systemic lack of access to rights and resources such as economic equity, adequate nutrition, and affordable healthcare (Gravlee 2020; Krieger 2020). Yet, the process of producing racialized health disparities can be even more insidious, as daily experiences of racism and other social inequities have the potential to become physiologically incorporated. In this ecosocial process, called *embodiment*, social factors become biological, as the bodies of marginalized peoples are disproportionately affected by a range of acute and chronic stressors experienced through that marginalization (Krieger and Davey Smith 2004; Gravlee 2009; Simons et al. 2016). One potential way in which this occurs—particularly relevant to forensic anthropologists generating a biological profile—is through *weathering*, or the premature biological aging that can occur as a consequence of these cumulative effects (Geronimus 1992). In this section, we first describe structural inequity, embodiment, and the health consequences disproportionately experienced among BIPOC. Following that, we describe the weathering hypothesis in more detail.

Health Outcomes and Mechanisms of Embodiment

Structural inequity exists in segregated or otherwise oppressive societies in which socioeconomic systems are developed and maintained in order to advantage one group(s) over others. The embodiment of structural inequity has been linked with increased risks of hypertension (Gravlee, Dressler, and Bernard 2005), cardiovascular disease (Calvin et al. 2003), later-life disability (Taylor 2008), impaired immune function (McDade 2002), Type II diabetes (Smith-Morris 2008; Mendenhall 2012), and maternal and fetal mortality (MacDorman et al. 2016) in BIPOC populations. These health disparities have been observed both within and outside of the United States, and among BIPOC of varying socioeconomic positions, indicating that the experience of social marginalization, not only the experience of poverty, is the driving factor (Geronimus 2001; Gravlee, Dressler, and Bernard 2005).

Physiologically, the disproportionate detrimental impacts on the bodies and bodily systems of socially marginalized individuals are consequences of acute and chronic stress. Stress is, simply, the process by which a stimulus provokes a behavioral, emotional, psychological, and/or physiological response (Ice and James 2006). Although activation of the stress response may equally result from distinct scenarios, the majority of physical stressors require similar reactions from the body—specifically, the suppression of bodily systems that are non-vital to immediate survival and the heightening of those that are (e.g., blood pressure, heart rate, immune defenses; Sapolsky 2004; Wiley and Allen 2017). For humans, merely imagining a stressful situation can elicit a stress response, allowing more frequent opportunities to continue stress response activation (Wiley and Allen 2017). The human experience of stress is also mediated by personal, biological, and cultural factors, meaning what one individual perceives as a threat may not produce the same response in another. Individuals living with social, economic, and political marginalization experience more extreme stressors, including uncertainties surrounding job, housing, and food insecurities, as well as disproportionately violent interactions and both individual-level and systemic racism (Gravlee 2009; Sapolsky 2004, 2005; Marmot 2004).

To use an example from the United States, a safe space to be White (e.g., a coffee shop in a gentrified neighborhood) may not be a safe space to be Black. As a response to the constant psychosocial stressors inherent in *living-while-Black* (Gabbidon and Peterson 2006), Black Americans physiologically adapt via repetitive and excessive activation of the body's stress response. However, the human stress response evolved not to mitigate long-term psychosocial stressors but to allow the body to mobilize rapidly and effectively in times of acute, physical stress—a context in which it is adaptive (Wiley and Allen 2017; Sapolsky 2004). In contrast, a prolonged stress response will extensively deteriorate bodily systems, increasing individuals' risk for a range of adverse cardiovascular, digestive, and reproductive conditions, as well as their susceptibility to contagious diseases and even cognitive deterioration (Ice and James 2006; Sapolsky 2004). It is the chronicity of long-term activated stress responses that produces the long-term disruption of bodily equilibrium that has proven critically pathogenic to human health.

The Weathering Hypothesis

First proposed by Arline Geronimus (1992), the weathering hypothesis was originally conceived as a heuristic model to contextualize how the varied, lived experiences of social, economic, and political marginalization may adversely affect health throughout the life course, cumulatively producing ever-widening health differentials between social groups. The weathering hypothesis specifically examines population-level health indicators delineated by U.S. racial groups.

According to the weathering hypothesis, the health of Black Americans—especially Black women—begins to deteriorate earlier and faster than their White counterparts in early adulthood, producing pronounced, racialized health disparities by middle age (Geronimus et al. 2006; Geronimus 1992). Thus, Black Americans may undergo what can be physically and biologically traced as rapid, premature aging processes compared to White individuals of the same age. This trend was initially identified by Geronimus (1992, 1996) when analyzing the relationship between maternal age to birth outcomes for women in the United States. The prevailing model at the time assumed that high rates of Black teenage childbearing directly contributed to excess Black infant mortality rates, emphasizing personal responsibility rather than systems-level factors and relying on a monolithic, developmental concept of aging. In this paradigm, both biological and psychosocial developmental processes were falsely assumed universal stages—thus, all teen mothers were automatically "unfit" biologically and/or behaviorally to bear children, and all mothers in their twenties were mature and "low risk." Human development, however, does not follow rigid stages or steps, nor does every human age similarly. Indeed, as Geronimus (1992, 1996) revealed, neonatal mortality rates *increase* as maternal age increases for Black women, while White women experience the inverse. The weathering hypothesis has since been expanded to contexts beyond maternal and fetal mortality (e.g., Simons et al. 2016; Taylor 2008), though it is typically still examined within the context of demonstrated disparities between U.S. social races.

The biosocial weathering process even works at the molecular level. In contrast to genetic research focusing on inherited molecular variation, epigenetic research investigates how variation is created, beginning *in utero* and continuing into adulthood, in response to environmental factors—often resulting in varying genetic expressions with similar underlying genotypes

(Mulligan 2016; Entringer et al. 2011). Epigenetic research indicates that lived experiences of racism can accelerate aging at the cellular level (Carter et al. 2019) or even the chromosomal level, shortening the length of the telomeres that influence an individual's rate of aging and the onset of age-related diseases (Epel et al. 2004; Rej et al. 2020).

Mitigating Factors: Resilience and Resistance

Social, cultural, and environmental factors can also be protective, improving individual health and well-being. Social affiliation, integration, and support, in particular, are strongly linked with improved health outcomes (Berkman et al. 2000; Sapolsky 2006). For example, among children at risk for traumatic stressful events, parental responsiveness has been linked with longer telomeres, an indicator of resilience to stress (Asok et al. 2013). The cultural meaningfulness of healing practices may also show positive impacts on health and can potentially be harnessed to improve health outcomes (see Marten 2021). Further, when individuals who experience social inequity engage in acts of resistance to the oppressive social structures that serve to marginalize them, this may be cathartic and empowering (Godsay and Brodske 2018). While their agency may be constrained by the opportunities available to them, they are not powerless. Discussions of racialized and other societal health disparities must challenge the rhetoric of exploitation and victimization (Gamble 2014) to acknowledge that people have the capacity to be resilient even in the face of this oppression.

Resilience, as it is termed more generally in the social sciences, has been described as perseverance in the face of adversities and, to some degree, as a developed measure of resistance to the adverse effects of violence and stress (Panter-Brick 2014; Southwick et al. 2014). The concept of resilience can be exceedingly broad, encompassing a combination of biological, psychological, social, and cultural factors that interact and determine how an individual or group may respond to violent or stressful events (Southwick et al. 2014), or long-term exposure to chronic stressors (Panter-Brick 2014). Panter-Brick's (2014) description of resilience helpfully includes examples of biomarkers—including blood pressure, stress hormones, immune function, and gene methylation—that may inform how chronic stress and forms of systemic violence can be embodied, and further, how they may potentially be tracked. While it is difficult to imagine identifying the specific effects of resilience in the forensic anthropological context, we believe it is important to introduce the concept here, as an awareness of how bodies resist systemic violence and stress can inform interpretations of their effects on the human skeleton.

FORENSIC ANTHROPOLOGICAL EVIDENCE OF SOCIAL MARGINALIZATION: MECHANISMS AND MANIFESTATIONS

For each of the above theoretical constructs, we present hypothesized effects that may be visible in the hard tissues of the human body and associated materials. With few exceptions, these theories have not yet been applied specifically to the context of forensic anthropological analysis.

Forensic Anthropological Evidence of Structural Violence

As introduced in the opening vignette of the child from Flint, MI, structural-level inequities can have skeletal-level impacts. In this hypothetical case, the cariogenic effects of the child's lead exposure were visible in their extreme dental disease and confirmed at the elemental level through isotopic testing. Indeed, isotopic analyses have the potential to chronicle exposure to toxic elements among marginalized decedents, as lead and other harmful elements more frequently characterize the built environment of people who experience social marginalization (Hanna-Attisha et al. 2016; Richardson and Norris 2010). Lack of access to affordable dental care may also translate to periodontal differences between the hard-tissue remains of impoverished versus wealthy individuals, with the former exhibiting higher frequencies and greater severities of carious lesions, abscesses, and other dental diseases (Soler, Beatrice, and Martínez this volume). Structural inequities in food availability may also play a role in dental disease.

The characteristics of antemortem fractures (e.g., well versus poorly set; with or without evidence of surgical intervention) may also speak to a history of access to medical care, or lack thereof. The frequency, types, and locations of injuries sustained during life may also differ between socially privileged versus marginalized groups, tracking with lifestyle variables for the latter in a particular region (e.g., undertaking a particular type of labor, experiencing physical altercations; de la Cova 2012).

Above and beyond a lack of access to affordable healthcare to mitigate existing diseases, socially marginalized case decedents may have simply experienced higher disease loads (de la Cova 2011), particularly of cardiovascular disease and Type II diabetes. Cardiovascular disease can be interpreted from skeletal evidence, if calcifications indicative of atherosclerosis are present in association with the remains (Biehler-Gomez et al. 2018). Recent research has also proposed skeletal correlates for diabetes mellitus (Dupras et al. 2010).

The chronic stress of experiencing social marginalization may also result in what biological anthropologists frequently term *non-specific stress indicators.* Linear enamel hypoplasias, which can result from episodes of neonatal/maternal and childhood stress as well as congenital anomalies, result from disruptions to enamel deposition and often appear as horizontal lines, grooves, pits, or sections of missing enamel (Armelagos et al. 2009; Hillson and Bond 1997; Goodman and Rose 1990; Soler and Beatrice 2018; Beatrice and Soler 2016). Porotic lesions of the cranium (i.e., cribra orbitalia and porotic hyperostosis) can result from respiratory infections and various forms of anemia, all of which may be seen in higher frequencies in individuals lacking access to nutritive food sources and/or healthcare (Mensforth et al. 1978; O'Donnell et al. 2020; Walker et al. 2009). In non-adults, vertebral neural canal dimensions have been invoked as indicative of periods of stress or other growth disruptions (Newman and Gowland 2015). Fluctuating asymmetry in the human skull, reflective of developmental instability, has also been linked with poor nutrition or systemic stress (DeLeon 2007).

Structural violence is often invoked in studies of non-specific stress indicators, but political, symbolic, and everyday violence typically are not. It is certainly the case that structural-level factors lead to the lived experiences of social and/or economic inequity for individuals whose remains bear these indicators. However, it is also possible that the other violences—in particular, everyday violence—also play a role in normalizing these inequities. In order to untangle these various violences, case data in the form of depositional context, associated material evidence, and evidence of the location and nature of perimortem trauma would prove essential, in addition to the embodied skeletal indicators discussed above.

Finally, although it is outside the scope of embodied hard-tissue impacts, an individual's risk of becoming a forensic case in the first place is both non-random and structurally dictated. For socially marginalized individuals, chances are higher of dying of homicidal violence, using drugs that might lead to an accidental overdose, and/or dying in a location or context that would delay the recovery of their remains and increase their chances of decomposing to the point of skeletonization (e.g., while experiencing housing insecurity). The intersection of marginalization with mortality is disproportionate for members of marginalized versus privileged social groups. This means that there is a high chance that forensic anthropologists will encounter case decedents whose remains bear evidence of the lived experiences of social marginalization, highlighting the importance of understanding the intersecting violences and how they are embodied (Moore and Kim this volume).

Forensic Anthropological Evidence of Everyday Violence

The vignette in which the cases of sex workers remained unidentified presented one major ramification of everyday violence: disproportionate chances of becoming a cold case for individuals whose premature deaths are normalized. When case decedents show evidence of having died in a context of sexual violence, if they are estimated to be females and/or women, and particularly, if they are transwomen of color, this constitutes evidence of everyday violence. Recent research centering transgender and gender-nonconforming persons in forensic anthropological analysis might be productively applied in such a context (Cirillo et al. 2020; Schall, Rogers, and Deschamps-Braly 2020; Tallman, Kincer, and Plemons 2022). For these decedents, along with all individuals against whom violence has been societally normalized, frequencies of antemortem injury and importantly, rates of injury recidivism may be elevated (Prince-Buitenhuys et al. 2017); and fracture patterning may differ, perhaps reflecting different forms or frequencies of interpersonal violence (de la Cova 2012). Traditionally, everyday violence is analyzed via ethnographic evidence, so, as noted above, contextual data will be important for differentiating everyday violence from other components of the violence continuum.

While housing insecurity was mentioned above under structural violence, it may be considered largely through the lens of everyday violence. Housing insecurity has been so normalized in the United States that people without houses are often "unseen in plain sight." An individual experiencing housing insecurity might be expected to manifest some of the skeletal evidence of structural violence discussed above (e.g., periodontal disease, fracture healing indicating lack of access to medical care). They might also exhibit indicators of weathering discussed below (e.g., osteoarthritis, antemortem tooth loss). Further evidence regarding their lack of housing might be provided by the material context of their recovery, if their remains are associated with bedding, multiple items of clothing, and/or other necessities. Dying in a remote or marginal location, particularly in absence of a social network, also has associated ramifications for delayed recovery and identification.

Forensic Anthropological Evidence of Symbolic Violence

It is challenging to identify this complicated form of violence even among the living. The type of case narratives and witness statements necessary to identify the subtle, "invisible" effects of symbolic violence on a decedent are typically not available to forensic anthropologists. Further, it is difficult to see how it would be productive to point out the "unwitting consent" of a marginalized case decedent in the events leading to their own death (Bourdieu 2001, 8).

However, collaboration with cultural anthropologists working with living populations in local areas of interest may be an important way to interrogate the potential effects of symbolic violence on community health. For example, in the introductory vignette of the Guatemalan *desaparecidos*, cultural anthropologists may help describe their families' and communities' lived experiences of traumatic military oppression. Further, medical and psychological anthropologists may shed light on the ways in which embodied trauma is culturally expressed (Abramowitz 2010), as well as potential means of healing.

Forensic Anthropological Evidence of Direct Political Violence

As introduced in the vignette of the mass grave excavation, targeted violence perpetrated by governmental or oppositional forces is perhaps most relevant to contexts in which forensic anthropologists analyze victims of human rights abuses. It also overlaps and interacts with structural violence, for example when groups that are already marginalized by societal structures experience disproportionate police brutality. Direct political violence may be evidenced on human remains in terms of the type, nature, and location of perimortem trauma. In the grave-excavation vignette, the remains of the *desaparecidos* consistently bore evidence of occipital gunshot trauma, consistent with a context of execution rather than armed combat (Baraybar and Gasior 2006). Methods used to perpetrate mass killings will differ depending on cultural context and whether the perpetrators are governmental, oppositional, or members of the citizenry at large (Komar and Lathrop 2012), underscoring the importance of a fine-grained understanding of the nature of the conflict under investigation.

Material evidence and other non-biological contextual data may also inform a determination that direct political violence was a factor in a decedent's death. In the hypothetical Guatemalan example, textiles indicated the Indigenous heritage of the targeted individuals. The presence of ligatures, or archaeological evidence of body positioning indicating that they had once been present, is another example of material evidence indicating a context of execution.

Forensic Anthropological Evidence of Weathering

The premature aging identified in living people experiencing social injustice may also be discernible in skeletal remains from the same groups. If the socially marginalized body "ages faster" than expected, the typical age indicators utilized in forensic anthropological age estimation may fail to provide accurate age-at-death estimates for these individuals, instead generating estimates that are erroneously high. This may lead to methodological inability of the biological profile to accurately narrow the universe of missing persons and contribute to an identification.

In order to resolve this disconnect, the applicability of indicators such as the acetabula, fourth ribs, and pubic symphyses to estimating age within marginalized populations should be tested (*sensu* İşcan, Loth, and Wright 1987)—and the results explicitly contextualized in terms of weathering rather than attributed by default to the "heritable differences between human ancestral populations" that are often implicit in such studies (Winburn et al. 2022, 146). More general age indicators like osteoarthritis might also be observed in higher frequencies among marginalized versus more privileged individuals (Watkins 2012)—particularly those whose lives included hard physical labor. Traits like antemortem tooth loss, potentially affected by socioeconomic and healthcare inequities, may also be prematurely advanced in individuals without access to dental care, along with the mandibular morphological changes correlated with antemortem tooth loss (Parr, Passalacqua, and Skorpinski 2017).

Intergenerational weathering effects may also be visible. Prenatal and perinatal stressors, as evidenced by developmental enamel defects, have been shown to correlate with adolescent or young-adult mortality in bioarchaeological contexts (Armelagos et al. 2009). In the forensic context, instances of nutritional stress during development may also be identifiable via the analysis of dental anomalies or ratios of informative stable isotopes (Burt 2013).

Forensic Anthropological Evidence of Resilience

Per the osteological paradox (Wood et al. 1992), skeletal lesions cannot always be interpreted as straightforward evidence of health versus disease, as the weakest, sickest individuals may die before their bones show evidence of lesions, and the strongest and healthiest may survive to show extreme skeletal involvement in disease or stress processes. In the forensic context, we must also acknowledge that the presence of the above-posited indicators of marginalization could be interpreted as evidence of resistance to adversity, rather than victimization by it. The non-specific stress indicators discussed above are expressions of a person's ability and will to persevere despite considerable disadvantages. As such, it may be productive to frame any correlations between experiences of marginalization and skeletal and dental lesions as possible evidence of resilience, not victimization. Contextual data from cultural anthropologists, as described above, may also be important to generate insights into these differences.

METHODOLOGICAL RECOMMENDATIONS

A Multidisciplinary Toolkit for Identifying Marginalization

We propose that the discipline of forensic anthropology move toward developing a theoretically sound toolkit for investigating skeletal impacts of marginalization. This toolkit must be multidisciplinary, including collaboration with chemists to enable the identification of structurally influenced exposures to toxic elements and consultation with cultural and medical anthropologists familiar with the lived signatures of marginalization, who may themselves be embedded within communities experiencing its effects.

The toolkit will rely on context. Developed through epidemiological and ethnographic research, the theoretical frameworks discussed in this chapter rely on richly contextualized accounts of the experiences of social inequity. If we wish to identify the causes and kinds of violence experienced by forensic case decedents, we will need not only medicolegal information about their deaths but also sociocultural information about their lives. Going forward, we anticipate that consensually collected, anonymized CT data either from living or deceased individuals with documented life histories and diverse life experiences (Edgar and Berry 2019) will be vital to testing whether signatures of marginalization are discernable in forensic case decedents.

Rigorous recovery standards are also necessary for contextualized analyses of forensic anthropological casework. In many of the above examples, preserving contextual physical data—including atherosclerotic calcifications, textiles, ligatures, and other material evidence—could mean the difference between correct and flawed interpretations of which violence(s) are embodied and why, in addition to what the ultimate causes of morbidity and mortality may be. Finding and thoroughly documenting this evidence *in situ* is essential.

We acknowledge that years of collaborative research are necessary before markers of marginalization could be deployed in actual forensic casework. To that end, for each of our above-posited links between different types of violence and their possible manifestations in skeletal, dental, isotopic, and material cultural/contextual data, we challenge researchers to see a testable hypothesis. If future research indeed produces the anticipated toolkit for deducing forensic anthropological evidence of marginalization, we must then take a step beyond the context of research. In the spirit of Farmer and colleagues' (2013) call for a faithful accounting of the means and causes of death and poor health, where structural and systemic marginalization occurs, it must be documented officially. We envision an analytical future in which forensic anthropologists who identify traits indicating a decedent's lived experiences of social marginalization would report these findings in the work products they provide to medicolegal and law enforcement agencies. We argue that a profile indicating structural vulnerability could prove equally powerful as the traditional biological profile in narrowing searches for missing persons to include individuals with the most relevant life experiences.

Cognitive Bias Mitigation

The proposed sensitive and contextualized biosocial analyses present a problem for a forensic-science discipline currently grappling with its long-standing commitment to positivist-style objectivity in the face of mounting evidence of its susceptibility to cognitive bias (Nakhaeizadeh, Dror, and Morgan 2014; Nakhaeizadeh, Hanson, and Dozzi 2014; Nakhaeizadeh et al. 2018; Nakhaeizadeh, Dror, and Morgan 2020; Winburn 2018; Winburn and Clemmons 2021). *Cognitive bias* refers to the implicit biases that practitioners may hold about the remains under study, influenced by anything from their training, mentorship, and analytical experiences to inadvertently biasing information introduced by collaborators (e.g., medical examiner personnel using gendered pronouns or mentioning a particular trauma modality during a field recovery; Winburn 2018). Indeed, knowing contextual case data that is extraneous to the particular analyses being conducted has been shown to affect expert decision-making processes in many forensic science disciplines (e.g., Dror et al. 2021a, b; Hamnett and Dror 2020). Further, there is the potential that forensic scientists' analyses may be influenced not only by implicit (i.e., unknown/uninterrogated) biases, but also by explicit (i.e., known/overt) biases. This could potentially form another layer of structural or everyday violence if those biases translate to gendered or racialized disparities in terms of which cases are resolved and which are deprioritized (Bethard and DiGangi 2020; DiGangi and Bethard 2021).

In order to mitigate the effects of cognitive bias while allowing for analysis of embodied social marginalization, we argue for the utility of quality control protocols like blended-blind analysis and linear sequential unmasking (LSU). In blended-blind analysis, the case analyst may be blinded to non-skeletal case data, while the peer reviewer possesses information vital to understanding the social context of the decedent's life and death. In LSU, analyses are initially completed "in the blind," but case context is gradually unmasked as analyses progress (Dror et al. 2015). Both reduce case analysts' exposure to biasing data and enable them to approximate *mitigated objectivity*—a realistic form of attempted objectivity that acknowledges the theory-ladenness of anthropological data and attempts to constrain it with strong method, theory, research design, and quality control (Winburn 2018; Wylie 1992).

CONCLUSION

With this chapter, we have strived to bridge medical anthropological and social epidemiological theory and forensic anthropological method by highlighting possible mechanisms and manifestations for social inequity to become embodied within human hard-tissue remains. For each construct or framework detailed above—the ecosocial theories of embodiment and weathering and the continuum of structural, everyday, symbolic, and direct political violence—we present possible pathways for skeletal embodiment and impacts that may be discernible postmortem in bones and teeth. We also note the potential for the context provided by archaeologically sound field recoveries to complement these analyses.

We challenge our readers to treat each of our above-posited links as a hypothesis to be tested. Recent forensic anthropological research indicates the utility some of the above traits hold for differentiating between people who faced extreme social adversity and those who did not (e.g., linear enamel hypoplasia, porotic hyperostosis; Beatrice and Soler 2016). We envision the development of a holistic, biocultural forensic anthropological toolkit for the analysis and identification of such a life history, and we hope that our posited connections will inspire research forming its basis.

Some of the protocols we propose (e.g., isotopic analyses) may rarely be realistic within forensic anthropologists' financial and timeline strictures. Yet, others, including archaeological recovery protocols, bias mitigation, collaboration with medical anthropologists, and the development of a skeletal profile indicative of marginalization are imminently applicable to the context of routine forensic anthropological casework. We anticipate that all will play a role as we work toward bringing evidence of violence to light in socially marginalized casework decedents. There is much that we do not yet know about the myriad ways in which various forms of violence may affect the human skeleton, and in many cases, we may not be able to pinpoint exactly which type(s) of violence are responsible. Yet, if we do not consider the possibility that skeletal tissues can embody social inequity, we run the risk of methodological failure and, potentially, fewer identifications.

Perhaps more insidiously, if we continue to normalize the suites of traits visible in socially marginalized case decedents as *status quo*, rather than making explicit the possibility of embodied violence, we are complicit with the forces that create and perpetuate these forms of violence. In the United States, forensic anthropologists tend to think of structural violence as something that happens to "other people." We use the presence of non-specific stress indicators, for example, to inform a determination of a non-U.S. origin for Latinx decedents recovered from the region of the U.S.-Mexico border. Yet, it is possible that similar impacts may be visible in the hard tissues of people marginalized by our own societal context. We must make explicit and test the hypothesis that social inequity may be embodied among all individuals who live with social marginalization—including those born on our own soil. We must also consider that observed skeletal differences that seem to track along the lines of U.S. social races (e.g., in stature, rates or patterns of aging) may actually reflect biologized social factors, not innate hereditary differences in skeletal biology. Support for these hypotheses would be very powerful in taking down the typological and racialized approaches that have long plagued our discipline.

REFERENCES

Abramowitz, Sharon Alane. 2010. "Trauma and humanitarian translation in Liberia: The tale of open mole." *Culture, Medicine, and Psychiatry* 34, no. 2: 353–79. https://doi.org/10.1007/s11013-010-9172-0

Armelagos, George J., Alan H. Goodman, Kristin N. Harper, and Michael L. Blakey. 2009. "Enamel hypoplasia and early mortality: Bioarcheological support for the Barker hypothesis." *Evolutionary Anthropology: Issues, News, and Reviews* 18, no. 6: 261–71. https://doi.org/10.1002/evan.20239

Asok, Arun, Kristin Bernard, T. L. Roth, J. B. Rosen, and Mary Dozier. 2013. "Parental responsiveness moderates the association between early-life stress and reduced telomere length." *Development and Psychopathology* 25, no. 3: 577–85. https://doi.org/10.1017/S0954579413000011

Baraybar, José Pablo, and Marek Gasior. 2006. "Forensic anthropology and the most probable cause of death in cases of violations against International Humanitarian Law: An example from Bosnia and Herzegovina." *Journal of Forensic Sciences* 51, no. 1: 103–8. https://doi.org/10.1111/j.1556-4029.2005.00035.x

Beatrice, Jared S., and Angela Soler. 2016. "Skeletal indicators of stress: A component of the biocultural profile of undocumented migrants in southern Arizona." *Journal of Forensic Sciences* 61, no. 5: 1164–72. https://doi.org/10.1111/1556 -4029.13131

Bellinger, David C. 2016. "Lead contamination in Flint—an abject failure to protect public health." *New England Journal of Medicine* 374, no. 12: 1101–3. https://doi .org/10.1056/NEJMp1601013

Berkman, Lisa F., Thomas Glass, Ian Brissette, and Teresa E. Seeman. 2000. "From social integration to health: Durkheim in the new millennium." *Social Science & Medicine* 51, no. 6: 843–57. https://doi.org/10.1016/s0277-9536(00)00065-4

Berkman, Lisa F., and Ichirō Kawachi. 2014. "A historical framework for social epidemiology: Social determinants of population health." In *Social Epidemiology*, 2nd edition, edited by Lisa F. Berkman, Ichirō Kawachi, and M. Maria Glymour, 1–16. Oxford: Oxford University Press. https://doi.org/10.1093/med/9780195377903 .003.0001

Bethard, Jonathan D., and Elizabeth A. DiGangi. 2020. "Letter to the editor—Moving beyond a lost cause: Forensic anthropology and ancestry estimates in the United States." *Journal of Forensic Sciences* 65, no. 5: 1791–92. https://doi.org/10.1111 /1556-4029.14513

Biehler-Gomez, Lucie, Annalisa Cappella, Elisa Castoldi, Laurent Martrille, and Cristina Cattaneo. 2018. "Survival of atherosclerotic calcifications in skeletonized material: forensic and pathological implications." *Journal of Forensic Sciences* 63, no. 2: 386–94. https://doi.org/10.1111/1556-4029.13592

Blakey, Michael L. 2021. "Understanding racism in physical (biological) anthropology." *American Journal of Physical Anthropology* 175, no. 2: 316–25. https://doi.org/10.1002/ajpa.24208

Boas, Franz. 1912. "Changes in the bodily form of descendants of immigrants." *American Anthropologist* 14, no. 3: 530–62. https://doi.org/10.1525/aa.1912.14.3.02a00080

———. 1940. *Race, language, and culture.* New York: Macmillian.

Bourdieu, Pierre. 1984. *Distinction: A Social Critique of the Judgment of Taste.* Translated by Richard Nice. Routledge.

———. 2001. *Masculine Domination.* Translated by Richard Nice. Stanford: Stanford University Press.

Bourgois, Philippe. 2003. *In Search of Respect: Selling Crack in El Barrio*, 2nd edition. Cambridge University Press.

———. 2004. "The continuum of violence in war and peace: Post-Cold War lessons from El Salvador." In *Violence in War and Peace: An Anthology*, edited by Nancy Scheper-Hughes and Philippe Bourgois, 425–34. Malden: Wiley-Blackwell.

Burt, Nicole M. 2013. "Stable isotope ratio analysis of breastfeeding and weaning practices of children from medieval Fishergate House York, UK." *American Journal of Physical Anthropology* 152, no. 3: 407–16. https://doi.org/10.1002/ajpa.22370

Calvin, Rosie, Karen Winters, Sharon B. Wyatt, David R. Williams, Frances C. Henderson, and Evelyn R. Walker. 2003. "Racism and cardiovascular disease in African Americans." *The American Journal of the Medical Sciences* 325, no. 6: 315–31. https://doi.org/10.1097/00000441-200306000-00003

Carter, Sierra E., Mei Ling Ong, Ronald L. Simons, Frederick X. Gibbons, Man Kit Lei, and Steven R. H. Beach. 2019. "The effect of early discrimination on accelerated aging among African Americans." *Health Psychology* 38, no. 11: 1010–13. https://doi.org/10.1037/hea0000788

Cirillo, Laura A., J. C. Deschamps-Braly, Kyra E. Stull, Marin A. Pilloud. 2020. "Cranial feminization surgery methods and Osteological identification of post-operative individuals." In *Proceedings of the 72nd Annual Meeting of the American Academy of Forensic Sciences*, A128: 172.

Clancy, Kathryn B. H. and Jenny L. Davis. 2019. "Soylent is people, and WEIRD is white: Biological anthropology, whiteness, and the limits of the WEIRD." *Annual Review of Anthropology* 48: 169–86. https://doi.org/10.1146/annurev-anthro-102218-011133

Cooper, Alexia, and Erica L. Smith. 2011. *Homicide Trends in the United States, 1980–2008.* Bureau of Justice Statistics. https://bjs.ojp.gov/content/pub/pdf/htus8008.pdf

Crenshaw, Kimberlé W. 1991. "Mapping the margins: Intersectionality, identity politics, and violence against women of color." *Standard Law Review* 43, no. 6: 1241–99.

Cunningham, Stewart, Teela Sanders, Lucy Platt, Pippa Grenfell, and P. G. Macioti. 2018. "Sex work and occupational homicide: Analysis of a UK murder database." *Homicide Studies* 22, no. 3: 321–38. https://doi.org/10.1177%2F1088767918754306

de la Cova, Carlina. 2011. "Race, health, and disease in 19th-century-born males." *American Journal of Physical Anthropology* 144, no. 4: 526–37. https://doi.org/10.1002/ajpa.21434

———. 2012. "Patterns of trauma and violence in 19th-century-born African American and Euro-American females." *International Journal of Paleopathology* 2, nos. 2–3: 61–68. https://doi.org/10.1016/j.ijpp.2012.09.009

DeLeon, Valerie B. 2007. "Fluctuating asymmetry and stress in a medieval Nubian population." *American Journal of Physical Anthropology* 132, no. 4: 520–34. https://doi.org/10.1002/ajpa.20549

Dennis, Rutledge M. 1995. "Social Darwinism, scientific racism, and the metaphysics of race." *Journal of Negro Education* 64, no. 3: 243–52. https://psycnet.apa.org/doi/10.2307/2967206

DiGangi, Elizabeth A., and Jonathan D. Bethard. 2021. "Uncloaking a lost cause: Decolonizing ancestry estimation in the United States." *American Journal of Physical Anthropology* 175, no. 2: 422–36. https://doi.org/10.1002/ajpa.24212

Dinno, Alexis. 2017. "Homicide rates of transgender individuals in the United States: 2010–2014." *American Journal of Public Health* 107, no. 9: 1441–47. https://doi.org/10.2105/AJPH.2017.303878

Dror, Itiel, Judy Melinek, Jonathan L. Arden, Jeff Kukucka, Sarah Hawkins, Joye Carter, and Daniel S. Atherton. 2021a. "Cognitive bias in forensic pathology decisions." *Journal of Forensic Sciences* 66, no. 5: 1751–57. https://doi.org/10.1111/1556-4029.14697

Dror, Itiel E., Kyle C. Scherr, Linton A. Mohammed, Carla L. MacLean, and Lloyd Cunningham. 2021b. "Biasability and reliability of expert forensic document examiners." *Forensic Science International* 318: 110610. https://doi.org/10.1016/j.forsciint.2020.110610

Dror, Itiel E., William C. Thompson, Christian A. Meissner, Irv Kornfield, Dan Krane, Michael Saks, and Michael Risinger. 2015. "Letter to the editor-context management toolbox: A Linear Sequential Unmasking (LSU) approach for minimizing cognitive bias in forensic decision making." *Journal of Forensic Sciences* 60, no. 4: 1111–12. https://doi.org/10.1111/1556-4029.12805

Dupras, Tosha L., Lana J. Williams, Harco Willems, and Christoph Peeters. 2010. "Pathological skeletal remains from ancient Egypt: The earliest case of diabetes mellitus?." *Practical Diabetes International* 27, no. 8: 358–363a. https://doi.org/10.1002/pdi.1523

Edgar, Heather J.H., and Daneshvari Berry S. 2019. "NMDID: A new research resource for biological anthropology." *American Journal of Physical Anthropology* 168, no. S68: 66.

Entringer, Sonja, Elissa S. Epel, Robert Kumsta, Jue Lin, Dirk H. Hellhammer, Elizabeth H. Blackburn, Stefan Wüst, and Pathik D. Wadhwa. 2011. "Stress exposure in intrauterine life is associated with shorter telomere length in young adulthood." *Proceedings of the National Academy of Sciences* 108, no. 33: E513–18. https://doi.org/10.1073/pnas.1107759108

Epel, Elissa S., Elizabeth H. Blackburn, Jue Lin, Firdaus S. Dhabhar, Nancy E. Adler, Jason D. Morrow, and Richard M. Cawthon. 2004. "Accelerated telomere shortening in response to life stress." *Proceedings of the National Academy of Sciences* 101, no. 49: 17312–15. https://doi.org/10.1073/pnas.0407162101

Farmer, Paul. 2004. "An anthropology of structural violence." *Current Anthropology* 45, no. 3: 305–25. https://doi.org/10.1086/382250

Farmer, Paul, Jim Yong Kim, Arthur Kleinman, and Matthew Basilico. 2013. "Introduction: A biosocial approach to global health." In *Reimagining Global Health: An Introduction,* edited by Paul Farmer, Jim Yong Kim, Arthur Kleinman, and Matthew Basilico, 1–14. University of California Press. https://doi.org/10.1525/9780520954632-003

Gabbidon, Shaun L., and Steven A. Peterson. 2006. "Living while Black: A state-level analysis of the influence of select social stressors on the quality of life among Black Americans." *Journal of Black Studies* 37, no. 1: 83–102. https://doi.org/10.1177%2F0021934705277475

Galtung, Johan. 1969. "Violence, peace, and peace research." *Journal of Peace Research* 6, no. 3: 167–91.

Gamble, Vanessa Northington. 2014. *"The immortal life of Henrietta lacks* reconsidered." *Hastings Center Report* 44, no. 1. https://doi.org/10.1002/hast.239

Geronimus, Arline T. 1992. "The weathering hypothesis and the health of African-American women and infants: evidence and speculations." *Ethnicity & Disease* 2, no. 3: 207–21.

———. 1996. "Black/white differences in the relationship of maternal age to birthweight: A population-based test of the weathering hypothesis." *Social Science & Medicine* 42, no. 4: 589–97. https://doi.org/10.1016/0277-9536(95)00159-x

———. 2001. "Understanding and eliminating racial inequalities in women's health in the United States: The role of the weathering conceptual framework." *Journal of the American Medical Women's Association* 56, no. 4: 133–36, 149–50.

Geronimus, Arline T., Margaret Hicken, Danya Keene, and John Bound. 2006. ""Weathering" and age patterns of allostatic load scores among blacks and whites in the United States." *American Journal of Public Health* 96, no. 5: 826–33. https://doi.org/10.2105/AJPH.2004.060749

Goad, Gennifer. 2020. "Expanding humanitarian forensic action: An approach to US cold cases." *Forensic Anthropology* 3, no. 1: 50–58. https://doi.org/10.5744/fa.2020.1006

Godsay, Surbhi, and Anne E. Brodsky. 2018. "'I believe in that movement and I believe in that chant': The influence of Black Lives Matter on resilience and empowerment." *Community Psychology in Global Perspective* 4, no. 2: 55–72. https://doi.org/10.1285/i24212113v4i2p55

Goodman, Alan H., and Jerome C. Rose. 1990. "Assessment of systemic physiological perturbations from dental enamel hypoplasias and associated histological structures." *American Journal of Physical Anthropology* 33, no. S11: 59–110. https://doi.org/10.1002/ajpa.1330330506

Goodman, Alan H., Yolanda T. Moses, and Joseph L. Jones. 2020. *Race: Are We So Different?* Chichester: John Wiley & Sons.

Gravlee, Clarence C. 2009. "How race becomes biology: embodiment of social inequality." *American Journal of Physical Anthropology* 139, no. 1: 47–57. https://doi.org/10.1002/ajpa.20983

————. 2020. "Systemic racism, chronic health inequities, and COVID-19: A syndemic in the making? *American Journal of Human Biology* e23482. https://doi.org /10.1002/ajhb.23482

Gravlee, Clarence C., H. Russell Bernard, and William R. Leonard. 2003. "Boas's changes in bodily form: The immigrant study, cranial plasticity, and Boas's physical anthropology." *American Anthropologist* 105, no. 2: 326–32. https://doi.org/10 .1525/aa.2003.105.2.326

Gravlee, Clarence C., William W. Dressler, and H. Russell Bernard. 2005. "Skin color, social classification, and blood pressure in southeastern Puerto Rico." *American Journal of Public Health* 95, no. 12: 2191–97. https://doi.org/10.2105/ AJPH.2005.065615

Hamnett, Hilary J., and Itiel E. Dror. 2020. "The effect of contextual information on decision-making in forensic toxicology." *Forensic Science International: Synergy* 2: 339–48. https://doi.org/10.1016/j.fsisyn.2020.06.003

Hanna-Attisha, Mona, Jenny LaChance, Richard Casey Sadler, and Allison Champney Schnepp. 2016. "Elevated blood lead levels in children associated with the Flint drinking water crisis: A spatial analysis of risk and public health response." *American Journal of Public Health* 106, no. 2: 283–90. https://doi.org/10.2105/ AJPH.2015.303003

Hillson, Simon, and Sandra Bond. 1997. "Relationship of enamel hypoplasia to the pattern of tooth crown growth: A discussion." *American Journal of Physical Anthropology* 104, no. 1: 89–103. https://doi.org/10.1002/(SICI)1096-8644 (199709)104:1%3C89::AID-AJPA6%3E3.0.CO;2-8

Hoke, Morgan K., and Lawrence M. Schell. 2020. "Doing biocultural anthropology: Continuity and change." *American Journal of Human Biology* 32, no. 4: e23471. https://doi.org/10.1002/ajhb.23471

Holmes, Seth M. 2013. *Fresh Fruit, Broken Bodies: Migrant Farmworkers in the United States*. Berkeley and Los Angeles: University of California Press.

Human Rights Campaign Foundation. 2018. "A national epidemic: Fatal anti-transgender violence in America 2018." https://assets2.hrc.org/files/assets/resources /AntiTransViolence-2018Report-Final.pdf?_ga=2.64681327.1191269802 .1570129723- 2062334073.1570129723

Ice, Gillian H., and Gary D. James. 2006. *Measuring Stress in Humans*. New York: Cambridge University Press.

İşcan, Mehmet Yaşar, Susan R. Loth, and Ronald K. Wright. 1987. "Racial variation in the sternal extremity of the rib and its effect on age determination." *Journal of Forensic Sciences* 32, no. 2: 452–66. https://doi.org/10.1520/JFS11147J

Kimmerle, Erin H., Anthony Falsetti, and Ann H. Ross. 2010. "Immigrants, undocumented workers, runaways, transients and the homeless: Towards contextual identification among unidentified decedents." *Forensic Science Policy and Management* 1, no. 4: 178–86. https://doi.org/10.1080/19409041003636991

Komar, Debra A., and Sarah Lathrop. 2012. "Patterns of trauma in conflict victims from Timor Leste." *Journal of Forensic Sciences* 57, no. 1: 3–5. https://doi.org/10 .1111/j.1556-4029.2011.01931.x

146   *Allysha P. Winburn et al.*

Krieger, Nancy. 2001. "Theories for social epidemiology in the 21st century: An ecosocial perspective." *International Journal of Epidemiology* 30, no. 4: 668–77. https://doi.org/10.1093/ije/30.4.668

———. 2003. "Does racism harm health? Did child abuse exist before 1962? On explicit questions, critical science, and current controversies: An ecosocial perspective." *American Journal of Public Health* 93: 194–99. https://doi.org/10.2105/AJPH.93.2.194

———. 2020. "ENOUGH: COVID-19, structural racism, police brutality, plutocracy, climate change—and time for health justice, democratic governance, and an equitable, sustainable future." *American Public Health Association* 110, no. 11: 1620–23. https://doi.org/10.2105/AJPH. 2020.305886

Krieger, Nancy, and George Davey Smith. 2004. "'Bodies count,' and body counts: Social epidemiology and embodying inequality." *Epidemiologic Reviews* 26, no. 1: 92–103. https://doi.org/10.1093/epirev/mxh009

Krieger, Nancy, Diane L. Rowley, Allen A. Herman, Byllye Avery, and Mona T. Phillips. 1993. "Racism, sexism, and social class: Implications for studies of health, disease, and well-being." *American Journal of Preventive Medicine* 9, no. 6: 82–122. https://doi.org/10.1016/S0749-3797(18)30666-4

Lett, Elle, Emmanuella Ngozi Asabor, Theodore Corbin, and Dowin Boatright. 2020. "Racial inequity in fatal US police shootings, 2015–2020." *Journal of Epidemiology & Community Health* 75, no. 4: 394–97. http://dx.doi.org/10.1136/jech-2020-215097

Lucchesi, Anita, and Abigail Echo-Hawk. 2018. "Missing and murdered indigenous women & girls: A snapshot of data from 71 urban cities in the United States." The *Urban Indian Health Institute.* http://www.uihi.org/wp-content/uploads/2018/11/Missing-and-Murdered-Indigenous-Women-and-Girls-Report.pdf

MacDorman, Marian F., Eugene Declercq, Howard Cabral, and Christine Morton. 2016. "Is the United States maternal mortality rate increasing? Disentangling trends from measurement issues." *Obstetrics and Gynecology* 128, no. 3: 447–55. https://doi.org/10.1097/AOG.0000000000001556

Marmot, Michael. 2004. "Status syndrome." *Significance* 1, no. 4: 150–54. https://doi.org/10.1111/j.1740-9713.2004.00058.x

Marten, Meredith G. 2021. "The countersyndemic potential of medical pluralism among people living with HIV in Tanzania." *Global Public Health*: 1–14. https://doi.org/10.1080/17441692.2021.1882529

McDade, Thomas W. 2002. "Status incongruity in Samoan youth: A biocultural analysis of culture change, stress, and immune function." *Medical Anthropology Quarterly* 16, no. 2: 123–50. https://doi.org/10.1525/maq.2002.16.2.123

Mendenhall, Emily. 2012. *Syndemic Suffering: Social Distress, Depression, and Diabetes among Mexican Immigrant Women.* Walnut Creek: Left Coast Press.

Mensforth, Robert P., C. Owen Lovejoy, John W. Lallo, and George J. Armelagos. 1978. "Part two: The role of constitutional factors, diet, and infectious disease in the etiology of porotic hyperostosis and periosteal reactions in prehistoric infants and children." *Medical Anthropology* 2, no. 1: 1–59. https://doi.org/10.1080/01459740.1978.9986939

Mulligan, Connie J. 2016. "Early environments, stress, and the epigenetics of human health." *Annual Review of Anthropology* 45: 233–49. https://doi.org/10.1146/annurev-anthro-102215-095954

Nakhaeizadeh, Sherry, Itiel E. Dror, and Ruth M. Morgan. 2014. "Cognitive bias in forensic anthropology: Visual assessment of skeletal remains is susceptible to confirmation bias." *Science & Justice* 54, no. 3: 208–14. https://doi.org/10.1016/j.scijus.2013.11.003

———. 2020. "Cognitive bias in sex estimation: The influence of context on forensic decision-making." In *Sex Estimation of the Human Skeleton*, edited by Alexandra R. Klales, 327–42. Academic Press. https://doi.org/10.1016/B978-0-12-815767-1.00020-1

Nakhaeizadeh, Sherry, Ian Hanson, and Nathalie Dozzi. 2014. "The power of contextual effects in forensic anthropology: A study of biasability in the visual interpretations of trauma analysis on skeletal remains." *Journal of Forensic Sciences* 59, no. 5: 1177–83. https://doi.org/10.1111/1556-4029.12473

Nakhaeizadeh, Sherry, Ruth M. Morgan, Carolyn Rando, and Itiel E. Dror. 2018. "Cascading bias of initial exposure to information at the crime scene to the subsequent evaluation of skeletal remains." *Journal of Forensic Sciences* 63, no. 2: 403–11. https://doi.org/10.1111/1556-4029.13569

Newman, Sophie L., and Rebecca L. Gowland. 2015. "The use of non-adult vertebral dimensions as indicators of growth disruption and non-specific health stress in skeletal populations." *American Journal of Physical Anthropology* 158, no. 1: 155–64. https://doi.org/10.1002/ajpa.22770

O'Donnell, Lexi, Ethan C. Hill, Amy S. Anderson Anderson, and Heather J.H. Edgar. 2020. "Cribra orbitalia and porotic hyperostosis are associated with respiratory infections in a contemporary mortality sample from New Mexico." *American Journal of Physical Anthropology* 173, no. 4: 721–33. https://doi.org/10.1002/ajpa.24131

Packard, Randall M. 2016. *A History of Global Health: Interventions into the Lives of Other Peoples*. Baltimore: Johns Hopkins University Press.

Panter-Brick, Catherine. 2014. "Health, risk, and resilience: Interdisciplinary concepts and applications." *Annual Review of Anthropology* 43: 431–48. https://doi.org/10.1146/annurev-anthro-102313-025944

Parr, Nicolette M., Nicholas V. Passalacqua, and Katie Skorpinski. 2017. "Investigations into age-related changes in the human mandible." *Journal of Forensic Sciences* 62, no. 6: 1586–91. https://doi.org/10.1111/1556-4029.13475

Prince-Buitenhuys, Julia R., Heather L. MacInnes, Colleen F. Milligan, and Eric J. Bartelink. 2017. "An exploration of skeletal evidence of injury recidivism in cases of transients and homelessness from Northern California." In *Broken Bones, Broken Bodies: Bioarchaeological and Forensic Approaches for Accumulative Trauma and Violence*, edited by Caryn E. Tegtmeyer and Debra L. Martin, 183–200. Lanham: Lexington Books.

Rej, Peter H., HEAT Steering Committee, Clarence C. Gravlee, and Connie J. Mulligan. 2020. "Shortened telomere length is associated with unfair treatment attributed to race in African Americans living in Tallahassee, Florida." *American Journal of Human Biology* 32, no. 3: e23375. https://doi.org/10.1002/ajhb.23375

Richardson, Lynne D., and Marlaina Norris. 2010. "Access to health and health care: How race and ethnicity matter." *Mount Sinai Journal of Medicine* 77, no. 2: 166–77. https://doi.org/10.1002/msj.20174

Sapolsky, Robert M. 2004. "Social status and health in humans and other animals." *Annual Review of Anthropology* 33: 393–418. https://doi.org/10.1146/annurev.anthro.33.070203.144000

———. 2005. "Sick of poverty." *Scientific American* 293, no. 6: 92–99. https://doi.org/10.1038/scientificamerican1205-92

———. 2006. "Culture in animals: The case of a non-human primate culture of low aggression and high affiliation." *Social Forces* 85, no. 1: 217–33. https://doi.org/10.1353/sof.2006.0142

Schall, Jenna L., Tracy L. Rogers, and Jordan C. Deschamps-Braly. 2020. "Breaking the binary: The identification of trans-women in forensic anthropology." *Forensic Science International* 309: 110220. https://doi.org/10.1016/j.forsciint.2020.110220

Scheper-Hughes, Nancy. 1993. *Death Without Weeping: The Violence of Everyday Life in Brazil*. University of California Press.

———. 2013. "No more angel babies on the Alto do Cruzeiro." *Natural History* 121, no. 5: 28–38.

Scheper-Hughes, Nancy, and Philippe Bourgois, editors. 2004. *Violence in War and Peace: An Anthology*. Malden: Wiley-Blackwell.

Scheper-Hughes, Nancy, and Margaret M. Lock. 1987. "The mindful body: A prolegomenon to future work in medical anthropology." *Medical Anthropology Quarterly* 1, no. 1: 6–41. https://doi.org/10.1525/maq.1987.1.1.02a00020

Simons, Ronald L., Man Kit Lei, Steven R.H. Beach, Robert A. Philibert, Carolyn E. Cutrona, Frederick X. Gibbons, and Ashley Barr. 2016. "Economic hardship and biological weathering: The epigenetics of aging in a US sample of black women." *Social Science & Medicine* 150: 192–200. https://doi.org/10.1016/j.socscimed.2015.12.001

Singer, Merrill, and Hans Baer. 2018. *Critical Medical Anthropology*. Routledge.

Smith-Morris, Carolyn. 2008. *Diabetes among the Pima: Stories of Survival*. University of Arizona Press.

Snow, Clyde C., Fredy A. Peccerelli, José S. Susanávar, Alan G. Robinson, and Jose Maria Najera Ochoa. 2008. "Hidden in plain sight: X.X. burials and the desaparecidos in the department of Guatemala, 1977–1986." In *Statistical Methods for Human Rights*, edited by Jana Asher, David Banks, and Fritz J. Scheuren, 89–116. New York: Springer. https://doi.org/10.1007/978-0-387-72837-7_5

Soler, Angela, and Jared S. Beatrice. 2018. "Expanding the role of forensic anthropology in a humanitarian crisis: An example from the USA-Mexico border." In *Sociopolitics of Migrant Death and Repatriation*, edited by Krista E. Latham and Alyson J. O'Daniel, 115–28. Cham: Springer. https://doi.org/10.1007/978-3-319-61866-1_9

Southwick, Steven M., George A. Bonanno, Ann S. Masten, Catherine Panter-Brick, and Rachel Yehuda. 2014. "Resilience definitions, theory, and challenges: Interdisciplinary perspectives." *European Journal of Psychotraumatology* 5, no. 1: 25338. https://doi.org/10.3402/ejpt.v5.25338

Tallman, Sean, and Cate Bird. 2022. "Diversity and inclusion in forensic anthropology." *Forensic Anthropology* 5, no. 2: 84–101. https://doi.org/10.5744/fa.2020.3001

Tallman, Sean, Caroline Kincer, and Eric Plemons. 2022. "Centering transgender individuals in forensic anthropology and expanding binary sex estimation in casework and research." *Forensic Anthropology* 5, no. 2: 161–80. https://doi.org/10.5744/fa.2020.0030

Taylor, Miles G. 2008. "Timing, accumulation, and the black/white disability gap in later life: A test of weathering." *Research on Aging* 30, no. 2: 226–50. https://doi.org/10.1177%2F0164027507311838

Wacquant, Loic. 2004. "Response to Paul Farmer in 'An anthropology of structural violence.'" *Current Anthropology* 45, no. 3: 322. http://www.jstor.org/stable/10.1086/382250?origin=JSTOR-pdf

Walker, Phillip L., Rhonda R. Bathurst, Rebecca Richman, Thor Gjerdrum, and Valerie A. Andrushko. 2009. "The causes of porotic hyperostosis and cribra orbitalia: A reappraisal of the iron-deficiency-anemia hypothesis." *American Journal of Physical Anthropology* 139, no. 2: 109–25. https://doi.org/10.1002/ajpa.21031

Watkins, Rachel. 2012. "Variation in health and socioeconomic status within the W. Montague Cobb skeletal collection: Degenerative joint disease, trauma and cause of death." *International Journal of Osteoarchaeology* 22, no. 1: 22–44. https://doi.org/10.1002/oa.1178

———. 2018. "Anatomical collections as the anthropological other: Some considerations." In *Bioarchaeological Analyses and Bodies: New Ways of Knowing Anatomical and Archaeological Skeletal Collections*, edited by Pamela K. Stone, 27–47. Cham: Springer. https://doi.org/10.1007/978-3-319-71114-0_3

Wiley, Andrea S., and John S. Allen. 2017. *Medical Anthropology: A Biocultural Approach*, 3rd edition. New York: Oxford University Press.

Winburn, Allysha P. 2018. "Subjective with a capital S? Issues of objectivity in forensic anthropology." In *Forensic Anthropology: Theoretical Framework and Scientific Basis*, edited by C. Clifford Boyd Jr. and Donna Boyd, 21–38. New York: Wiley. https://doi.org/10.1002/9781119226529.ch2

Winburn, Allysha P., and Chaunesey M.J. Clemmons. 2021. "Objectivity is a myth that harms the practice and diversity of forensic science." *Forensic Science International: Synergy* 3: 100196. https://doi.org/10.1016/j.fsisyn.2021.100196

Winburn, Allysha P., Antaya Jennings, Dawnie W. Steadman, and Elizabeth A. DiGangi. 2022. "Ancestral diversity in skeletal collections: Perspectives on African American body donation." *Forensic Anthropology* 5, no. 2: 141–52. https://doi.org/10.5744/fa.2020.1023

Wood, James W., George R. Milner, Henry C. Harpending, Kenneth M. Weiss, Mark N. Cohen, Leslie E. Eisenberg, Dale L. Hutchinson et al. 1992. "The osteological paradox: Problems of inferring prehistoric health from skeletal samples [and comments and reply]." *Current Anthropology* 33, no. 4: 343–70. https://doi.org/10.1086/204084

Wylie, Alison. 1992. "On 'heavily decomposing red herrings': Scientific method in archaeology and the ladening of evidence with theory." In *Metaarchaeology*, edited by Lester Embree, 269–88. Dordrecht: Springer. https://doi.org/10.1007/978-94-011-1826-2_12

Chapter 6

Disability, Disaster, Demography, and the Camp Fire Fatalities

Samuel Mijal and P. Willey

In this chapter, we argue that the intersectional identities of those who were considered impaired and old/elderly contributed to their marginalized status within the Camp Fire Communities (CFC) and subsequently made them more vulnerable during the catastrophic 2018 Northern California wildfire.[1] Members of those groups were more likely to die and become the focus of forensic anthropologists and other death investigators. To contextualize those assertions, we present concepts of disability and impairment as well as discuss principles of demography and disaster mortality. We depict the Camp Fire tragedy, describe the pre-fire CFCs' demography, and compare it with those of California and the United States. Then, we present and interpret the Camp Fire fatalities, discussing the decedents' impairments and vulnerabilities. Our goals are to view the Camp Fire as a catastrophic event and explore characteristics that caused members of vulnerable groups to die disproportionately and require attention from forensic anthropologists. This work lies at the intersection of public health, concepts of disability and impairment, and disaster anthropology.

IMPAIRMENT AND DISABILITY CONCEPTS

Discussions about disability and impairment within anthropology rely on terminology and models drawn from critical disability studies. Critical disability studies emerged with the publication of the cornerstone work *Fundamental Principles of Disability* in 1976, which posited that disablement was primarily a product of socially constructed barriers rather than personal impairments (Oliver 2013; Union of the Physically Impaired Against Segregation 1976). Prior to this development, the medical model dominated disability thought.

Couched in Industrial Revolution-era thinking, the medical model focused on diagnosis and treatment of the individual (Oliver 2013; Siebers 2008). This perspective established an implicit mandate to cure people with disabilities (Murphy et al. 1988; Shuttleworth and Kasnitz 2004). Although this model is still utilized to some extent in the medical field, it has fallen from favor within anthropology because it fails to account for sociocultural factors that can drastically impact the debilitating power of impairment upon an individual (Byrnes and Muller 2017).

Unlike the medical model, the social model of disability conceptualized disability as a social category imposed on individuals by society. In this model, societies establish and reinforce what is "normal," shaping public spaces and social expectations to these norms (Oliver 2004). Society therefore disables individuals with physical and mental impairments by restricting their ability to move in public spaces and interact with other members of that society (Barnes 1991; Oliver 1990). Under this model, society also bears the responsibility of providing accessibility, accommodations, and equitable treatment (Oliver 2004).

Central to the social model is the distinction between impairment and disability. While these terms have multiple definitions, for the purposes of this chapter *impairment* is defined as the experience or perceived experience of physiological or behavioral statuses or processes that are socially identified as problems (Kasnitz and Shuttleworth 2001). They include illnesses, conditions, disorders, syndromes, and other similarly negatively valued differences, distinctions, or characteristics. They could be congenital or acquired, wholly aesthetic or functionally limiting, temporary or permanent. Impairments often carry an ethnomedical diagnostic category or label. Disability, on the other hand, is the experience of discrimination on the basis of perceived functional limitations of impairments (Kasnitz and Shuttleworth 2001). This discrimination is socially constructed and takes many forms, but all are rooted in the conceptualization of what is "normal" in a society.

However, the social model is not without criticism. The most glaring fault in the social model is essentially the same as the medical model—the apparent disconnect between biological and sociocultural influences on the individual (Shakespeare 2013; Goodley, Hughes, and Davis 2012; Siebers 2008). While the medical model focuses solely on the biological factors impacting the individual, the social model has been criticized for emphasizing the sociocultural factors of disability to the point that it risks ignoring the challenges that biological factors can present (Shakespeare 2006). Consequently, if disability is defined only in terms of social discrimination and oppression, then definitions of impairment should acknowledge the physical pain and limiting effects it can place on daily activity (Thomas 2004). Furthermore, implicit in the social model is the idea that social discrimination is the ultimate impediment preventing a barrier-free society. While the adaptation of environments and services wherever possible is a worthy endeavor, practical constraints, such as cost or even competing accommodations (e.g., curb cuts to accommodate wheelchair users versus defined curbs to accommodate the visually impaired), can limit the access of individuals with impairments even if social stigmatization is not a factor (Shakespeare 2006).

More recent models, such as the biopsychosocial model, have been utilized to accommodate these issues by taking a wholistic perspective. This model focuses on the individual, their health and bodily function while still considering personal and environmental factors. Since 2001, the World Health Organization (WHO) has published evolving recommendations based on the biopsychosocial model through the International Classification of Function, Disability and Health (ICF) (WHO 2001). However, this model is not without its critics, who note the ICF's oversimplification of contextual factors within the model and who challenge the model's holistic claims (Kumar and Smith 2005; Roush and Sharby 2011; Solli and Barbosa da Silva 2012). To combat this, the WHO has continuously updated the ICF to take these critiques into consideration (2018). Crucial to disability studies is the idea that impairment separates those people with perceived impairments into a group apart from those considered "normal" (Ablon 1995). This form of stigmatization is unique. Unlike gender, ethnic, or religious stigmatization, anyone can become disabled at any time, whether through disease, illness, accident, or age (McDermott and Varenne 1995). The probability of acquiring these impairments increases for older adults, defined for our purposes as sixty-five years or older. This definition follows the Centers for Disease Control definition and conforms to conceptualizations of old age in the United States (Centers for Disease Control and Prevention 2015). However, old age, as with other age categories, is a social construct influenced by customs, practice, and perceived role within a community. For older adults, risk of impairment is twofold. First, age-related changes contribute to many physical and mental impairments such as hearing loss, and decreases in visual acuity and cognitive function. Second, as individuals age, they are at increased exposure to environmental contributors to impairment, such as disease, illness, and accident (Berg and Cassells 1992). These compounding factors contribute to older adults being the fastest growing demographic group at high risk for impairment. With an average lifespan for Americans of 78.7 years (Xu et al. 2020), most Americans will experience some form of age-related impairment.

Stigmatization of older adults in the United States often results in social isolation (Berg and Cassells 1992; National Academies of Sciences, Engineering, and Medicine 2020). For the purposes of this chapter, *social isolation* is defined as "the absence of social interactions, contacts, and relationships with family and friends, with neighbors on an individual level, and with 'society at large' on a broader level" (Berg and Cassells 1992, 243). The causes and effects of social isolation are numerous, including depression, illness, injury, and domestic violence. Socially isolated individuals have difficulty making or maintaining social relationships. Adults older than sixty-five years are more likely to be impacted by social isolation than younger people. Among older adults, isolation often results from the inability to leave their residences. One study estimated that 24 percent of independently living older adults in the contiguous United States (approximately 7.7 million people) were socially isolated and 4 percent (approximately 1.3 million people) could be characterized as severely socially isolated (Cudjoe et al. 2020). Given this high rate of social isolation among older adults, it follows that these groups have a greater difficulty utilizing social networks in the face of catastrophic events, such as a wildfire.

This chapter approaches the analysis of Camp Fire victims through the perspective of the social model. There are several social factors at play that must be explored to understand why Camp Fire victims were on average older and more likely to be impaired than the pre-fire CFC population. The fast-moving Camp Fire strained established social systems such as the CodeRED emergency alert system and community social networks to the point of failure. These failures disproportionately impacted the people who needed them most—older and impaired individuals relying on accommodations from public safety agencies and fellow community residents to escape natural disasters.

These accommodations come about as a result of three partnerships: namely, agency-agency partnerships, agency-resident partnerships, and resident-resident partnerships (Kolden and Henson 2019). Each of these interactions is socially prescribed and exists both within and outside of disaster contexts. Agency-agency partnerships describe collaboration between various agencies who, in part or in whole, manage disaster response mitigation, planning, and execution. Agency-resident partnerships are primarily concerned with developing relationships between the community and disaster planning and response agencies. This relationship describes both the communication of disaster safety precautions, updates, and evacuation planning to community residents and also the communication of specific needs of residents to these agencies. Finally, resident-resident partnerships, the most subtle and informal relationship type, operate along social networks to plan for and mitigate disasters on the household level. The strength of these three relationships within a community, especially agency-resident and resident-resident partnerships, impact the sensitivity of vulnerable portions of the population to catastrophic events, such as a wildfire (Kolden and Henson 2019; Wigtil et al. 2016).

In summary, physical and cognitive impairments, and the stigmatization associated with such differences, create vulnerable groups within a population. Many Americans will enter these groups as they move into older-age categories, with their related impacts upon physical and cognitive functions. One result of advanced age and impairment is social isolation, which can leave individuals bereft of support from the greater community. This isolation makes impaired individuals especially vulnerable during catastrophic events.

DEMOGRAPHY, DEATHS, AND DISASTERS

Marginalized and disadvantaged people are often unduly impacted by exposure to illness and hunger, those issues arising from and further exacerbated by having limited access to political and economic power. The impact of marginalization and its consequences become all the more apparent in differential mortality during catastrophic events.

Disasters consist of economically, politically, physically, and socially catastrophic events that have long-lasting impacts. Disasters include technological crises (e.g., nuclear meltdowns), famine, severe storms, emigrants under duress, earthquakes, landslides, volcanic eruptions, floods, tsunamis, epidemic diseases, hostile conflicts, (Chamberlain 2006, 69–80) and wildfires (Barrios 2017). Deaths during catastrophes have been claimed to affect all segments of the population equally, not just the most vulnerable members of the population. Because disasters are overwhelmingly devastating events across the entire population spectrum, the reasoning goes, catastrophic death profiles parallel the age structure of the parent population (Lyman 1987). Also called crisis, mass and living mortality, catastrophic events cause deaths resulting in a unimodal, positively skewed, L-shaped mortality distribution. Catastrophic mortality profiles differ from the more common attritional mortality distributions (Lyman 1987). In attritional mortality, group members die from more typical causes: those processes that disproportionately affect the young and old. The resulting attritional mortality distribution is bimodal, with more deaths at the two age extremes, forming a U-shaped curve. Even in catastrophic events, however, rarely—if ever—do all members of a population experience the same vulnerability and suffer similar mortality rates. Mortality in disasters is discriminating and non-random with some groups impacted more than others.

Disaster anthropology takes a nuanced, historical, and holistic perspective on catastrophic events and their demographic impact. According to this perspective, the potential for disaster lies at the juncture of physical and environmental forces, social and cultural institutions, and vulnerability and exposure to risk (Oliver-Smith 1999; Oliver-Smith and Hoffman 2002). Disasters further involve human-environment interaction, historical embeddedness, adaptations, and social inequality. During and following a disaster, the most vulnerable individuals and groups suffer the most.

Wildfires, in particular, demonstrate the intersection of natural hazards, social institutions, and vulnerabilities. In the past, wildfires were considered natural hazards that surround and threaten people, property, and communities. Now they are considered natural events that humans interpret, exacerbate, interact, and actively engage with. It is another repercussion of the Anthropocene (Barrios 2017), the proposed most recent geological epoch hallmarked by humans' overwhelming impact on the Earth and its ecosystems. Closer to home, California wildfires have worsened in recent decades due to climate change, increased fuel loads, and increased human development in the urban-wildland interface. These factors collided in the 2018 Camp Fire, directly causing eighty-five deaths, making it the deadliest fire in California history.

CAMP FIRE

At approximately 6:30 a.m. PST on Thursday, November 8, 2018, something that had long been feared occurred on Camp Creek Road near Pulga, California (figure 6.1). Prolonged drought, high winds, and arid conditions collided (Brewer and Clements 2020; Mass and Ovens 2021). High-speed winds snapped a worn C-hook holding a Pacific Gas and Electric 115kV

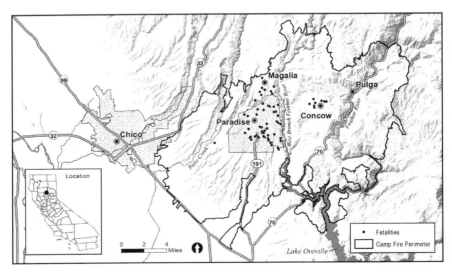

Figure 6.1   Map showing area burned by the 2018 Camp Fire, communities involved, and locations of fatalities. Map Credit: Judy Stolen.

electric transmission line, sending it arcing into a steel tower and showering the grass and brush below with sparks (Cal Fire 2019; Ramsey 2020). Less than half an hour after the fire began, sustained high winds, some exceeding 50mph (80 kph), sweep the fire from Pulga in the Feather River Canyon more than 4 miles (6.4km) into the town of Concow. From there, the Camp Fire ascended the side of the West Branch of the Feather River Canyon, striking the town of Paradise by 8:00 a.m. PST and Magalia shortly after. A few hours after its ignition, much of Concow, Paradise and Magalia were ablaze.

Early in this disaster, many residents made evacuation decisions lacking accurate, specific, up-to-date information on the fire. Even the fire's location and rate of spread were uncertain; this resulted in part from the Butte County emergency notification system failing (Todd, Trattner, and McMullen 2019). At 7:13 a.m., a Butte County Sheriff Office (BCSO) staff member issued evacuation orders to the first of fourteen zones in Paradise through the CodeRED software. This software package was recently purchased by BCSO to manage evacuations in the area, but the software and its application was flawed. First, by issuing sequential zone-by-zone notifications, some residents did not receive immediate notifications, and some failed to receive them at all (Moffitt 2019). Furthermore, CodeRED was an optional service. At the time of the fire, less than half of the CFCs' residents had chosen to participate in the notification system. Of the approximately 15,000 residents who might have been notified, only a third received calls, another third received voicemails and the remaining possible calls (approximately 5,400 phones, 36%) were never made (Moffitt 2019). A blanket warning was issued later though CodeRED via the national Integrated Public Alert and Warning System, which sends wireless emergency text alerts to mobile devices. Although 5,900 texts and emails were sent, not a single message was delivered because of an as-yet unidentified error (Moffitt 2019; Todd, Trattner, and McMullen 2019). To compound matters, the fire destroyed many cellphone towers and power and phone lines. With most residents receiving no emergency notification, many hoped that the fire would not jump from the West Branch of the Feather River Canyon onto the Paradise Ridge, as some previous wildfires had failed to do.

Of those people who received evacuation notices, most fled, others chose to ignore the dire circumstances in the hopes of defending their homes, while some lacked transportation to evacuate. As the chaotic evacuation began, informal community support networks fractured. These failures disproportionately affected the more vulnerable portions of the CFCs. Residents, who had known and assisted their neighbors for years, were unable to help them in the midst of the fire; either they were too busy saving themselves or they could not move against the flow of traffic during the evacuation (Chico Enterprise-Record 2019; Gee and Anguiano 2020). The flight of residents quickly became complicated because few roads led away from the fire toward safety. Evacuation traffic soon congested and clogged those roads, forcing some evacuees to abandon their vehicles.

Within two days, the Camp Fire had torn through the CFCs. Thousands of missing persons reports were established, most concerning the well-being of elderly relatives and those with mobility and cognitive impairments (Domonoske, Campbell, and Gonzales 2018). By the time the fire was contained seventeen days later, it had burned 153,336 acres (62,053 hectares), destroyed 18,804 structures, killed eighty-five people, and non-fatally injured three (Cal Fire 2019).

Following the fire, the BCSO had the responsibility for finding, recovering, and identifying the dead. Their efforts were supplemented by other law enforcement agencies, coroners from other counties, National Guard, as well as search and rescue, and anthropology teams. As they began the difficult task of sifting through the ruins of thousands of homes and hundreds of vehicles, the reality of the situation became clear and the anthropologists' support became even more critical.

During the twenty-one days of intense searching, nearly seventy-five anthropologists aided BCSO authorities in locating, confirming, and recovering remains (Milligan et al. ms; Pilloud et al. 2020). As recovery efforts developed, anthropology teams stood on alert while search and rescue teams scoured burned structures and vehicles. When putative human remains were discovered, anthropologists were deployed to those scenes. Anthropologists

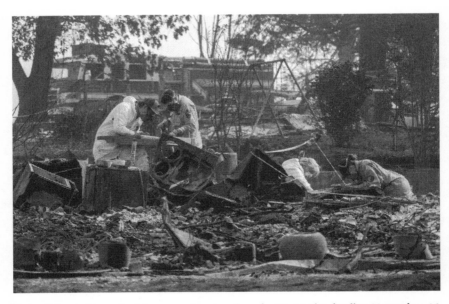

Figure 6.2   Anthropologists recovering remains of a Camp Fire fatality, November 16, 2018. Photograph courtesy of Jason Halley and Chico State.

determined if the suspected remains were human, and if they proved to be human whether they were of forensic significance. Thus, a few burnt archaeological and anatomical specimens were excluded from further forensic investigation. Using expedited archaeological techniques, anthropologists recovered the more thoroughly burnt (often calcined) remains as well as associated orthopedic devices and personal effects (figure 6.2). Coroners documented the scenes and recovered corpses that were less burnt and more complete. Recovered human remains were transferred to a morgue for identification by pathologists, odontologists, anthropologists, and DNA specialists (Gin et al. 2020).

METHODS

Pre-Fire Census and Disabilities

Demographic data for the CFCs are described and compared with California and U.S. data (U.S. Census and American Community Survey). Living demographic age and sex data for the CFCs, California and the United States were derived from the 2010 census (U.S. Census Bureau 2010). "Disability levels" and household data were estimated in 2017, the year preceding the fire (U.S. Census Bureau 2017). For population estimations, comparisons involving the California and U.S. figures also were from 2017 rather than 2010. Economic data came from the American Community Survey (2017).

The 2017 American Community Survey posed six questions to the head-of-households concerning the disability of each household member (U.S. Census Bureau 2017).

Hearing Difficulty (asked of all ages):
16a. Is this person deaf or does he/she have serious difficulty hearing?
Visual Difficulty (asked of all ages):
16b. Is this person blind or does he/she have serious difficulty seeing even when wearing glasses?
Cognitive Difficulty (asked of persons ages 5 and older):
17a. Because of a physical, mental, or emotional condition, does this person have serious difficulty concentrating, remembering, or making decisions?
Ambulatory Difficulty (asked of persons ages 5 or older):
17b. Does this person have serious difficulty walking or climbing stairs?
Self-care Difficulty (asked of persons ages 5 or older):
17c. Does this person have difficulty dressing or bathing?
Independent Living Difficulty (asked of persons ages 15 years or older):

18. Because of a physical, mental, or emotional condition, does this person have difficulty doing errands alone such as visiting a doctor's office or shopping?

Note that the Census used the term "difficulty" in these questions as an alternative for "disability," but the U.S. Census referred to responses to these questions as disability characteristics (Yang and Tan 2018). We use "difficulty" when referring specifically to these categories and the data generated from them.

Demography and Locations of the Camp Fire Fatalities

The BCSO provided the Camp Fire fatalities' demographic and location information such as the victims' age, sex, and death locations (BCSO Camp Fire Data Sheets CSUC 2019). Ages were recorded to the most recently completed whole year. Information concerning the victims' impairments and households came from BCSO, reminiscences by families and friends published in a local newspaper (Chico Enterprise-Record 2019), the Butte County District Attorney's legal brief (Ramsey 2020), and additional internet sources. Using the six difficulty categories from the 2017 American Community Survey, the Camp Fire fatalities were evaluated. Due to the ambiguous accounts concerning some fatalities, a seventh general difficulty category was added. This last category included individuals who were described as disabled but lacked information specific enough to categorize their situations as one of the six categories.

Altogether, eighty-five people died from the Camp Fire, all of whom but one have been identified. The one person who remains unidentified is believed to have been male; therefore he is omitted from the difficulties and age assessments but included in the demographic sex comparisons. Locations where each of the eighty-five died are known. However, one fatality had a Chico address and is excluded from our spatial assessments. In addition, two fatalities initially survived the fire, were evacuated, but later died from fire-related causes while under medical care in other locations; we included the locations where they sustained their injuries in our assessments. Of the eighty-five fatalities, seventy-three (85.9%) were found in or near homes, ten (11.8%) in or near vehicles, and two (2.3%) escaped and were hospitalized but later died from fire-related injuries.

RESULTS

Demography of Camp Fire Communities before the Fire

To understand the vulnerabilities of those who died in the Camp Fire, pre-fire demographic and economic foundations involving the three communities impacted by the Camp Fire needs to be established. Approximately 38,000 inhabitants lived in the CFCs (U.S. Census Bureau 2010). The CFCs have been characterized as retirement destinations (Kaiser Health News 2018; Newberry 2019). As retirement destinations, seniors lived largely independent lives, usually not in specifically designated residential or housing complexes designed for the elderly or infirm. As retirement communities, it is expected that they have greater proportions of older individuals, more females than males, lower household incomes, and greater frequencies of solitary living and impairment. To test the accuracy of those assumptions and establish a pre-fire base, census data were used.

Consistent with the older-age stereotype, the pre-Camp Fire CFCs tended to have a greater proportion of older adults. The combined CFCs' median age (49.8 years) was more than a decade older than the rest of California (35.2 years) as well as the United States (37.2 years). Comparing census data from the CFCs with California and the United States, as expected the communities had proportionately fewer subadults (<18 years) as well as fewer young and middle-aged adults and proportionately more older adults (≥65 years).

The pre-fire CFCs' sex ratio also differed from the California and U.S. figures. The CFCs' sex ratio of 51.8:48.2 females to males was skewed toward more females when compared to California (50.3: 49.7) or the United States (50.8: 49.1). Statistically, the CFCs had a significantly greater proportion of females than California ($\chi^2 = 35.11$, df = 1, P < 0.001) and the United States ($\chi^2 = 14.32$, df = 1, P < 0.001). Because females tend to outlive males, they become proportionately more frequent in older age groups. In part because of this demographic trend, the CFCs' older age distribution, as noted earlier, and their greater proportions of females were probably related.

Also consistent with that retirement stereotype, the pre-fire CFCs' median household annual income fell below the medians for both California and United States. The CFCs' annual median household income was $47,743, almost $20,000 below the California median of $67,139, and $10,000 below the U.S. median of $57,652. Presumably, many CFCs' residents lived on fixed incomes, such as Social Security and pensions, and/or inhabited one-income households. Concerning household makeup, 31.74 percent of CFCs' residents lived alone, with individuals over the age of sixty-five constituting 18 percent of single-person households (US Census Bureau 2017). These figures were greater than the 23.9 percent of California residents who live alone, 9.1 percent of whom are over sixty-five. Compared to the CFCs, the United States also had a lower rate of single households at 27.7 percent, with residents over the age of sixty-five constituting 10.5 percent of the total.

In addition to demographic and household information and most germane to this work, the pre-fire CFCs showed a greater frequency of difficulty than either California or the United States (table 6.1). The CFCs had significantly

Table 6.1 Comparisons of Camp Fire Communities, California and United States of America Rates of Disability

Disability Category	Communities	California	United States
Hearing Difficulty	8.1%	3.0%	3.6%
Vision Difficulty	2.0%	2.0%	2.3%
Cognitive Difficulty	5.9%	4.3%	5.1%
Ambulatory Difficulty	13.8%	5.9%	7.0%
Self-care Difficulty	4.1%	2.6%	2.7%
Independent Living Difficulty	9.2%	5.5%	5.8%

Source: Data from United States Census Bureau (2017).

greater proportions of overall difficulty (one or more disabilities) than both the United States and California ($\chi^2 = 1.72644E+17$, df=2, P<0.0001).

To summarize the CFCs' demographic and social parameters, these assessments provide support for the characterization that they served as retirement destinations. Compared with figures for California and the United States, the CFCs had an older population, proportionally more females, lower median household incomes, greater frequency of single-person households, and higher rates of impairments. On the other hand, it is important to note that the CFCs also served as homes and workplaces for other groups of people, just in smaller proportions when compared with California and the United States.

Camp Fire Fatalities

Having presented background to the CFCs, we now examine the Camp Fire's fatalities and their demography.

Demography of Camp Fire Fatalities

The ages of the Camp Fire fatalities varied, with older adults representing a disproportionate segment of victims from the overall CFCs population. The ages of fatalities ranged from 20 to 99 years with a mean of 72.06 years and median and mode of 72 years. Pronounced skewness was observed in the age data; no infants, children, or adolescents died in the blaze, those who would have comprised the left half of a U-shaped mortality curve. In general, young and middle-aged adults fared well too. At the upper-age extreme, however, more fatalities occurred among older individuals. This negative skewedness is the reverse of the typical L-shaped mortality distribution, which is positively skewed.

When examining sex, Camp Fire female fatalities exceeded male fatalities with forty-one males versus forty-four females, or a sex ratio of 100:107.3. When examining the fatality age distribution by sex, it proved to be statistically similar (T=1.605, df=82, P=0.112). However, when the four individuals who represented age outliers were excluded from the data set (two younger outliers of each sex), then a statistically significant difference emerged (T=2.158, df=78, P=0.034). With the outliers excluded, female fatalities averaged five years older than males.

Of the seventy-one Camp Fire fatalities with available information, thirty-three (46.5%) were reported to have lived alone, while thirty-eight (53.5%) lived with at least one other person (e.g., a parent, child, significant other, or roommate). The household composition of the remaining fourteen victims was unknown. An independent samples *t* test compared ages between fatalities who lived alone (mean=76.36 years) and those who lived with at least one other person (mean=67.08 years) and showed a statistically significant difference (T=2.770, df=69, P=0.007). Older fatalities were, therefore, more likely to have lived alone.

Comparing where fatalities occurred by separate communities (fatalities' residences for those two dying later during hospitalization) with pre-fire census information for the CFCs, a statistically significant difference was evident (χ^2=29.47, df=4, P<0.001). Contributing most to the difference was the greater than expected frequency of fatalities in Concow; to a lesser extent, fewer than expected fatalities occurred in Magalia, and Paradise had about the expected number of fatalities. These different fatality rates probably resulted from the Camp Fire striking the residential portion of Concow earliest and most completely and Magalia later with proportionately less destruction.

Disability and Camp Fire Fatalities

The fatalities' difficulties by census category are presented in table 6.2. Overall, thirty-six (42.9%) of the eighty-four identified individuals fell into at least one of the census categories. Among the identified fatalities, ambulatory difficulties were the most prevalent disability, being present in 34.5 percent (*n*=29) of the Camp Fire fatalities. Examples of ambulatory difficulties in the Camp Fire fatalities included an amputated leg, reliance on a walker, and sprained ankle. As a specific example, one eighty-year-old male had a severely sprained ankle, which had temporarily limited his mobility. Although the morning of the fire he made several phone calls requesting aid, his rescue did not occur, and his remains were found inside his residence (Ramsey 2020, 11).

Cognitive and independent living difficulties were the two next most common disabilities (both n=5, 6%). Dementia was the most common cognitive difficulty mentioned. As an example, the remains of an eighty-six-year-old female, who had dementia and was in failing health, were discovered in her Paradise home (Ramsey 2020, 17). The most common independent living difficulty involved the need for a caretaker.

Table 6.2   Disability difficulties among Camp Fire fatalities by American Community Survey categories (2017)[a]

Disability Category	Number	Percentage of total fatalities
Difficulty in one or more categories	36	42.9%
Ambulatory difficulty	29	34.5%
Cognitive difficulty	5	6.0%
Independent living difficulty	5	6.0%
General, nondescript difficulty	3	3.6%
Self-care difficulty	2	2.4%
Hearing difficulty	1	1.2%
Vision difficulty	1	1.2%

[a] The one unidentified Camp Fire fatality was excluded from these calculations, reducing the total to 84 fatalities.
Sources: Butte County Sheriff's Office (2019), Chico Enterprise-Record (2019), Ramsey (2020)

In addition, three (3.6%) individuals were noted as having been "handicapped" or "debilitated" by recent medical procedures (Chico Enterprise-Record 2020; Ramsey 2020). As an example, remains of a seventy-eight-year-old male who was recovering from heart surgery were found in his Paradise residence (Ramey 2020, 15). Although they did not fit existing categories, the mention of their impairments by family members and BCSO was important. Two (2.4%) individuals suffered self-care difficulty associated with immobility. As an example, the body of an eighty-one-year-old female, who had a caregiver from 9 a.m. until 9 p.m. daily, was found in her Paradise home (Ramsey 2020, 12). Hearing and vision difficulties were each observed in one (1.2%) fatality.

Comparing the frequency of difficulties among the Camp Fire decedents to that of the CFCs Survey census data revealed a marked difference in ambulatory difficulties. The rate of ambulatory difficulties among the Camp Fire fatalities (34.5%) was more than double the rate of the CFCs (13.8%). As expected, this difference in ambulatory rates between the Camp Fire fatalities and the CFCs proved statistically significant (χ^2=35.4192, df=1, P<0.00001). Hearing and vision difficulties among Camp Fire fatalities were much lower than the CFCs and lower even than the California and U.S. rates. Independent living difficulties among the Camp Fire fatalities were comparable to those of California and the United States, but lower than the CFCs. Cognitive and self-care difficulties among Camp Fire fatalities were roughly equal to the rates for California and the United States and between the low and high end of the CFCs.

DISCUSSION

This section presents comparisons and the broader implications of these results as well as the limitations of our approach. We consider fire deaths on the national level, Camp Fire survivors living in care facilities, the number of Camp Fire fatalities, sequelae following the fire, and the limitation of Camp Fire victims' disability information.

Comparisons with California and U.S. Studies

As has been demonstrated elsewhere previously and involving other kinds of disasters (e.g., Knowles and Garrison 2006, Mosby et al. 2021, Powell et al. 2009, Tokesky and Weston 2006), Camp Fire victims consisted of a disproportionate number of older adults and persons with impairments. The Camp Fire mortality data show similarities with fatalities of larger geopolitical units, including those in California and the United States. In a recent twenty-year review (2000–2020) of California wildfires, Masri et al. (2021) found larger areas being burned in recent decades. Those burnt areas had greater proportions of older inhabitants and lower income residents, including lower median household incomes, and lower property values. Thus, the Camp Fire's destruction of the CFCs was not an isolated event on the state level.

Examining U.S. mortality statistics during a recent ten-year period (2008-2017), fire deaths varied annually from 2855 to 3400 fatalities, increasing by 9.6 percent in that decade (U.S. Fire Administration 2019, 10). The report presents all fatalities related to burning, including deaths occurring in residences, non-residences, vehicles, outside, and "other" fires (U.S. Fire Administration 2019). Among these categories, the greatest number of fire fatalities occurred in residential structures (77.6%), followed by vehicle fires (15.2%), and outside fires trailing far behind (only 1.9%; U.S. Fire Administration 2019, 15, figure 3). "Wildland" fire fatalities constitute only a portion of the outside fires. Thus, as attention-getting as wildfires are and as much media coverage as they receive, they constitute only a small part of overall fire-related deaths at the national level. Nevertheless, outside fire fatalities, the category that includes wildland fires, increased markedly in the decade studied, more than doubling what it had been at the beginning of the study period (U.S. Fire Administration 2019, 36). Notably, the report highlighted outside/wildland fires as a topic of growing concern.

The report on the U.S. fire fatalities also assessed demographic data. Overall, the national report recognized that some groups of people have greater fire-related susceptibilities. Vulnerable groups included males, African Americans, Native Americans, the elderly, and those with limited physical and cognitive abilities (U.S. Fire Administration 2019, 4). Consequently, the report declared that all of those vulnerable groups deserve additional attention and should be emphasized in planning and protection. However, later in the report, when areas of particular concern were stressed (U.S. Fire Administration 2019, 5), all of those categories just listed were repeated *except* those individuals with limited physical and cognitive abilities. Accidental or purposeful, their omission was inexcusable.

"Institutionalized" Infirm and Elderly

For the more severely infirm members of the CFCs, institutional aid was available. "Institutionalized" members included people in the hospital (i.e., Feather River Hospital) and "nursing homes," "assisted living facilities," as well as in "elder care accommodations." Although according to our results, they should have been among the most vulnerable individuals and most prone to fire-related deaths, nearly all of the institutionalized people were evacuated safely and survived. The single exception to that generalization was an eighty-eight-year-old male who lived in a Paradise "retirement community" bungalow. He apparently slept through the staff's attempts to rouse him and perished (Gee and Anguiano 2020). With this exception, it was not the "institutionalized" impaired who perished in the Camp Fire. It was mostly the infirm and disabled living relatively independent lives who died.

Three possible explanations emerge for these observations. First, it may represent a continuum of vulnerability with the most vulnerable individuals being better cared for and more protected. Consequently, the most vulnerable were more likely to receive critical information about the fire's approach and be subject to mandatory evacuation. Second, socioeconomic status may explain the observations. People who are more prosperous have greater resources, and they can afford better care, including assisted-living attention. During catastrophic events, they may be better protected, more favored, and more likely to be evacuated. Lastly, independently oriented individuals may be at greater risk. They may resist "institutionalized" living, remain in private residences, live in single-person households, and may be more vulnerable during catastrophic events. Others, who are more socially engaged and/or more dependent on others, may fare better in disasters. They may receive more timely information, have greater social bonds that support them, and have essential decisions forced on them.

Counting Fatalities, Counting Victims

In this work, we have studied the official eighty-five Camp Fire fatalities, and we have excluded other unofficial deaths as well as long-term injuries and displacements that the wildfire caused. Beyond the eighty-five Camp Fire deaths, media sources claimed that an additional fifty lives were lost, many of them elderly or ill (Von Kaenel 2020). For the purposes of legal proceedings and other official listings, however, those additional fifty were excluded as Camp Fire fatalities. In some wildfires, fatalities attributed to those other fires have sometimes included persons dying from causes indirectly related to a fire or from stress related to the event in addition to those dying directly from thermal injuries received from the fires. Examples of indirect associated fatalities include firefighters dying in a helicopter crash (Iron Alps Complex Fire 2010) as well as evacuees dying of an apparent heart attack or post-evacuation fall (Harris Fire 2007). Re-defining the Camp Fire fatalities beyond the official count would have cast a larger net and may have indicated even greater vulnerabilities among the disabled and elderly.

In additional to the Camp Fire fatalities, another parameter that should be considered is fire-related non-fatal injuries and fire-related sequelae. Officially, three people were injured in the Camp Fire and survived (Cal Fire 2019). However, they constituted the mere tip of the injury and casualty iceberg. Subsequent challenges for people who survived the Camp Fire included cramped evacuation centers and exposure to illness while there. As a particularly telling example, in the days following their escape from the fire, some Camp Fire evacuees were exposed to norovirus while staying in shelters. In one shelter, more than 25 percent of the evacuees suffered from the disease (Karmarkar et al. 2020). Although that report did not document the socioeconomic status, age, sex, or disability of the evacuees, we suspect the same characteristics of the Camp Fire fatalities would have made similar evacuees more vulnerable to becoming ill and its severity. The poor, elderly, socially isolated, and disabled would be the most susceptible among the evacuees, both immediately following the fire as well as during the longer recovery period.

Limitations of Disability Data for Camp Fire Victims

This analysis is limited by its ability to identify impairment among the Camp Fire fatalities. Our information came from two main sources. After the fire, family and friends recounted their loved one's lives in published reminiscences, some of which included incidental information about impairment. We did not systematically survey or query loved ones concerning disability of the deceased. As the second major source, the medical records available through BCSO were limited to information that could assist in identification of the unknowns, such as the use of hearing aids or an amputated limb. Neither source serves as an adequate substitute for detailed assessment or thorough medical documentation. Consequently, it is likely that the impairment data we used substantially undercounted the actual rate of impairment among the Camp Fire fatalities. In all likelihood, the frequency of impairment was probably far greater among the victims than we were able to document.

CONCLUSION

The purpose of this chapter was to establish the most vulnerable groups in the CFCs by examining traits that occur in higher-than-expected rates among the Camp Fire fatalities. In that process, we showed which CFCs' members were most likely to require the services of forensic anthropologists. Of the many possible vulnerabilities, older-aged residents and those with ambulatory impairments emerged as the most at risk of dying. Camp Fire victims were on average two decades older than overall community members and one-third of the victims had ambulatory difficulties, over twice the rate found in the community. In terms of their age profile, they displayed neither the classic U- or L-shaped mortality distributions, but instead a reverse L-shaped curve.

In addition to widely recognized difficulty categories, old age often includes impairments. We suspect that the ailments and challenges faced by most elderly adults have been overlooked or diminished as impairments, including hearing, vision, self-care, cognitive, and mobility issues that may go unreported by the sufferer. Those impairments are often considered a normal part of the aging process, emerging slowly over many years. But even this predictable process alone may impede a person's ability to prepare for and escape from catastrophic events.

In addition to age and mobility vulnerabilities, we explored another, spatial avenue to understand vulnerabilities. The Camp Fire has been considered "Paradise's fire." Of the three settlements in the CFCs, Paradise sustained the greatest number of fatalities as well as the greatest property damage. However, Concow suffered a greater proportion of fatalities than either of the other two settlements. In addition to demographic and socioeconomic reasons, the Camp Fire struck Concow first (thirty minutes after ignition), giving residents little time for warnings and evacuations. As well, Concow had fewer escape routes than the other CFCs. Only later did the fire strike Paradise and Magalia, providing more time for those residents to become aware of the danger and flee along several major arterial roadways.

Wildfires in California and elsewhere will intensify as the climate warms, the environment dries, and urban expansion into wildland areas increases. Wildland-urban interface and population density are among the major factors in wildfire mortality (Chen et al. 2021). As an example, within the state, seven of the twenty deadliest wildfires in California history have occurred in the last five years (Cal Fire 2020). Failure to identify vulnerable groups and address their particular needs for emergency notifications, evacuation, and other assistance will cost additional lives.

To prepare for these eventualities, governmental policies for fire-prone areas must emphasize the most vulnerable residents. At the planning stage, people must be made aware of potential threats and prepare to act when a disaster occurs. Having reliance in the warning system, knowing the responsibilities of agencies, and establishing "bridging actors" both before and during a catastrophe are essential (Faas et al. 2017). More effective emergency alert systems need to be installed, tested, used, and made available to all citizens. As with other hazards, individuals display complex and manifold reactions to, and interpretations of, wildfires (McCaffrey 2004). Wildfires are more than natural disasters; they include cultural dynamics involving economic, social, and political variables (Charnley et al. 2015).

Fortunately, there are some examples of success in organizing the diverse number of roles involved in disaster scenarios to mitigate loss of life and property. The 2017 Thomas Fire was at one time the largest wildfire in California history (now the seventh largest; Cal Fire 2021). Before that fire season, Montecito, California, had faced repeated wildfire exposure. The Montecito Fire Protection District embarked on a two-decade-long project to educate and promote community awareness of wildfire mitigation through increased engagement between community members and agencies. This undertaking included engaging in-person with older and disabled adults about how to best accommodate them in space clearing and evacuation efforts. These efforts reduced property damage and saved lives (Kolden and Henson 2019) and serve as a successful model to be emulated.

Since its inception, forensic anthropology has stood at the juncture of biological and social interests, applying the field's unique perspectives to broad, usually practical, matters. Recently, forensic anthropology has moved beyond its traditional emphasis on skeletons in civil cases and war dead into new realms and contributing to theoretical discourse. For example, migrant deaths, international concerns, crimes against humanity, and mass fatality incidents have emerged as focal points. Among those issues that have captured recent emphasis are fatalities resulting from wildfires. Forensic anthropologists can use their unique skills and perspectives to understand wildfires and their victims, identify the most vulnerable people in these circumstances, recommend steps to diminish wildfire deaths, and failing that, aid in finding, recovering, and identifying those who perished.

NOTE

1. Acknowledgments: Nearly seventy-five volunteer anthropologists labored on the Camp Fire recoveries and identifications. Most volunteers were Chico State faculty and staff members, and former and present undergraduate and graduate students. In addition to us in the direst of times, colleagues and students from Universities of Nevada, Las Vegas, and Reno as well as members of other outside agencies rushed to our aid. Once the embers cooled and thoughts turned to interpreting the disaster, Chico

State Merriam librarians aided our research. They included James Tyler, Pamela Nett Kruger, and especially George H. Thompson, who directed our census work. Butte County Sheriff Office officials provided much-needed information. In particular, we thank Investigative Assistant Jen Celentano and Investigative Sergeant Steve Collins for their support and access to the Camp Fire fatality data. Ashley Kendell, Colleen Milligan, and Alison Galloway included our Camp Fire demography research in their 2020 American Academy of Forensic Sciences symposium and gave us permission for its elaboration into the area of disability and impairment. Cartographer Judy Stolen drew the map of the Camp Fire region. Casey Hegel worked closely with us concerning the locations and demography of the Camp Fire fatalities and double-checked much of our data. We look forward to her thesis mapping the Camp Fire and its victims. Two anonymous peer reviewers provided much-appreciated criticisms and suggestions on an earlier and much rougher draft manuscript. Finally, our thanks go to Jennifer Byrnes and Iván Sandoval-Cervantes for including this work in their volume.

REFERENCES

Ablon, Joan. 1995. "The Elephant Man's 'Self' and 'Other': The Psycho-Social Costs of a Misdiagnosis." *Social Science & Medicine* 40 (11): 1481–1489.

Barnes, Colin. 1991. *Disabled People in Britain and Discrimination: A Case for Anti-Discrimination Legislation*. London: Hurst & Co.

Barrios, Roberto E. 2017. "What Does Catastrophe Reveal for Whom? The Anthropology of Crises and Disasters at the Onset of the Anthropocene." *Annual Review of Anthropology* 46: 151–166.

Berg, Robert, and Joseph S. Cassells. 1992. "Social Isolation among Older Individuals: The Relationship to Mortality and Morbidity." In *The Second Fifty Years: Promoting Health and Preventing Disability*, edited by Robert L. Berg and Joseph Cassells, 243–262. Washington, DC: National Academies Press.

Brewer, Matthew J., and Craig B. Clements. 2020. "The 2018 Camp Fire: Meteorological Analysis Using In Situ Observations and Numerical Simulations." *Atmosphere* 11 (1): 47.

Butte County Sheriff's Office. 2019. "Camp Fire Data Sheets." Excel spreadsheet titled "CAMP FIRE DATA SHEETS CSUC 2019."

Byrnes, Jennifer F., and Jennifer L. Muller. 2017. "Mind the Gap: Bridging Disability Studies and Bioarchaeology—An Introduction." In *Bioarchaeology of Impairment and Disability*, edited by Jennifer F. Byrnes and Jennifer L. Muller, 1–15. Cham: Springer.

Cal Fire. 2019. "Camp Fire. November 15, 2019." California Department of Forestry and Fire Protection. https://fire.ca.gov/incident/?incident=75dafe80-f18a-4a4a-9a37-4b564c5f6014. Accessed February 27, 2021.

———. 2020. "Top 20 Deadliest California Wildfires." California Department of Forestry and Fire Protection. https://www.fire.ca.gov/media/lbfd0m2f/top20_deadliest.pdf. Accessed December 15, 2020.

————. 2021. "Top 20 Largest California Wildfires." California Department of Forestry and Fire Protection. https://www.fire.ca.gov/media/4jandlhh/top20_acres .pdf. Accessed May 4, 2021.

Centers for Disease Control and Prevention. 2015. "Indicator Definitions." In *Chronic Disease Indicators.* https://www.cdc.gov/cdi/definitions/older-adults .html. Accessed May 22, 2021.

Chamberlain, Andrew. 2006. *Demography in Archaeology.* Cambridge: Cambridge University Press.

Charnley, Susan, Melissa R. Poe, Alan A. Ager, Thomas A. Spies, Emily K. Platt, and Keith A. Olsen. 2015. "A Burning Problem: Social Dynamics of Disaster Risk Reduction through Wildfire Mitigation." *Human Organization* 74 (4): 329–340.

Chen, Bin, Yufang Jin, Erica Scaduto, Max A. Moritz, Michael L. Goulden, and James T. Randerson. 2021. "Climate, Fuel, and Land Use Shaped the Spatial Pattern of Wildfire in California's Sierra Nevada." *Journal of Geophysical Research: Biogeosciences* 126 (2): e2020JG005786.

Chico Enterprise-Record. 2019. "85 Lives, 85 Stories: These Are the Lives that Ended in California's Deadliest Wildfire." *Chico Enterprise-Record.* 2019. https:// extras.chicoer.com/campfireremembrances/. Accessed January 14, 2020.

Cudjoe, Thomas K. M., David L. Roth, Sarah L. Szanton, Jennifer L. Wolff, Cynthia M. Boyd, and Roland J. Thorpe, Jr. 2020. "The Epidemiology of Social Isolation: National Health and Aging Trends Study." *Journals of Gerontology: Social Sciences* Series B 75 (1): 107–113.

Domonoske, Camila, Barbara Campbell, and Richard Gonzales. 2018. "More than 1,000 People Now Listed as Missing in California's Deadliest Fire." National Public Radio, November 16, 2018. https://www.npr.org/2018/11/16/668552010 /more-than-600-people-now-missing-in-californias-deadliest-fire. Accessed January 28, 2021.

Faas, A. J., Anne-Lise K. Velez, Clare FitzGerald, Branda L. Nowell, and Toddi A. Steelman. 2017. "Patterns of Preference and Practice: Bridging Actors in Wildfire Response Networks in the American Northwest." *Disasters* 41 (3): 527–548.

Gee, Alistair, and Dani Anguiano. 2020. *Fire in Paradise: An American Tragedy.* New York: W W Norton.

Gin, Kim, Jason Tovar, Eric J. Bartelink, Ashley Kendell, Colleen Milligan, P. Willey, James Wood, Eugene Tan, Rosemary S. Turingan, and Richard F. Selden. 2020. "The 2018 California Wildfires: Integration of Rapid DNA to Dramatically Accelerate Victim Identification." *Journal of Forensic Sciences* 65 (3): 791–799.

Goodley, Dan, Bill Hughes, and Lennard Davis, eds. 2012. *Disability and Social Theory: New Developments and Directions.* New York: Springer.

Kaiser Health News. 2018. "The Paradise Wildfire's Harm to Senior Citizens." November 20, 2018. https://www.usnews.com/news/healthiest-communities/ articles/2018-11-20/paradise-camp-fire-pushes-seniors-from-retirement-homes-to -field-hospitals. Accessed May 22, 2021.

Karmarkar, Ellora, Seema Jain, Jeff Higa, Jazmin Fontenot, Regina Bertolucci, Thalia Huynh et al. 2020. "Outbreak of Norovirus Illness among Wildfire Evacuation Shelter Populations — Butte and Glenn Counties, California, November 2018."

Morbidity and Mortality Weekly Report 69: 613–617. http://dx.doi.org/10.15585/mmwr.mm6920a1.

Kasnitz, Devva, and Russell P. Shuttleworth. 2001. "Anthropology in Disability Studies." *Disability Studies Quarterly* 21 (3): 2–17.

Knowles, R., and B. Garrison. 2006. "Planning for Elderly in Natural Disasters." *Disaster Recovery Journal* 19 (4): 1904–1907.

Kolden, Crystal A., and Carol Henson. 2019. "A Socio-Ecological Approach to Mitigating Wildfire Vulnerability in the Wildland Urban Interface: A Case Study from the 2017 Thomas Fire." *Fire* 2 (1): 1–19.

Kumar, Anand, and Barry Smith. 2005. "The Ontology of Processes and Functions: A Study of the International Classification of Functioning, Disability and Health." In *Proceedings of the AIME 2005 Workshop on Biomedical Ontology Engineering, Aberdeen, Scotland.*

Lyman, R. Lee. 1987. "On the Analysis of Vertebrate Mortality Profiles: Sample Size, Mortality Type, and Hunting Pressure." *American Antiquity* 52 (1): 125–142.

Masri, Shahir, Erica Scaduto, Yufang Jin, and Jun Wu. 2021. "Disproportionate Impacts of Wildfires among Elderly and Low-Income Communities in California from 2000–2020." *International Journal of Environmental Research and Public Health* 18 (8): 3921–3939. https://doi.org/10.3390/ijerph18083921.

Mass, Clifford F., and David Ovens. 2021. "The Synoptic and Mesoscale Evolution Accompanying the 2018 Camp Fire of Northern California." *Bulletin of the American Meteorological Society* 102 (1): E168–E192.

McCaffrey, Sarah. 2004. "Thinking of Wildfire as a Natural Hazard." *Society and Natural Resources* 17 (6): 509–516.

McDermott, Ray, and Hervé Varenne. 1995. "Culture as Disability." *Anthropology & Education Quarterly* 26 (3): 324–348.

Milligan, Colleen, Alison Galloway, Ashley Kendell, Lauren Zephro, P. Willey, and Eric Bartelink. MS "Recovery and Identification of Fatal Fire Victims from the 2018 Northern California Camp Fire Disaster." For *The Forensic Analysis of Burned Human Remains*, edited by Sarah Ellingham, Joe Adserias, Sara C. Zapico and Doug Ubelaker. New York: Wiley. Manuscript submitted April 2021.

Moffitt, Bob. 2019. "Many Residents Did Not Receive Emergency Alerts During the Camp Fire. Will You Be Warned If A Disaster Is Heading Your Way?" Capradio, July 11, 2019. https://www.capradio.org/articles/2019/07/11/emergency-alert-will-you-be-notified-if-a-wildfire-is-heading-toward-your-town/. Accessed January 28, 2021.

Mosby, Kim, Traci Birch, Aimee Moles, and Katie E. Cherry. 2021. "Disasters." In *Handbook of Rural Aging*, edited by Lenard W. Kaye, 111–115. Milton Park, UK: Routledge.

Murphy, Robert, Jessica Sheer, Yolanda Murphy, and Richard Mack. 1988. "Physical Disability and Social Liminality: A Study in the Rituals of Adversity." *Social Science & Medicine* 26 (2): 235–242.

National Academies of Sciences, Engineering, and Medicine. 2020. *Social Isolation and Loneliness in Older Adults: Opportunities for the Health Care System.* Washington, DC: The National Academies Press. https://doi.org/10.17226/25663.

Newberry, Laura. 2019. "Poor, Elderly and Too Frail to Escape: Paradise Fire Killed the Most Vulnerable Residents." *Los Angeles* Times, February 10, 2019. https://www.latimes.com/local/lanow/la-me-ln-camp-fire-seniors-mobile-home-deaths-20190209-story.htmlParadise. Accessed May 22, 2021.

Oliver, Michael. 1990. *The Politics of Disablement.* Basingstoke: Macmillan.

———. 2004. "The Social Model in Action: If I Had a Hammer." *Implementing the Social Model of Disability: Theory and Research* 2: 18–31.

———. 2013. "The Social Model of Disability: Thirty Years On." *Disability & Society* 28 (7): 1024–1026. https://doi.org/10.1080/09687599.2013.818773.

Oliver-Smith, Anthony. 1999. "What Is a Disaster? Anthropological Perspectives on a Persistent Question." In *The Angry Earth: Disaster in Anthropological Perspective*, edited by Anthony Oliver-Smith and Susanna M. Hoffman, 18–34. Milton Park: Routledge.

Oliver-Smith, Anthony, and Susanna M. Hoffman. 2002. "Introduction: Why Anthropologists Should Study Disasters." In *Catastrophe and Culture: The Anthropology of Disaster*, edited by Susanna M. Hoffman and Anthony Oliver-Smith, 3–22. Santa Fe, NM: School of American Research Press.

Pilloud, Marin A., Eric J. Bartelink, Ashley Kendell, and Colleen Milligan. 2020. "Forensic Anthropology in a Changing Climate." *Anthropology News* website, April 22, 2020. https://doi.org/10.1111/AN.1388.

Powell, Simone, Louise Plouffe, and Patti Gorr. 2009. "When Ageing and Disasters Collide: Lessons from 16 International Case Studies." *Radiation Protection Dosimetry* 134 (3–4): 202–206.

Ramsey, Michael L. 2020. "The Camp Fire Public Report: A Summary of the Camp Fire Investigation. June 16, 2020." Butte County District Attorney's Office, Oroville, California. PGE-the-CAMP-FIRE-PUBLIC-REPORT.pdf. Accessed December 15, 2020.

Roush, Susan E., and Nancy Sharby. 2011. "Disability Reconsidered: The Paradox of Physical Therapy." *Physical Therapy* 91: 1715–1727.

Shakespeare, Tom. 2006. "The Social Model of Disability." *The Disability Studies Reader* 2: 197–204.

———. 2013. *Disability Rights and Wrongs Revisited.* Milton Park: Routledge.

Shuttleworth, Russell P., and Devva Kasnitz. 2004. "Stigma, Community, Ethnography: Joan Ablon's Contribution to the Anthropology of Impairment-Disability." *Medical Anthropology Quarterly* 18 (2): 139–161.

Siebers, Tobin. 2008. *Disability Theory.* Ann Arbor: University of Michigan Press.

Solli, Hans M., and António Barbosa da Silva. 2012. "The Holistic Claims of the Biopsychosocial Conception of WHO's International Classification of Functioning, Disability, and Health (ICF): A Conceptual Analysis on the Basis of a Pluralistic-Holistic Ontology and Multidimensional View of the Human Being." *Journal of Medicine and Philosophy* 37 (3): 277–294.

Thomas, Carol. 2004. "Developing the Social Relational in the Social Model of Disability: A Theoretical Agenda." In *Implementing the Social Model of Disability: Theory and Research*, edited by Colin Barnes and Geof Mercer, 32–47. Leeds: The Disability Press.

Todd, Zoe, Sydney Trattner, and Jane McMullen. 2019. "Ahead of Camp Fire Anniversary, New Details Emerge of Troubled Evacuation." October 25, 2019. https://www.pbs.org/wgbh/frontline/article/camp-fire-anniversary-new-details -troubled-evacuation/. Accessed January 28, 2021.

Tokesky, G., and M. Weston. 2006. "Impacts and Contributions of Older Persons in Emergency Situations: A Case Study of Hurricane Katrina in the United States of America." Unpublished report. Geneva: World Health Organization.

Union of the Physically Impaired Against Segregation. 1976. *Fundamental Principles of Disability*. London: Union of the Physically Impaired Against Segregation.

United States Census Bureau. 2010. "P12: Sex by Age." 2010 Census. U.S. Census Bureau. https://data.census.gov/cedsci/. Accessed January 28, 2021.

———. 2017. "S1810: Disability Characteristics." 2017 American Community Survey. U.S. Census Bureau's American Community Survey Office. https://data .census.gov/cedsci/. Accessed January 28, 2021.

United States Fire Administration. 2019. "Fire in the United States 2008-2017." https://www.usfa.fema.gov/data/statistics/reports/fius_2008-2017.html. Accessed November 12, 2020.

Von Kaenel, Camille. 2020. "Official Camp Fire tally is 85 deaths, but we found 50 more". *The Mercury News*, February 15, 2020. https://www.mercurynews. com/2020/02/15/official-camp-fire-tally-is-85-deaths-but-we-found-50-more/ Accessed February 27, 2021.

Wigtil, Gabriel, Roger B. Hammer, Jeffrey D. Kline, Miranda H. Mockrin, Susan I. Stewart, Daniel Roper, and Volker C. Radeloff. 2016. "Places Where Wildfire Potential and Social Vulnerability Coincide in the Coterminous United States." *International Journal of Wildland Fire* 25: 896–908.

World Health Organization. 2001. International Classification of Functioning, Disability and Health (ICF). https://apps.who.int/iris/handle/10665/42407. Accessed January 3, 2022.

———. 2018. International Classification of Functioning, Disability and Health (ICF). http://www.who.int/classifications/icf/en/. Accessed May 22, 2021.

Xu, Jiaquan, Sherry L. Murphy, Kenneth D. Kochanek, and Elizabeth Arias. 2020. "Mortality in the United States, 2018." National Center for Health Statistics Data Brief, no. 355. Hyattsville, Maryland: National Center for Health Statistics.

Yang, K. Lisa, and Hock E. Tan. 2018. "Disability Statistics." https://disabilitystatis-tics.org/sources-DS.cfm. Accessed December 19, 2020.

Chapter 7

Gender Identities and Intersectional Violence within Forensic Anthropology

Jaxson D. Haug

INTRODUCTION

It is understood that the gender-diverse population is socially positioned for structural vulnerability and an extremely high risk of facing numerous levels of violence (Meyer 2008; Stotzer 2009; Quesada, Hart, and Bourgois 2011; James et al. 2016; Rodriguez, Agardh, and Asomoah 2018). Organizations such as Trans Murder Monitoring (TMM) have been focusing on the murders of gender-diverse individuals across the globe and their findings show that 3,314 gender-diverse individuals were killed between January 2008 and September 2019 (Fedorko, Kurmanov, and Berredo 2020). Violence is typically thought of as strictly physical, yet violence has many layers beyond physicality (Krug et al. 2002). Violence can be broken down into three categories: self, interpersonal, and collective (Krug et al. 2002). Each one of those categories can further be broken down, which will be explained later in this chapter. Using an understanding of Kimberlé Crenshaw's intersectionality theory, this work touches on how forensic anthropologists may be inadvertently perpetuating violence toward the gender-diverse population. An understanding of intersectional violence will allow forensic anthropology to break the pattern and move forward as a more inclusive field.

An ever-growing challenge within the field of forensic anthropology is the application and understanding of gender identities. There has been a lack of formalized attempts to include gender within a biological profile. However, there have been recent studies that have taken place to help create a more gender-diverse forensic anthropology (e.g., Buchanan 2014; Bouderdaben 2019; Cirillo et al. 2020; Haug 2020a and b; Kincer 2020; Michael et al. 2020; Schall, Rogers, and Deschamps-Braly 2020; Tallman, Kincer, and

Plemons 2022). Currently, there are no distinct methods available to positively identify an individual as transgender within forensic anthropology. In one sense, this arguably makes sense, as gender identity is not a biological classification; however, the absence of methods leaves anthropologists complicit in rendering gender-diverse people invisible. In short, the exclusion of gender identity within the biological profile and the resulting invisibility of gender-diverse identities help perpetuate the cycle of violence experienced by the community.

These issues are complex, and understandings of identity are constantly evolving. The goal of this chapter is to highlight the unintentional violence being perpetrated by forensic anthropologists through the current discourse of gender within the biological profile and how forensic anthropology can move forward as a field. It is argued that the ways in which forensic anthropologists employ sex needs to be reconceptualized to include discussions on gender to properly halt the perpetuation of violence toward the gender-diverse community. To truly understand the importance of reconceptualization in reporting sex, forensic anthropologists need to utilize understandings of intersectionality, violence, and the cycle of socialization.

Sex, often discussed as *biological sex*, is a well-known and understood portion of the forensic anthropology biological profile. While it is typically referred to as *biological sex* within anthropology, this work will be using the term based on the standards set out by the World Professional Association of Transgender Health (WPATH), which is assigned sex at birth (Bouman et al. 2017). *Gender* and *assigned sex at birth* are frequently confused and used interchangeably which, as this chapter will further discuss, is problematic. Within this chapter, the terms *transgender* and *gender-diverse* will be used interchangeably.

Ultimately, what should be taken away from this chapter is that there needs to be acknowledgment and movement within forensic anthropology past the current binary notions of sex and gender. The emphasis within forensic anthropological casework should be on acknowledgment past the binary and not on gender estimation as this cannot be done. As a field, forensic anthropology needs to reconceptualize its binary assessment of sex and gender within forensic casework.

TERMINOLOGY

Language is complex, and meanings are consistently changing throughout space and time (Bouman et al. 2017). This is seen in cases where once acceptable terms, such as *hermaphrodite* or *transexual*, are viewed as pejorative and although they are occasionally still used in certain localities and fields, they are generally understood to be negative (Bouman et al. 2017). In relation to the discussion at hand, language and terminology deeply permeate spaces both within and outside forensic anthropology. Language use can and often historically has been utilized as a weapon of systemic oppression of marginalized groups, as well as a tool to fuel stereotypes (Bouman et al. 2017). This permeation of anthropological research into popular society can be seen in such discussions where binary language use fueled gendered stereotypes, such as "man the hunter" and "woman the gatherer" (Slocum 1975).

It is important to recognize the weight that language holds as forensic anthropologists move forward with research and recommendations of gender diversity within casework. While this work attempts to follow WPATH language recommendations, these terms may not be the only ways or the best way to address certain aspects now or in the future. What is currently understood as "gender," the social aspects of assigned sex at birth, did not come into popular language until the 1950s (Hausman 1995). The current accepted umbrella term *transgender* was not applied to popular use until the 1990s (Weismantel 2013). Even currently, many terms are contested within the gender-diverse community and what is an appropriate term for some may not be appropriate for others. For example, individuals may choose to identify as transsexual even if others in the community associate negative connotations with this term. It is important to recognize these differences when moving forward with research and recommendations for the inclusion of gender diversity within forensic casework.

IDENTITIES

The term *identity*, while usually broadly defined, lacks a strict agreed upon definition. Here, *identity* is defined as an individual's sense of belonging to particular broader groups. Specifically, it is a sense of identification with certain groups for how the individual and that group perceives them (Díaz-Andreu et al. 2005). Identities are not always static and can be defined by individual agency (Díaz-Andreu et al. 2005).

While identity is multidimensional, the primary identity of focus here is gender. Much like gender identity and sex get confused, gender identity and sexual orientation are frequently conflated. In short, sexual orientation, or sexuality, is not the same as gender identity and is the spectrum of attraction an individual has for other individual(s), such as homosexual, bisexual, heterosexual, queer, and pansexual (APA 2015; Fausto-Sterling 2012; Nanda 2014). While it can be part of an intersecting portion of an individual's identity, it is not gender identity nor is it assigned sex at birth.

Individuals have many dimensions of identity, and those dimensions overlap. In this case, the overlap, or intersectionality, plays a role in the violence experienced by members of the gender-diverse community. Gender identity is individual, yet it is developed within the confines of a particular culture, making it complex and situational (Fausto-Sterling 2012). In this sense, what is important for forensic anthropology is to understand the ways in which gender intersects with assigned sex at birth and violence.

For most, gender identity begins based on assigned sex at birth, designated by a physicians' perception of a newborn's external genitalia (Fausto-Sterling 2012). This designation is either male or female. If a newborn has ambiguous genitalia, the physician and family often decide on what is an appropriate external sex based on available tissues, often during the first few weeks of life (Money, Hampson, and Hampson 1955; Karkazis 2008). This is the start of gendered socialization and the beginnings of understanding the complexity of comprehending the differences of sex and gender (Fausto-Sterling 2012).

Gender

Much of the Western world has boiled gender down to the binary oppositions of male or female. Gender, however, does not exist in a binary vacuum; it is a fluid spectrum. While many people identify as male or female, there are numerous other gender identities. Cross-cultural comparison reveals considerable non-binary variability. We see counters to the gender binary in various cultures across the globe, such as the Hijras in India (Nanda 2014). Gender, unlike assigned sex at birth, cannot be determined through biology. Gender is a social category with constraints rooted in any culture at any point in time (Butler 2004; Mardell 2016; Nanda 2014). What one culture emphasizes about gender may not be the same as another, nor do all cultures place gender as an important category of social position (Nanda 2014). Meaning, gender categories are not universal and in short, not as cut and dry as they are made out to be.

Binary gender is argued to be colonialist and capitalist—a means of oppression for systems of power (Oyewumi 1998; Lugones 2007; Nanda 2014; Lugones 2020). Indigenous sex, gender roles, and ideologies were affected with the introduction of European encounters, practically destroying this diversity (Nanda 2014). This can be seen in locations such as the pre-Euro-American contact Philippines, where gender roles had been largely complimentary and egalitarian, as were various other Southeast Asian cultures (Peletz 2009; Nanda 2014). Tables 7.1 and 7.2 illustrate some examples of cultures with more than two genders, as well as the spectrum of gender identities. This is not an exhaustive list of cultures with non-binary genders or identities, but merely illustrative of known cultural forms of gender identity.

Table 7.1 Examples of Cultures with Nonbinary Genders

Category	Location of Origin
The Alyha and Hwame	Indigenous Mohave/Mojave-of the Mojave Desert
Fa'afafine and Fa'afatama	Samoa
Hijras and Sādhin	Hindu India
Waria and Bissu	Indonesia
Māhū	Native Hawaii
Suku	Maidu of Northern California

Source: Nanda 2014.

Table 7.2 Spectrum of Gender Identities

Identity	Definition
Agender	Gender Neutral or lack of a gender
Bigender	Fluctuation of both "male" and "female" genders
Cisgender	Congruence of given sex and gender identity
Gender Variant	Individuals who do not match societal gender expectations
Genderqueer	Umbrella term for gender non-conforming/non-binary individuals
Non-binary	Umbrella term for genders that don't fall under exclusive "masculinity/femininity."
Transgender	Umbrella term for individuals with an incongruence between their given sex and gender presentation. Can include but not limited to identities such as: genderqueer, non-binary, gender fluid, among others.
Two-Spirit	Traditionally used in Indigenous cultures in recognition of individuals who have "male" and "female" qualities.

Sources: APA 2015; Garofalo et al. 2006; Haug 2020a; Hayon and Stevenson 2019; Human Rights Campaign 2019; Mardell 2016; Stotzer 2009.

Lorber (1994) placed gender into two categories: as a social institution and as expressed by an individual. This conceptualization of gender helps to understand the intersectionality of the identity itself, as it is both social and individual. In relation to the subject of this chapter, gender is in reference to both social institutions and individual self. The lack of gender within forensic identification could be understood at both a social-institution level and at an individual level. The effects of the exclusion of gender identity within forensic anthropology, however, are seen at a social-institution level.

Gender identity is structured by an individual's culture and society (Fausto-Sterling 2012; Nanda 2014). What is considered masculine in America is not necessarily masculine elsewhere. The ideas of what is masculine/feminine at one point in history may not be considered masculine/feminine at a separate point in time. Gendered socialization begins at birth, and culture plays a large role in how an individual is socialized throughout life (Harro 2000; Fausto-Sterling 2012; Reby et al. 2016). Gender identity, like many other identities, has a complex relationship with power in societies. Part of the problem with transgender-based violence is rooted in the Cycle of Socialization, which is a theoretical framework that can be used to understand social identities and their intersectional roles in the world (Harro 2000).

The number of terms involved when discussing gender identity can be overwhelming (see table 7.2), especially with the continual introduction of new terms and definitions. In general, *cisgender* refers to any individual who identifies with their assigned sex at birth, male or female. The definitions for transgender have been contested, but unlike cisgender, it is more of an umbrella term which encompasses various identities such as *genderqueer*, *non-binary*, and *gender fluid*. Here, the term *transgender* covers anyone who does not identify with their assigned sex at birth and will be used interchangeably with gender-diverse individuals.

Transgender people are frequently conceptualized as necessarily desiring, participating in, or having completed medical transition. Not all transgender individuals, however, need, can, or want to medically transition. Medical transition encompasses a significant variety of approaches, including hormone replacement therapy (HRT) and surgical procedures designed to reshape both hard and soft tissues (Hayon and Stevenson 2019). Some transgender individuals socially transition but see no need for medical transition and some are precluded by underlying medical conditions. Studies suggest that between 20 percent and 40 percent of transgender individuals want surgical interventions (Grant et al. 2011; Bradford et al. 2013; Canner et al. 2018). These study estimates are limited, as they were opportunistic samples of transgender individuals. However, they show that not all transgender people want surgical interventions (Grant et al. 2011; Bradford et al. 2013; Canner et al. 2018).

Because gender is internally and culturally rooted, the expression of gender identity encompasses a vast array of lived experiences. Importantly, transgender experience is not unitary, and anthropologists should not compartmentalize those lived experiences into another binary of pre-transition or transitioned. If forensic anthropologists compartmentalize individual transitions to another binary, they are further othering and boxing transgender individuals. The pre- and post-transition binary would also place normalcy on transgender individuals needing medical interventions to prove "trans-ness." Understanding that not all transgender individuals want or need medical interventions further explains how a pre- and post-transition binary would only be harmful.

ASSIGNED SEX AT BIRTH

Assigned sex at birth is often conflated as an uncomplicated, biologically determined binary of males and females. However, sex, like gender, is exhibited on a broad spectrum (Hayon and Stevenson 2019). Further, the factors that influenced the development of physical characteristics that result in a sex being assigned at birth are complex, layered, and interact with each other during development (Fausto-Sterling 2012). Here genetic, anatomical, and hormonal systems that influence assigned sex at birth will be reviewed.

Genetic

It is generally understood that an individual's genetic sex or their sex chromosomes are more than likely going to fall either as male (XY) or female (XX). While these two arrangements of sex chromosomes are common, variation exists in the numbers of sex chromosomes, referred to as *sex chromosome aneuploidies*. Variability in chromosome numbers is more commonly seen than was once assumed (Skuse, Printzlau, and Wolstencroft 2018).

Common sex chromosome aneuploidies include, but are not limited to, Klinefelter syndrome (XXY) and Triple X syndrome (XXX). Klinefelter syndrome is seen in individuals often assigned male at birth. They typically have lowered levels of testosterone than most XY men and are frequently infertile (Fausto-Sterling 2012). Triple X syndrome is seen in individuals assigned female at birth. They may be taller than average with "normal" development; however, triple X syndrome is associated with a higher rate of learning disabilities (Fausto-Sterling 2012; Skuse, Printzlau, and Wolstencroft 2018). These aneuploidies occur at rates of 1:750 and 1:1000, respectively, making them rare but not uncommon (Morris et al. 2008; Ratcliffe 1999; Skuse, Printzlau, and Wolstencroft 2018). Thus, genetic sex is not binary in humans.

Anatomic

In many jurisdictions, doctors are required to give a binary assignment of sex based on external genitalia at birth (Bauer et al. 2017). Having only two sex assignment options leads many surgeons and families to pick a sex assignment for intersex individuals with fairly ambiguous genitalia. Genetics and hormones often play a role in anatomical sex, with certain aneuploidies and disorders affecting internal and external genitalia. For example, in Androgen insensitivity syndrome (XY), people are born with what are considered male sex chromosomes, but because they do not have receptors for testosterone, they develop feminized genitalia (Fausto-Sterling 2012). Anatomic variations can be seen with individuals having a masculinized vulva or a large clitoris or having internal sex organs that are inconsistent with their external sex organs (e.g., penis and testis with ovaries) (Fausto-Sterling 2012).

Hormonal

Hormones are regulatory molecules that convey signals in the body, and some classes are important to physiological sex development. Even hormones have general variations, such as genetic and anatomic sex; this is seen with differences in hormone ranges which are affected by genetics and developmental experiences (Fausto-Sterling 2012; Worthman 2003). It was previously understood that female was the *in utero* default, and that male sex difference is brought on by genetic differences. However, that has shifted with a deeper understanding of the SRY gene or sex reversal on the Y chromosome. With the early activation of the SRY gene, cells start to differentiate to testes that secrete testosterone and Müllerian inhibiting factor, leading to a development of male characteristics. For females, the autosomal gene Z allows female sex differentiation through the absence of the SRY gene. The sex hormones testosterone/dihydrotestosterone and estrogen/estradiol play important roles in the development of secondary sexual characteristics during adrenarche and puberty (Fausto-Sterling 2012).

Sex hormones are essential for far more than just morphological differences. Testosterone and estrogen/estradiol are both found and necessary in all human bodies and play roles in regulating mood, energy, and other non-sexed biological systems (Crocetti 2013). While they may assist in making an individual feel more at ease in their body, it is essential to understand that even though these hormones play a role in secondary sex characteristics they have nothing to do with gender identity. Androgens have been used to treat depression in women with no effect on their personal gender identity (Crocetti 2013). These hormones do have an active role in what we consider gendered bodies, which is in part how hormones have come to be seen as sexed/gendered (Crocetti 2013). The truth, however, is that these hormones play far greater roles outside of sex development and should not be viewed as binary.

INTERSEX

Individuals who are diagnosed with intersex conditions or as clinically described, disorders of sex development (DSD), are situated in a complex place, especially in relation to biological understandings of intersex diagnoses in forensic anthropology and beyond. *Intersexuality* is described as individuals born with a combination of genital, gonadal, and chromosomal male/female traits (Karkazis 2008; Reis 2009; Nanda 2014). It is important to note here that while DSD is used frequently in the medical community, many within the intersex community find the classification to be demeaning as it negatively pathologizes and others intersex bodies (Lee et al. 2016; Carpenter 2018). *Intersex* as a term is often used by advocacy groups and the intersex community as a non-pathological term so it has been argued that there may be a more appropriate clinical umbrella term, so that intersex does not become pathologized (Carpenter 2018). As there are over forty known congenital variations, neutral terminology such as congenital variations of sex development or differences of sex development are more appropriate in clinical settings as opposed to ones that are disordered and negative (Carpenter 2018).

In some cases, individuals may never know that they are intersex, or may find out later in life. Socialization and the normative ideals of binary sex and gender play large roles in the medical outcomes of intersex individuals (Karkazis 2008). Largely, medical and social interventions on intersex lives have historically been attempts to root binary notions of sex and gender within societies (Karkazis 2008). In this sense, the labeling of intersex bodies can be understood through normative ideals of what is naturally male or female (Karkazis 2008). Intersex bodies challenge normative ideals of the male/female dichotomy; therefore, society has deemed that they need to be fixed by placing them into a singular box of male/female. Through labeling and assigning intersex bodies into binary classifications, physicians and family members socially reinforce heteronormative bodies, thus continuing to other a large spectrum of individuals and continuing to play into the notion that sex is binary (Karkazis 2008).

In the past, many physicians did not discuss congenital variations of sex development with patients or families, leaving these individuals without appropriate knowledge or resources for understanding these variations (Lee et al. 2016). The labeling of intersex individuals with ambiguous genitalia at birth can also lead to various issues later in life. In particular, while not all individuals are incorrectly assigned a sex/gender, it is not rare to have intersex individuals seek gender-affirming treatment (Lee et al. 2016). While an intersex individual may be transgender or gender diverse, not all intersex individuals would classify themselves in that manner.

Human rights defenders have argued that the forced sex assignment violates human rights norms and are considered unnecessary medical procedures (Carpenter 2018). It has even been argued that the World Health Organization (WHO) should modify its International Classification of Diseases (ICD) to the neutral terminology as well as ensuring that any codes in relation to variations in sex development do not allow for violations of human rights in the form of unnecessary surgeries (Carpenter 2018).

GENDER AND ASSIGNED SEX AT BIRTH: METHODS WITHIN FORENSIC ANTHROPOLOGY

Methods for estimating assigned sex at birth are relatively straightforward and understood with metric and morphological methods for estimation. It is understood that nearly every element of the human skeleton has potential to be used in estimating assigned sex at birth; however, the two most common skeletal elements for estimation are the cranium and the *os coxa*, with accuracy rates of 80–90 percent and 96 percent, respectively (Phenice 1969; Buikstra and Ubelaker 1994; Walker 2005; Klales, Ousley, and Vollner 2012).

Most of these methods are based on size differences deriving from sexual dimorphism. Already rooted in gendered ideals, gracile features are considered distinctly feminine, and robust features are distinctly masculine; gracile typically being deemed smaller and less protuberant. Because sex differences lie on a spectrum, and are not binary, they are not always accurate. An individual can have a robust cranium, while their pelvis might show what are considered feminine traits. Sometimes, the analysis is ambiguous, and the anthropologist is left trying to draw conclusions from skeletal traits that are only minutely considered more masculine or feminine for an estimate or leaving the estimate as indeterminate.

Forensic anthropology currently lacks robust methods for estimating if a decedent may have been gender diverse. Some studies have emphasized that the skeletal markers of facial feminization surgeries (FFS) can be used as a strategy to assist with identifying transgender women postmortem (Buchanan 2014; Cirillo et al. 2020; Haug 2020a and b; Schall, Rogers, and Deschamps-Braly 2020). Their utility is undermined by the tremendous variation in pathways to transition. FFS is an expensive and time-consuming set of procedures that is not always accessible to every transgender person who might want it. Further, its use is not limited to the transgender community.

It is notable that the individuals who can afford to undergo FFS typically are not the same individuals that experience fatal violence. Transgender women of color are at the highest risk of facing fatal violence. A study looking at temporal trends in gender-affirming surgery noted that most individuals self-identified as White (Canner et al. 2018). This study also found that the number of individuals having to pay completely out-of-pocket has been steadily decreasing, but in 2014 it was around 39 percent (Canner et al. 2018). Intersectional thinking is important here. At the intersection of race and class, the healthcare disparity within the transgender community shows that these often life-saving procedures are still inaccessible to the most vulnerable individuals within the community.

As noted, assigned sex at birth and gender are not synonymous and gender is not biological. It is clear that forensic anthropologists cannot and should not assume an individual's gender identity through skeletal elements (Klales 2020; Garofalo and Garvin 2020). So why is the inclusion of gender identity important to forensic anthropology? It is not necessarily the inclusion, but the exclusion that makes a difference.

THE CYCLE OF SOCIALIZATION

Forensic anthropologists need to critically examine the harm being committed through the exclusion of gender identity with the perpetuation that assigned sex at birth is an immutable binary. Anthropologists are socialized in various settings, and therefore, are not immune to their own implicit and cognitive biases (Nakhaeizadeh, Dror, and Morgan 2014; Nakhaeizadeh, Dror, and Morgan 2020). Bobbie Harro (2000) argued that humans are born into specific unequal social identities. They further argue that individuals are socialized to these roles in the system of oppression throughout life. These roles are defined as "dominant/agent" groups being the "norm" and "subordinate/target" groups being minorities or others (Harro 2000, 17).

Harro asserts that cultures already have functioning structures of oppression in place and that individuals merely fall into this system of agent or target in each area of their identities. That is, a White, middle-class, cisgender woman would find herself in the dominant group for most of her social identities. However, intersectionality shows us that the addition of being a woman places her in an othered space in that facet of her identity. These intersections largely effect how individuals are treated within a society. For example, Crenshaw (1991) showed that intersecting racism and sexism shaped the experiences of Black women, and these experiences were often filled with disparities that White women, even those of similar identities outside of race, such as socioeconomic backgrounds, did not experience.

Harro (2000) breaks this cycle of socialization up into three main categories surrounding a core rooted in ignorance and fear: the beginning, institutional and cultural socialization, and results. This framework is used to assert that socialization of oppression is cyclical and starts off unconsciously leading individuals either to stick with the *status quo* or to disrupt the norm. This cycle beautifully illustrates how prejudice and ignorance have inherently fueled societies to maintain oppressive systems. Harro (2000) asserts that the only true way to make positive change is through those in power to act as allies to minority groups. It is important, however, to recognize the neatness of this framework. Institutionalized power is cyclical, but real experiences cannot be as clear-cut when it comes to individual lives; intersectional thinking is important here when it comes to unpacking personal biases. Understanding that everyone holds multiple ways in which they were socialized within their own societies can help forensic anthropologists work on creating more unbiased work.

Judith Butler's (2004) *Undoing Gender* attempts to find solutions for expanding the ways in which the gender-diverse community is socially recognized. This is done in two processes that are intertwined but require separate work. The first being the need to change individual thought processes to understand the ethical importance of recognizing gender-diverse and intersex bodies as being valid and important. The second process is to unravel or undo binary assumptions about gender (Butler 2004; Elliot 2016). These processes are part of undoing the teachings of normative Western socialization that the world of sex and gender are binary and anything outside of that binary is abnormal or less than (Butler 2004; Elliot 2016). In this case, forensic anthropologists must unpack their socialized biases and work to "undo" current binary assumptions toward sex and gender.

Forensic anthropologists are at a place in history where they are being directed to disrupt the norm or to continue the *status quo* of binary thinking. This can only take place if forensic anthropologists are willing to do the work to look at their own socialization and implicit biases that can, and do, find their way into even the most objective scientists' work. Anthropologists have the opportunity to take agency of their actions and have the capability to move from the *status quo* to make positive change. This is especially so when looking at the privileged status of a relatively homogenous forensic anthropology community (Tallman and Bird 2022).

WHAT IS INTERSECTIONAL VIOLENCE?

The World Health Organization (WHO) provides a useful definition of *violence*:

> the intentional use of physical force or power, threatened or actual, against oneself, another person, or against a group or community, that either results in or has a high likelihood of resulting in injury, death, psychological harm, maldevelopment, or deprivation. (Krug et al. 2002, 5)

In the World Report on Violence and Health (WRVH) (Krug et al. 2002), *violence* is broken down into three categories: *self-directed violence*, *interpersonal violence*, and *collective violence*. Each category is further subdivided based on the nature of the violence: physical, sexual, psychological, and depravation/neglect (Krug et al. 2002). While this typology is not universally accepted or perfect, it is useful in helping us understand the intersectionality of violence.

It is largely understood that violence cannot be explained away by merely biological and evolutionary theories (Accomazzo 2012). It is important to further recognize that much, like gender, colonialism has played a large role in the acts and studies of violence. Violence can only be understood when looking through multiple lenses, and part of that is understanding that implicit biases need to be considered when studying violence (Accomazzo 2012).

Violence

Self-directed violence is when the perpetrator and victim are the same. The WHO separates self-directed violence into two categories: self-abuse and suicide (Krug et al. 2002). In the case of transgender individuals within the United States, self-directed violence is largely seen through suicide where suicide attempts are significantly higher than the rate of attempts by the general U.S. population (James et al. 2016). According to the 2015 U.S. Transgender Survey, 40 percent of respondents had attempted suicide in their lifetime; at the time, this was nine times the rate of the U.S. population (James et al. 2016).

Interpersonal violence is violence between individuals. The WHO separates interpersonal violence into family/intimate partner and community violence (Krug et al. 2002). *Family/intimate partner violence* is divided into violence against a child, a partner, or an elder. *Community violence* is subcategorized depending on whether the victim is known to the perpetrator or not.

Collective violence is considered to be perpetrated by a larger group of individuals. The WHO separates collective violence into social, political, and economic. Bourdieu (1977) and Bourdieu and Wacquant (2003) explored the concept of symbolic violence, helping to frame the theories behind structural violence (Accomazzo 2012). The symbolic violence theory was so appealing because it incorporated an understanding of the dynamics of victims, perpetrators, and witnesses (Accomazzo 2012). *Structural violence* is a form of *collective violence*, defined as "a host of offenses against human dignity: extreme and relative poverty, social inequalities ranging from racism to gender inequality, and the more spectacular forms of violence that are uncontestedly human rights abuses" (Farmer 2005, 8). This violence is on a large, institutional scale and it is primarily fueled by normative social forces (Accomazzo 2012). Structural violence describes the institutionalized discrimination faced by gender-diverse individuals on a daily basis. This is the level of violence in which forensic anthropology is implicated.

Intersectionality

The term *intersectionality* was coined by Kimberlé Crenshaw in her 1989 and 1991 works, although as she notes, it was not a new theory of identity. In "Mapping the Margins," Crenshaw discussed the ways identity categories have been treated in the mainstream as non-overlapping phenomena when they are intertwined with one another. For Crenshaw, and here, this compartmentalizing approach creates otherness and builds distance, thereby marginalizing the other (Crenshaw 1991). Crenshaw used violence against women to discuss intersectionality of identities. Thus, Crenshaw argued that treating women as a homogenous whole against whom violence is perpetuated ignores aspects of identity, such as race and class, that affect the likelihood of violent experiences (Crenshaw 1991). Her work focused on showing that multiple areas of identity need to be considered to understand how "the social world is constructed" (Crenshaw 1991, 2).

Intersectionality conceptualizes the ways in which power structures are not mutually exclusive when it comes to reinforcing oppressive systems within societies (Meyer 2008). Understanding that these oppressive processes are intertwined means that forensic anthropologists need to take into account various structures in order to comprehend both their implicit biases and the reasons behind violence toward gender-diverse individuals (Meyer 2008).

While her focus did not explicitly include the gender-diverse community, Crenshaw's intersectionality theory is instructive. The gender-diverse community, too, is not defined along a single axis. Age, race, ethnicity, class, disability status, and HIV status are just some of the dimensions along which gender-diverse people exhibit variability (Open Society Foundation Public Health Program 2013). For example, the lived experiences of an upper-class, White, transgender man will not be the same as those of a poor, Black, transgender woman. In the case of this example, the intersections of race, gender identity, and socioeconomic status each apply different levels of structural inequalities on these individuals. For the Black transgender woman, statistically, her lived experiences would likely feature a larger range of structural and physical violence (Meyer 2008; James et al. 2016). Forensic anthropologists need to take into account varying aspects of an individual's identity in order to truly understand the violence being perpetuated.

How is Violence Intersectional?

All violence is intersectional, and understanding violence requires a holistic lens (Englander 2003; Meyer 2008). The WHO describes this lens as an ecological framework that helps break down violent outcomes at multiple levels (Krug et al. 2002). Victims' experiences with violence are shaped by the systems of oppression in their societies (Meyer 2008). The big picture is revealed when anthropologists take the time to look through multiple lenses. Employing a biocultural framework that encompasses theories such as intersectionality allows anthropologists to achieve this broader view. A clear grasp of these frameworks allows for the understanding that violence is perpetuated in various ways not merely through physicality.

Effects of Violence

Violence is a public health problem that impacts both society and individuals (Krug et al. 2002; Rutherford et al. 2007). Due to the intersectional nature of violence, the effects often blanket the lives of the gender-diverse community with self-directed, interpersonal, and collective violence making them structurally vulnerable. Physical violence is arguably the easiest way to see the effects of violence, but often physical violence is experienced concurrently with other layers of violence. If we use an understanding of intersectionality, then we cannot look at biology and the environment as separate variables when it comes to the health effects of violence (Singer 2001; Page-Reeves et al. 2013; Singer et al. 2017).

The effects of violence toward the gender-diverse community could easily be described as a syndemic (Singer et al. 2017). *Syndemics* are defined as "the aggregation of two or more diseases or other health conditions in a population in which there is some level of deleterious biological or behavior[al] interface that exacerbates the negative health effects of any or all of the diseases involved" (Singer et al. 2017, 941). All levels of violence are associated with deeper health effects, including depression, disabilities, and high-risk sexual behavior (WHO 2014; Divan et al. 2016). It has been seen that the collective violence stemming from structural biases have negative health effects on those experiencing it (Open Society Foundation Public Health Program 2013; Divan et al. 2016). These health effects even have the potential to be passed down generationally (Crews et al. 2014; Zuk and Spencer 2020).

Anti-Transgender Violence

While it is nearly impossible to achieve an accurate census of the gender-diverse community, it is estimated that there are more than 25 million individuals globally (Somenek 2019). Those who do not have a gender identity congruent with their assigned sex at birth are significantly more likely to experience violence than the rest of the community (Stotzer 2009; James et al. 2016). In the United States, compared to cisgender counterparts, gender-diverse individuals were found to be over four times as likely to experience acts of violent crime (Dowd 2021). Although a lack of accurate record keeping poses an ongoing problem, there are growing efforts to research violence against gender-diverse individuals. Transgender Europe has set up a monitoring system to track murders of transgender people worldwide through their "Transrespect vs. Transphobia" program. The gathered data from the year 2020 showed that, worldwide, 350 trans- and gender-diverse individuals were murdered by Friday, November 20, the International Transgender Day of Remembrance, an increase of 6 percent over the 2019 rate (Transrespect vs. Transphobia 2020). In the United States alone, 271 transgender individuals were murdered between 2008 and 2019. Homicide is better reported and recorded than other forms of violence against transgender people. However, the absence of comprehensive statistics on the non-homicidal violence experienced compounds the structural and systematic violence. Through the lack of comprehensive statistics, the community's suffering is rendered invisible, and thereby rendered inconsequential.

Structural violence is enacted through legal and bureaucratic systems, and manifests in economic disadvantages and in inequitable access to housing and healthcare (Harper and Schneider 2003; James et al. 2016; Rodriguez, Agardh, and Asomoah 2018; Griner et al. 2020). The resulting economic necessity drives transgender and gender-diverse individuals into the underground economy, which further increases risk of violence due to high-risk behaviors and survival crimes such as sex work. Participation in the underground economy can lead to increased health problems, such as HIV/AIDS. The 2015 U.S. Transgender survey found that one in five transgender individuals had to resort to the underground economy at some point in their lives (James et al. 2016). Further still, nine out of ten transgender individuals who relied on underground economy work were either attacked or discriminated against by police (James et al. 2016).

The structural violence that shapes interactions with the healthcare system also leads to the large health disparities that we see within the gender-diverse community (Open Society Foundation Public Health Program 2013; Divan et al. 2016; Hayon and Stevenson 2019). One case study saw a White transgender man who had been diagnosed with ovarian cancer unable to secure appropriate care. He was pushed from doctor to doctor, with one even telling him that it would be embarrassing for the women sitting around him at a gynecologic practice. He died a year after his diagnosis (Open Society Foundation Public Health Program 2013).

In the 2013 study, Transforming Health, it was noted that even though levels of physical and structural violence are staggering, there are very few protections for gender-diverse individuals and even where they exist, they are seldom enforced (Open Society Foundation Public Health Program 2013). These inequities that have been normalized through our social institutions help institutionalize violence and discrimination toward the gender-diverse community (Kritz 2020).

HOW ARE FORENSIC ANTHROPOLOGISTS COMPLICIT IN INTERSECTIONAL VIOLENCE?

Gender-diverse individuals are already subjected to misgendering and a myriad of violence in life, and are frequently misrepresented by families, forensics, and journalistic work in death. Misgendering, deadnaming, and re-enforcing the sex/gender binary are all violent acts toward the transgender community. *Deadnaming* is the act of referring to a transgender person as the name given at birth that they no longer identify with. It may seem small to an outsider especially in relation to a decedent, but in life, publicly misgendering or deadnaming an individual could be a death sentence. Forensic anthropologists work diligently to assess biological profiles of decedents for positive identification. Again, gender is not biological, but it can play a role in the positive identification of a decedent.

The American Anthropological Association (2009) and the American Association of Biological Anthropologists (2003) both place "do no harm" high within their ethical codes. This code is arguably being broken every time a transgender individual gets misgendered. In short, misgendering is violence. The problem here is that when forensic anthropologists do not include gender within the casework, or tacitly conceptualize sex as binary, they are at risk of inadvertently misgendering a decedent. While the gender-diverse population is much smaller than the cisgender population, it has been displayed repeatedly that they are more likely to become victims to physical and fatal violence (Stotzer 2009; James et al. 2016). Largely, the gender-diverse community is tasked with speaking up about the misgendering of one of their own in death, while simultaneously mourning. Therefore, while gender-diverse people are a relatively small percentage of the total population, their disproportionate risk of violence means that forensic anthropologists cannot ignore the possibility of their presence in their casework. Misgendering people in death amplifies the violence they have experienced in life.

It has been pointed out that ethical considerations have not been placed at the forefront of the field (Passalacqua and Pilloud 2018). Forensic anthropologists across the globe do not follow one specific code of ethics, nor is there an overarching code for the whole of forensic sciences. The codes followed are association specific and are not uniform across the board (Passalacqua and Pilloud 2018). For American anthropologists, the overarching association that covers all subfields of anthropology is the American Anthropological Association (AAA). The AAA has seven ethics codes, the first of which is "do no harm" (American Anthropological Association 2009). This code is arguably the most important in the discussion on inclusion of gender identity within forensic anthropology.

Many law enforcement agencies do not place differences in sex and gender in their categorization systems. It is also important to note that many coroners and medical examiners use the outward expressions of sex, such as genitalia, without focus on gender identity for the process of identification (Garofalo and Garvin 2020). As law enforcement can rely on a forensic anthropology case report, anthropologists must be cognizant of wording and the current binary of sex/gender is hurtful to the gender-diverse community even if superficially it appears helpful for identification.

Looking through lenses outside of casework, it is easy to understand how and why this is a problem within forensic anthropology. It appears that, for most forensic anthropologists, this is not a purposeful act of violence, but due to an institutionalization of implicit biases. Forensic anthropologists need to acknowledge that just because they are not purposefully creating violence does not mean they are not complicit.

RECOMMENDED STEPS FORWARD

Prevention of Violence

Forensic anthropologists become involved after a death has occurred. Consequently, forensic anthropologists are unlikely to contribute to the primary prevention of violence through casework, but secondary prevention and universal interventions actively help change the scope of violence. Forensic anthropologists need to be clear eyed about the violence suffered by the gender-diverse community. Gender-diverse decedents need to be counted. The reconceptualization of sex analysis within the biological profile to be broader than the binary makes the community visible and pays proper respect to the dignity of gender-diverse people both in life and in death. The start of these changes could be as simple as terminology switches within casework documentation. For example, instead of stating "sex" or "biological sex" one could use terms such as "assigned sex at birth" or "assigned skeletal sex."

Limitations

This is a growing area of research and while there are estimates, there are not accurate census information of gender-diverse individuals. There are not accurate available data sources to quantify violence in general, let alone the violence faced by gender-diverse individuals (Krug et al. 2002). The available data from sources such as the UCR are helpful, but do not provide accurate information about the number of gender-diverse individuals experiencing violence. Typically, collected data on violence are focused only on physical, not structural, violence.

As previously discussed, not every transgender individual is going to want or need medical intervention to transition or address their gender dysphoria. Although, not every gender-diverse individual will utilize medical transition, progressively more government agencies are allowing individuals to accurately be represented with their legal identification. This puts an increased likelihood of leaving an individual unidentified when family members, law enforcement, or media misgender a person when reporting their disappearance.

It should be stressed that identity is internal, and while it may have some external or physiological signs, it cannot be determined simply by looking at an individual. Living individuals may be non-binary but were assigned male at birth and present as traditionally masculine within a society; however, their physical presentation may not dictate their gender identity.

Forensic anthropologists should understand gender identities and the features of gender- or sex-affirming surgeries. Even an introductory understanding of these can help point law enforcement in the right direction for a positive identification. While having a strong understanding of gender-affirming surgeries is a helpful tool for any forensic anthropologist, it cannot be used as a positive determination. For example, in facial feminization surgeries, there are various surgeries that may be conducted together but it is dependent on the patient's skeletal features, so some may be performed, and others may be unnecessary. These surgeries are not strictly performed for facial feminization surgeries; some of these procedures, like mid-face osteotomies, may be performed for facial traumas. Facial feminization procedures are also used by cisgender women because they may feel that their face is too masculine. Thus, the presence of these surgeries is not an unambiguous indicator of being transgender or gender diverse. However, knowledge of these procedures is helpful for forensic anthropologists when taking a biocultural approach to their casework as they can apply these and other variables to their case reports.

Increased Research

In general, we are seeing an increased effort for gender-diverse research within forensic anthropology (e.g., Buchanan 2014; Bouderdaben 2019; Cirillo et al. 2020; Haug 2020a and b; Kincer 2020; Michael et al. 2020; Schall, Rogers, and Deschamps-Braly 2020; Michael et al. 2021; Tallman, Kincer, and Plemons 2022). There have also been groups, such as Trans Doe Task Force, who have teamed up with forensic anthropologists and law enforcement departments in an effort to help identify potential gender-diverse cold cases. Forensic anthropologists also need to include gender-diverse individuals within the conversations and research. Forensic anthropologists cannot afford to exclude from the conversation the very individuals they are attempting to help.

In-Field Activism

There has been discussion on the place of activism within forensic anthropology. Activism does not have to be strictly protesting what is wrong but should be actively teaching and working toward changing those wrongs. For forensic anthropologists, this can come from various settings. As many forensic anthropologists are also academics, they can strive to use the most appropriate terms for those groups they are working with as they teach and undertake research. Within the medicolegal community, they can use their positions to educate. If members of the law enforcement community make incorrect statements about sex and gender, it would be appropriate to gently advise them that sex and gender are different. In general, it should be said that just speaking up can sometimes be the smallest, but most helpful, way of being an activist and ally to the transgender and gender-diverse community.

Again, it is often left to the gender-diverse community to correct the misgendering that occurs by the police, medical examiners, and media in cases of fatal violence. This is just one extra level of stress and violence faced by a community mourning the loss of yet another gender-diverse individual. It should not be up to the community experiencing violence to fix problems that are only theirs because years of institutionalized ideologies have forced it upon them.

CONCLUSION

It seems clear that forensic anthropologists are not actively attempting to harm or perpetuate violence toward the gender-diverse community, but it is happening, and it should be addressed. Sex and gender needs to be reconceptualized within forensic anthropological casework. While gender identity cannot be determined via physical elements, it cannot be ignored by forensic anthropology any longer. Intersectionality plays a large role in understanding violence toward the gender-diverse community, as well as understanding violence as a whole. The most important understanding is that collective violence is being perpetuated by forensic anthropologists, which leads further to more collective, interpersonal, and even self-directed violence aimed toward the gender-diverse population. Acknowledging that forensic anthropology is taking part in perpetuating violence, and thereby violating anthropological ethics, is difficult but necessary work.

The gender-diverse community is full of varying identities but in general, just identifying as being gender diverse puts them in a position for experiencing higher levels of violence in any, or all, sectors of violence (Meyer 2008; Stotzer 2009; James et al. 2016). These intersecting identities are often what put individuals at risk for violence, and yet they can be sources for empowerment. Anthropologists hold the ability to transform the scope of sex and gender in forensic anthropology away from the current institutionalized binary conceptions. It has been said that once you know something you cannot unknow it, and anthropologists now know that they are taking part in perpetuating an oppressive system. It is at this crossroad in anthropological history that they make the choice to consciously continue the normative cycle or to make waves with reconceptualization. Understanding this, anthropologists can use their tools to help amplify and empower gender-diverse voices, even in death.

REFERENCES

Accomazzo, Sarah. 2012. "Anthropology of Violence: Historical and Current Theories, Concepts, and Debates in Physical and Socio-cultural Anthropology." *Journal of Human Behavior in the Social Environment* 22: 535–552. https://doi.org/10.1080/10911359.2011.598727

American Anthropological Association. 2009. "Code of Ethics of the American Anthropological Association Approved, June 1998." *Anthropology News* 39, no. 6: 19–20. https://doi.org/10.1111/an.1998.39.6.19.2

American Association of Biological Anthropology. 2003. "Code of Ethics of the American Association of Physical Anthropologists." https://physanth.org/documents/3/ethics.pdf

American Psychological Association. 2015. "Guidelines for Psychological Practice with Transgender and Gender Nonconforming People." *American Psychologist* 7, no. 9: 832–864. http://dx.doi.org/10.1037/a0039906

Bauer, Greta R., Jessica Braimoh, Ayden I. Scheim, and Christoffer Dharma. 2017. "Transgender-inclusive Measures of Sex/Gender for Population Surveys: Mixed Methods Evaluation and Recommendations." *PLoS ONE* 12, no. 5: 1–28. https://doi.org/10.1371/journal.pone.0178043

Bouderdaben, Fatimah A. 2019. "A Push for Trans-inclusive Language in Forensic Anthropology." In: Podium Abstract at the 88th Annual Meeting of the American Association of Physical Anthropologists Cleveland, OH.

Bouman, Walter Pierre, Amets Suess Schwend, Joz Motmans, Adam Smiley, Joshua D. Safer, Madeline B. Deutsch, Noah J. Adams, et al. 2017. "Language and Trans Health." *International Journal of Transgenderism* 18, no. 1: 1–6. https://doi.org/10.1080/15532739.2016.1262127

Bourdieu, Pierre. 1977. "Symbolic Power." In *Identity and Structure: Issues in the Sociology of Education*, edited by D. Gleeson, 112–122. Driffield: Studies in Education Ltd.

Bourdieu, Pierre and Loïc Wacquant. 2003. "Symbolic Violence." In *Violence in War and Peace*, edited by N. Scheper-Hughes and P. Bourgois, 272–274. Malden, MA: Blackwell Publishing.

Bradford, Judith, Sari L. Reisner, Julie A. Honnold, and Jessica Xavier. 2013. "Experiences of Transgender-Related Discrimination and Implications for Health: Results from the Virginia Transgender Health Initiative Study." *American Journal of Public Health* 103, no. 10: 1820–1829. https://doi.org/10.2105/AJPH.2012 .300796

Buchanan, Shelby. 2014. "Bone Modification in Male to Female Transgender Surgeries: Considerations for the Forensic Anthropologist." Master's Thesis, Louisiana State University. Retrieved from https://digitalcommons.lsu.edu/gradschool_theses/1290/

Buikstra, Jane E., and Douglas H. Ubelaker. 1994. *Standards for Data Collection from Human Skeletal Remains*. Fayetteville, Arkansas: Arkansas Archaeological Survey Report Number 44. https://doi.org/10.1002/ajhb.1310070519

Butler, Judith. 2004. *Undoing Gender*. New York and London: Routledge. https://doi .org/10.4324/9780203499627

Canner, Joseph K., Omar Harfouch, Lisa M. Kodadek, Danielle Pelaez, Devin Coon, Anaeze C. Offodile 2nd, Adil H. Haider, et al. 2018. "Temporal Trends in Gender-Affirming Surgery Among Transgender Patients in the United States." *JAMA Surg* 153, no. 7: 609–616. https://doi.org/10.1001/jamasurg.2017 .6231

Carpenter, Morgan. 2018. "Intersex Variations, Human Rights, and the International Classification of Diseases." *Health and Human Rights Journal* 20, no. 2: 205–214.

Cirillo, Laura, Jordan C. Deschamps-Braly, Kyra E. Stull, and Marin A. Pilloud. 2020. "Cranial Feminization Surgery Methods and Osteological Identification of Post-Operative Individuals." In Proceedings of the 72nd Annual Meeting of the American Academy of Forensic Sciences, February 17–22, 2020, Anaheim, CA.

Crenshaw, Kimberlé. 1989. "Demarginalizing the Intersection of Race and Sex: A Black Feminist Critique of Antidiscrimination Doctrine, Feminist Theory and Antiracist Politics." *University of Chicago Legal Forum* 1989, no. 1: 139–167.

———. 1991. "Mapping the Margins: Intersectionality, Identity Politics, and Violence against Women of Color." *Stanford Law Review* 43: 1241–1299. https:// doi.org/10.2307/1229039

Crews, David, Ross Gillette, Isaac Miller-Crews, Andrea C. Gore, and Michael K. Skinner. 2014. "Nature, Nurture and Epigenetics." *Molecular and Cellular Endocrinology* 398, no. 1 and 2: 42–52. https://doi.org/10.1016/j.mce.2014.07.013

Crocetti, Daniela. 2013. "Genes and Hormones: What Make Up an Individual's Sex." In *Challenging Popular Myths of Sex, Gender and Biology (Crossroads of Knowledge)*, edited by Malin Ah-King, 23–32. Springer. https://doi.org/10.1007 /978-3-319-01979-6_3

Díaz-Andreu, Margarita, Sam Lucy, Stasa Babic, and David N. Edwards. 2005. *The Archaeology of Identity: Approaches to Gender, Age, Status, Ethnicity and Religion*. New York: Routledge.

Divan, Vivek, Clifton Cortez, Marina Smelyanskaya, and JoAnne Keatley. 2016. "Transgender Social Inclusion and Equality: A Pivotal Path to Development." *Journal of the International AIDS Society* 19, no. 2: 1–6. https://doi.org/10.7448/ IAS.19.3.20803

Dowd, Rachel. 2021. "Transgender People Over Four Times More Likely Than Cisgender People to be Victims of Violent Crime." Press Release. Williams

Institute. UCLA School of Law. https://williamsinstitute.law.ucla.edu/press/ncvs -trans-press-release/. Accessed January 5, 2022.

Elliot, Patricia. 2016. *Debates in Transgender, Queer, and Feminist Theory*. New York: Routledge.

Englander, Elizabeth Kandel. 2003. *Understanding Violence*. 2nd ed. Mahwah, NJ: Lawrence Erlbaum Associates.

Farmer, Paul. 2005. *Pathologies of Power: Health, Human Rights, and the New War on the Poor*. Berkeley: University of California Press.

Fausto-Sterling, Ann. 2012. *Sex/Gender: Biology in a Social World*. New York: Routledge.

Fedorko, Boglarka, Sanjar Kurmanov, and Lukas Berredo. 2020. *A Brief Guide to Monitoring Anti-Trans Violence*. TGEU.

Garofalo, Evan M. and Heather M. Garvin. 2020. "The Confusion Between Biological Sex and Gender and Potential Implications of Misinterpretations." In *Sex Estimation of the Human Skeleton: History, Methods, and Emerging Techniques*, edited by Alexandra R. Klales, 35–52. London: Academic Press. https://doi.org/10 .1016/B978-0-12-815767-1.00004-3

Grant, Jaime M., Lisa A. Mottet, Justin Tanis, Jack Harrison, Jody L. Herman, and Mara Keisling. 2011. *Injustice at Every Turn: A Report of the National Transgender Discrimination Survey*. Washington, DC: National Center for Transgender Equality and National Gay and Lesbian Task Force. https://transe-quality.org/sites/default/files/docs/resources/NTDS_Report.pdf

Griner, Stacey B., Cheryl A. Vamos, Erika L. Thompson, Rachel Logan, Coralia Vázquez-Otero, and Ellen M. Daley. 2020. "The Intersection of Gender Identity and Violence: Victimization Experienced by Transgender College Students." *Journal of Interpersonal Violence* 35, nos. 23 and 24: 5704–5725. https://doi.org /10.1177/0886260517723743

Harper, Gary W. and Margaret Schneider. 2003. "Oppression and Discrimination Among Lesbian, Gay, Bisexual and Transgender People and Communities: A Challenge for Community Psychology." *American Journal of Community Psychology* 31, no. 3 and 4: 243–252. https://doi.org/10.1023/A:1023906620085

Harro, Bobbie. 2000. "The Cycle of Socialization." In *Readings for Diversity and Social Justice*, edited by M. Adams, W. Blumenfeld, R. Castaneda, H. Hackman, M. Peters, and X. Zuniga. New York: Routledge.

Haug, Jaxson. D. 2020a. "Gendered Faces: A Look at Male-to-Female Transgender Facial Feminization Surgeries and Their Relation to Sex Estimation in Forensic Anthropology." Master's Thesis. California State University, Los Angeles.

———. 2020b. *Applying Facial Feminization Surgery to Positive Forensic Identification*. In Proceedings of the 26th Scientific Symposium of the World Professional Association of Transgender Health, November 6–10, 2020, Virtual.

Hausman, Bernice. 1995. *Changing Sex: Transsexualism, Technology, and the Idea of Gender*. Durham: Duke University Press.

Hayon, Ronni and Kristin Stevenson. 2019. "Hormonal, Medical, and Nonsurgical Aspects of Gender Affirmation." *Facial Plastic Surgery Clinics of North America* 27, no. 2: 179–190. https://doi.org/10.1016/j.fsc.2018.12.001

Human Rights Campaign. 2019. *A National Epidemic: Fatal Anti-Transgender Violence in America in 2018*. https://www.hrc.org/resources/a-national-epidemic -fatal-anti-transgender-violence-in-america-in-2018. Accessed January 13, 2021.

James, Sandy E., Jody L. Herman, Susan Rankin, Mara Keisling, Lisa Mottet, and Ma'ayan Anafi. 2016. "The Report of the 2015 U.S. Transgender Survey." Washington, DC, National Center for Transgender Equality. https://transequality .org/sites/default/files/docs/usts/USTS-Full-Report-Dec17.pdf

Karkazis, Katrina. 2008. *Fixing Sex: Intersex, Medical Authority, and Lived Experience*. Durham: Duke University Press.

Kincer, Caroline D. 2020. "Centering Transgender Personhoods in Forensic Anthropology and Expanding Sex Estimation in Casework and Research." Master's Thesis. Boston University.

Klales, Alexandra R., ed. 2020. *Sex Estimation of the Human Skeleton: History, Methods, and Emerging Techniques*. London: Academic Press. https://doi.org/10 .1016/C2017-0-03550-4

Klales, Alexandra R., Stephen D. Ousley, and Jennifer N. Vollner. 2012. "A Revised Method of Sexing the Human Innominate using Phenice's Nonmetric Traits and Statistical Methods." *American Journal of Physical Anthropology* 149, no. 1: 104–114. https://doi.org/10.1002/ajpa.22102

Kritz, Brian. 2020. "Direct and Structural Violence against Transgender Populations: A Comparative Legal Study." *Florida Journal of International Law* 31: 211–237. https://scholarship.law.ufl.edu/fjil/vol31/iss2/2

Krug, Etienne G., Linda L. Dahlberg, James A. Mercy, Anthony B. Zwi, and Rafael Lozano. 2002. *World Report on Violence and Health*. Geneva: World Health Organization. https://apps.who.int/iris/handle/10665/42495

Lee, Peter A., Anna Nordenstrom, Christopher P. Houk, S. Faisal Ahmed, Richard Auchus, Arlene Baratz, and Katharine Baratz Dalke, et al. 2016. "Global Disorders of Sex Development Update since 2006: Perceptions, Approach and Care." *Hormone Research in Paediatrics* 85, no. 3: 158–180. https://doi.org/10.1159 /000442975

Lorber, Judith. 1994. *Paradoxes of Gender*. Yale University Press.

Lugones, Maria. 2007. "Heterosexualism and the Colonial/Modern Gender System." *Hypatia* 22, no. 1: 186–209. http://www.jstor.org/stable/4640051

———. 2020. "Gender and Universality in Colonial Methodology." *Critical Philosophy of Race* 8, nos. 1 and 2: 25–47. https://doi.org/10.5325/critphilrace.8 .1-2.0025

Mardell, Ashley. 2016. *The ABCs of LGBT+*. Mango Media Inc. Kindle.

Meyer, Doug. 2008. "Anti-Queer Violence: Race, Class, and Gender Differences Among LGBT Hate Crime Victims." *Race, Gender and Class* 15, nos. 3 and 4: 262–282. https://www.jstor.org/stable/41674664

Michael, Amy, Mariyam I. Isa, Anthony Redgrave, and Lee Redgrave. 2020. *Collaborative Approaches in the Identification of Transgender and Gender Variant Decedents*. In Proceedings of the 72nd Annual Meeting of the American Academy of Forensic Sciences, February 17–22, 2020, Anaheim, CA.

————. 2021. *Structural Vulnerability in Transgender and Non-Binary Decedent Populations: Analytical Considerations and Harm-Reduction Strategies*. In Proceedings of the 73rd Annual Meeting of the American Academy of Forensic Sciences. Virtual.

Money, John, Joan G. Hampson, and John L. Hampson. 1955. "Hermaphroditism: Recommendations Concerning the Assignment of Sex, Change of Sex, and Psychologic Management." *Bulletin of the Johns Hopkins Hospital* 97, no. 4: 284–300. PMID: 13260819.

Morris, Joan K., Eva Alberman, Claire Scott, and Patricia Jacobs. 2008. "Is the Prevalence of Klinefelter Syndrome Increasing?" *European Journal of Human Genetics* 16: 163–170. https://doi.org/10.1038/sj.ejhg.5201956

Nakhaeizadeh, Sherry, Itiel E. Dror, and Ruth M. Morgan. 2014. "Cognitive Bias in Forensic Anthropology: Visual Assessment of Skeletal Remains is Susceptible to Confirmation Bias." *Science and Justice* 54, no. 3: 208–214. https://doi.org/10.1016/j.scijus.2013.11.003

————. 2020. "Cognitive Bias in Sex Estimation: The Influence of Context on Forensic Decision-Making." In *Sex Estimation of the Human Skeleton: History, Methods, and Emerging Techniques*, edited by Alexandra R. Klales, 327–342. London: Academic Press. https://doi.org/10.1016/B978-0-12-815767-1.00020-1

Nanda, Serena. 2014. *Gender Diversity: Crosscultural Variations* (Second Edition). Waveland Press.

Open Society Foundation Public Health Program. 2013. *Transforming Health: International Rights-Based Advocacy for Trans Health*. https://www.opensociety foundations.org/publications/transforming-health

Oyewumi, Oyeronke. 1998. "De-confounding Gender: Feminist Theorizing and Western Culture, a Comment on Hawkesworth's 'Confounding Gender'." *Signs* 23, no. 4: 1049–1062. https://www.jstor.org/stable/3175203

Page-Reeves, Janet, Joshua Niforatos, Shiraz Mishra, Lidia Regino, Andrew Gingrich, and Robert Bulten. 2013. "Health Disparity and Structural Violence: How Fear Undermines Health Among Immigrants at Risk for Diabetes." *Journal of Health Disparities Research and Practice* 6, no. 2: 30–47. PMID: 24052924

Passalacqua, Nicholas V. and Marin A. Pilloud. 2018. *Ethics and Professionalism in Forensic Anthropology*. London: Academic Press.

Peletz, Michael G. 2009. *Gender Pluralism: Southeast Asia Since Early Modern Times*. New York: Routledge.

Phenice, T. W. 1969. "A Newly Developed Visual Method of Sexing in the Os Pubis." *American Journal of Physical Anthropology* 30: 297–301.

Quesada, James, Laurie K. Hart, and Philippe Bourgois. 2011. "Structural Vulnerability and Health: Latino Migrant Laborers in the United States." *Medical Anthropology* 30, no. 4: 339–362. https://doi.org/10.1080/01459740.2011.576725

Ratcliffe, Shirley G. 1999. "Long Term Outcome in Children of Sex Chromosome Abnormalities." *Archives of Disease in Childhood* 80: 192–195. http://dx.doi.org/10.1136/adc.80.2.192

Reby, David, Florence Levrero, Erik Gustafsson, and Nicolas Mathevon. 2016. "Sex Stereotypes Influence Adults' Perception of Babies' Cries." *BMC Psychology* 4, no. 19. https://doi.org/10.1186/s40359-016-0123-6

Reis, Elizabeth. 2009. *Bodies in Doubt: An American History of Intersex.* MD: Johns Hopkins University Press.

Rodriguez, Amanda, Anette Agardh, and Benedict Oppong Asamoah. 2018. "Self-Reported Discrimination in Health-Care Settings Based on Recognizability as Transgender: A Cross-Sectional Study Among Transgender U.S. Citizens." *Archives of Sexual Behavior* 47: 973–985. https://doi.org/10.1007/s10508-017-1028-z

Rutherford, Alison, Anthony B. Zwi, Natalie J. Grove, and Alexander Butchart. 2007. "Violence: A Glossary." *Journal of Epidemiological Community Health* 61: 676–680. https://doi.org/10.1136/jech.2005.043711

Schall, Jenna L., Tracy L. Rogers, and Jordan C. Deschamps-Braly. 2020. "Breaking the Binary: The Identification of Trans-women in Forensic Anthropology." *Forensic Science International* 309: 1–10. https://doi.org/10.1016/j.forsciint.2020.110356

Singer, Merrill. 2001. "Toward a Bio-cultural and Political Economic Integration of Alcohol, Tobacco and Drug Studies in the Coming Century." *Social Science and Medicine* 53, no. 2: 199–213. https://doi.org/10.1016/s0277-9536(00)00331-2

Singer, Merrill, Nicola Bulled, Bayla Ostrach, and Emily Mendenhall. 2017. "Syndemics and the Biosocial Conception of Health." *The Lancet* 389, no. 10072: 941–950. https://doi.org/10.1016/S0140-6736(17)30003-X

Skuse, David, Frida Printzlau, and Jeanne Wolstencroft. 2018. "Sex Chromosome Aneuploidies." *Neurogenetics* 147: 355–376. https://doi.org/10.1016/B978-0-444-63233-3.00024-5

Slocum, Sally. 1975. "Woman the Gatherer: Male Bias in Anthropology." In *Anthropological Theory: An Introductory History*, edited by Jon R. McGee and Richard L. Warms, 399–407. New York: McGraw Hill.

Somenek, Michael T. 2019. "Preface: Exploring Facial Gender Affirmation Surgery." *Facial Plastic Surgery Clinics of North America* 27, no. 2. https://doi.org/10.1016/j.fsc.2019.02.001

Stotzer, Rebecca L. 2009. "Violence Against Transgender People: A Review of United States Data." *Aggression and Violent Behavior* 14, no. 3: 170–179. https://doi.org/10.1016/j.avb.2009.01.006

Tallman, Sean D., and Cate E. Bird. 2022. "Diversity and Inclusion in Forensic Anthropology: Where We Stand and Prospects for the Future." *Forensic Anthropology* 5, no. 2: 84–101. https://doi.org/10.5744/fa.2020.3001

Tallman, Sean D., Caroline D. Kincer, and Eric D. Plemons. 2022. "Centering Transgender Individuals in Forensic Anthropology and Expanding Binary Sex Estimation in Casework and Research." *Forensic Anthropology* 5, no. 2: 161–180. https://doi.org/10.5744/fa.2020.0030

Transrespect versus Transphobia. 2020. "TMM Update Trans Day of Remembrance 2020." Transrespect vs. Transphobia Website, November 11, 2020. Accessed January 11, 2021. https://transrespect.org/en/tmm-update-tdor-2020/

Walker, Phillip L. 2005. "Greater Sciatic Notch Morphology: Sex, Age, and Population Differences." *American Journal of Physical Anthropology* 127, no. 4: 385–391. https://doi.org/10.1002/ajpa.10422

Weismantel, Mary. 2013. "Towards a Transgender Archaeology: A Queer Rampage Through Prehistory." In *The Transgender Studies Reader 2*, edited by Susan Stryker and Aren Z. Aizura, 319–334. New York: Routledge.

World Health Organization. 2014. "Global Status Report on Violence Prevention 2014." Luxembourg: WHO. https://www.who.int/publications/i/item/978924 1564793

Worthman, Carol M. 2003. "Hormones, Sex, and Gender." *Annual Review of Anthropology* 24, no. 1: 593–617. https://doi.org/10.1146/annurev.an.24.100195 .003113

Zuk, Marlene and Hamish G. Spencer. 2020. "Killing the Behavioral Zombie: Genes, Evolution, and Why Behavior Isn't Special." *BioScience* 70, no. 6: 515–520. https://doi.org/10.1093/biosci/biaa042

Chapter 8

Marginalization, Death, and Decline

The Role of Forensic Anthropology in Documenting the Osteology of Poverty and Evidence of Structural Violence in Detroit, Michigan in the Twenty-First Century

Megan K. Moore and Jaymelee J. Kim

INTRODUCTION

Being presented with an incomplete set of skeletonized human remains gathered by law enforcement, I (JJK) realized I needed to go to the scene to complete the recovery.[1] Cervical vertebrae two and three were missing but, given the notes in the initial report, it seemed likely they would be easily found at the scene. The case registration summary indicated that human remains accessioned in association with case 0001 had been found by a property owner in a "vacant building." At the time, I did not realize that so many of the death investigators' summaries would describe people found in empty lots, drainage ditches, and vacant buildings, nor did I fully grasp what the word "vacant" meant here in Detroit.

The vacant building was a garage situated on a residential property. The sergeant, local officer, and I approached the front door of the home for permission to access the building. A man opened the door to the modest home as children peered out at us from the living room. The gentleman did not speak English, so his young daughter translated. Given the age of our translator, we tactfully explained that the police had recently been in the garage investigating, and we needed to check the garage one more time. The resident agreed and we proceeded around the house down a small path, carelessly littered with used nitrile gloves of the team before us—each set folded into each other—as anyone who works in healthcare, scene recovery, or with human remains is taught to do. I followed the sergeant's lead, picking them up as we walked along. I thought again of the small children just a few feet away inside the home.

I rounded the corner and saw that the vacant garage stood, dilapidated, maybe twenty or thirty feet from the back door of the house. Windows no longer held glass, and I realized that I had erroneously interpreted "vacant" to mean empty. The garage was not empty; garbage and debris undulated in height from mid-calf to waist-high. When I mentioned this to the homicide sergeant, she affirmed that it was typical of "vacant" buildings. The officer motioned to what was left of a futon which lay crumpled amid the refuse where the remains had been found reportedly wrapped in an old blanket.

"We did not receive the scene photos?" inquired the sergeant behind me. I knew she shared my thought that scene photos would have been remarkably helpful now given the sheer magnitude of debris that lay before us.

"No. We did not take any."

I could feel my face reflecting my incredulity as I balanced myself carefully on unstable refuse and began to gently sift through mattress foam and springs, keenly aware that sharps or creatures might be present. For a good half hour we searched, flashlights in hand, heaving furniture and debris; I found a human tooth (#8) lost postmortem, but no vertebrae. Climbing out of the garage, we reconvened in the light, just outside the entrance to the vacant building.

"You should always take scene photos." I could hear the frustration in the sergeant's voice.

"There was no sign of foul play," replied the officer. To be fair, he had not been the one to work the scene, but I could feel the muscles in my face twitch at the admission. The remains were mummified and skeletal. Decomposition fluids had soaked through and discolored the sleeping area. The person was homeless and taking shelter in this squalor; the scene itself also would not give much indication of "disturbance," given its state.

"You know about the serial murders? Those women were found in vacant buildings, too." In her exasperated response, the sergeant referenced recent murders (Detroit News 2020). As she went on to impress upon him proper documentation and evidence collection, my eyes wandered across the green lawn, and I realized that a bone was on the ground just next to the officer's foot and embedded in mud. Within a few moments, the two missing cervical vertebrae, ostensibly dropped by crime scene investigators in the backyard of a family with young children. The sergeant and I exchanged looks, and I said my piece, emphasizing the need for proper remains recovery. It was not lost on me that two women of color were advocating for the fair treatment of someone haphazardly collected from the refuse. As I would find with cases to come, this man's bones embodied the poverty that I witnessed in his

last known home, without running water, electricity, or heat. Osteoarthritis, osteochondritis, diffuse idiopathic skeletal hyperostosis, ankylosing of ribs, ankylosing spondylitis and fusion of the sacroiliac joint were the more evident pathological conditions of the skeleton. While it may be determined that his death was not homicide, his body and location of his remains evidenced the violence he had experienced in life.

This is one of many cases encountered at scenes around Detroit. Having served as forensic anthropologists for southeastern Michigan since 2014 and 2019, respectively, both authors have collectively analyzed 141 cases as of the time of this writing. In this chapter, we present the skeletal and contextual evidence of structural violence as observed in the forensic anthropology casework for Detroit, MI from 2014 to 2021. Through the postmortem analysis of 128 adult individuals from the Wayne County Medical Examiner's Office (M.E.O.) and the context in which they were found, we provide a biology of poverty that is situationally specific. Here, we review the political and historical dynamics of Detroit, the role of "vacant" buildings, and health status of the living. We provide the case of Detroit within Wayne County, Michigan as an example of how structural violence theory can be applied to casework in the Global North, and to reveal how we can fulfill our obligation as forensic anthropologists to document evidence of all violence, even that which is often overlooked. To do this, we first define biology of poverty, and then historically and socially frame Detroit. Once the social variables are outlined, we present the postmortem evidence of trauma and pathology data along with contextual evidence from the forensic anthropology cases to highlight how the social arrangements of structural violence manifest in the remains and the contexts in which they are found, as well as the violence that often persists beyond death.

INTERPRETING A BIOLOGY OF POVERTY AND OSTEOLOGY OF STRUCTURAL VIOLENCE

Deborah Crooks (1998) encouraged the biological anthropology community to engage with a historically and situationally specific "biology of poverty." Such a framework would analyze human adaptations to specific environments and socially imposed constraints, which is an understudied phenomenon in wealthier countries such as the United States. While Crooks (1998) focuses on child development and well-being in Kentucky, we apply this model to the anthropological analysis of a mostly adult forensic skeletal sample. We go a step beyond the biology of poverty to discuss how lived experiences manifest in the remains and how the contexts in which they are found can be readily framed in terms of structural violence. This particular form of violence can be explained as a denial of access to resources (e.g., water, heat, healthcare, living wage, education, or home ownership) achieved by those in power through social mechanisms such as policies, practices, and beliefs in a given culture (Farmer 2003; Farmer et al. 2006; Rylko-Bauer and Farmer 2016). Unlike with international humanitarian and human rights interventions that interrogate physical violence in the contexts of war, there are not many clear political figures and military leaders to assign responsibility to, and there are no telltale forms of trauma to associate with extrajudicial killings (Kimmerle and Baraybar 2008). Social structures, rather than singular villains, keep the targeted group oppressed over time through inaccessibility woven into the fabric of society.

This lens contributes to emerging discussions in forensic anthropology. Beatrice and Soler (2016) complement Crooks's (1998) work, discussing how use of a biocultural profile can assist in the humanitarian crisis regarding border crossing deaths in the United States. The authors draw on stress indicator data from undocumented border crossers in Arizona's Pima County Office of the Medical Examiner. Their study reveals that skeletal stress indicators can assist in differentiating remains of American-born individuals from those of migrants due to the distinct skeletal responses to their respective environments. We adapt the structural violence framework similarly and apply it to the context of poverty in Detroit, Michigan in the United States. We frame certain pathological conditions as a physiological response to structural violence vis-à-vis limited access to resources such as healthcare, balanced nutrition, and access to heat and shelter during the harsh Michigan winters (Soler and Beatrice 2018; Soler, Beatrice, and Martínez this volume; Winburn et al. this volume).

Despite being in the Global North, the morbidity and mortality rates in Wayne County, Michigan, of which Detroit is the county seat, are high. For example, infant mortality rates in Detroit are 15 per 1000 live births, higher than that seen in Mexico, one of the more economically stable countries of the Global South (14 per 1000 live births), and they are well above the national U.S. rate (6 per 1000 live births) (CDC 2017a; Meyers and Hunt 2014; Plecher 2020). Limited access to water, another infringement on human rights, drew the attention of the United Nations when Detroit began a water shutoff program that left approximately 27,000 people without potable water (UN News 2014). UN Special Rapporteurs Catarina de Albuquerque and Leilani Farha stated: "the 'most vulnerable and poorest' of the city's population were being disproportionately affected, including a predominant number of African Americans" (UN News 2014). Diverse non-government organizations (NGOs) commonly use inability to access safe drinking water as an indicator of poverty and other health conditions (CDC 2017b). Access to water and infant mortality can serve as indicators of human rights concerns, suggesting the need for further investigation into structural factors that ultimately impact health and well-being (Winburn et al. this volume).

Responses of the body to the environment and its associated resources permeate deep-seated and longstanding literature that discusses the "embodiment" of inequality and the physiological effects of structural violence. While frequently discussed by other anthropological subdisciplines, such as bioarchaeology (See Klaus 2012; Nystrom 2014; Watkins 2012), this notion is only recently garnering attention from forensic anthropology (Gravlee 2009; Knudson and Stojanowski 2008; Tremblay and Reedy 2020; Wolputte 2004). However, recent critiques have suggested that forensic anthropologists have an obligation to document evidence of structural violence in casework, especially when considering the high number of unidentified cold cases in the United States, including those individuals who died migrating across the U.S. southwestern border (Beatrice et al. 2021; Bird and Bird this volume; Goad 2020; Reineke 2019; Soler and Beatrice 2018; Soler, Beatrice, and Martínez this volume). In these dialogues, scholars argue that power dynamics embedded in culture impact one's ascribed and achieved social identities and related access to resources. Ultimately, restricted access to resources and the chronic stress caused by structural violence will have a physical impact on the body.

For instance, from a biological and physiological perspective, it is well documented that the accumulated effects of stress can have a lasting impact on overall health and lower the body's immune response (Garland and Reitsema 2019; Juster, McEwen, and Lupien 2010; McEwen 2003). A physiological response to stress triggers the hypothalamic-pituitary-adrenal cortex or HPA complex, as the body tries to maintain stability, or allostasis (Schulz et al. 2012). This includes stress hormones such as cortisol and epinephrine, which are sensitive to social stressors. There are long-term impacts when children experience these stressors that subsequently carry into adulthood. Early trauma leads to HPA dysfunction, with children experiencing early family trauma having higher than average cortisol levels at the age of ten years and higher rates of morbidity compared to those not exposed to trauma (Flinn 2008). *Allostatic load*, the cumulative effects of stress causing wear and tear on the body's systems, increases as feelings of anxiety, loss, and fear accumulate and overwork the HPA complex. This leads to negative health outcomes such as higher blood pressure, higher rates of cardiovascular disease, negative effects on cognitive functioning, and higher mortality rates (Flinn 2008; Geronimus et al. 2020; Schulz et al. 2012; Winburn et al. this volume). The link between social stressors and physical manifestations in the body undergirds the application of structural violence theory.

As Mathena-Allen and Zuckerman (2020, 56) explain, "while populations on the receiving end of inequality, such as women, the poor, and other marginalized populations, may be obfuscated or invisible in the historical record, their lived experiences can be reconstructed through skeletal material." Just as the forensic humanitarian or human rights anthropologist reconstructs narratives of physical violence around the world enacted on marginalized peoples, there is an urgency to reconstruct narratives of structural violence and inequality experienced by the deceased within the United States. We recognize the need to contextualize our forensic anthropology cases more holistically in the broader sociopolitical history. To do this, we first situate the population of Detroit in its recent racial and economic history.

THE CASE OF WAYNE COUNTY, MICHIGAN

Historically Positioning Bodies and Poverty (1960s–Present)

Literatures interrogating osteological relationships to poverty posit that there must be contextualization of quantitative data, cultural processes, and historical backdrop (Beatrice et al. 2021; Crooks 1998; Goad 2020; Moore 2015; Nystrom 2014; Reineke 2019; Soler and Beatrice 2018; Watkins 2012; Williams 1992; Winburn et al. this volume). As recent scholarship in forensic humanitarian and human rights anthropology demonstrates, forensic science is not divorced from the political, social, and economic contexts in which it operates (Kim and Hepner 2019; Kim and Rosenblatt forthcoming; Rosenblatt 2015; Rosenblatt 2019; Wagner 2008), reinforcing the premise that contextualization of human remains cannot be overlooked, even in domestic casework of the Global North. The need for contextualization is emphasized by the contentious contribution of forensic anthropologists to colonially biased and racialized frameworks, with assessments of "ancestry" coming under critique (Bethard and DiGangi 2020; DiGangi and Bethard 2021). Rather than complying with marginalizing ideologies, there has been pressure in the field to dismantle methodologies that reinforce oppression of living populations. Considering the ethical duties of combating racist ideology and assisting in making the invisible visible, the lens of an osteology of structural violence within the biology of poverty framework facilitates our efforts. Stubblefield (2021) urges forensic anthropologists to engage with the communities they serve. Here, we offer a glimpse into the positionality of marginalized bodies in the historical context of Detroit, Michigan, and Wayne County.

From 1950 to 2015, Detroit experienced a dramatic 60 percent decrease in population; 90 percent decline in manufacturing work; 70 percent decline in businesses; and 55 percent median income decrease (Eisinger 2014). Much of the population and economic decline began with "White Flight" after the Race Riots and Civil Rights Movement of the 1960s. From 1968 to 1969, 173,000 predominantly White residents left Detroit. There has been a steady outmigration to the present day, leading to economic collapse via a shrinking client base for businesses and job scarcity. In 1987, General Motors shut down its Clark and Fleetwood assembly plants, and laid off over 6,600 workers in the process, most of whom were Black (Thompson 2017). As of the 2010 Census, Detroit had 713,000 residents, but the city was built to support two million (Safransky 2014). This has had a lasting impact on the Detroit economy, particularly for minority groups (McClure et al. 2019). As is known through studies of redlining, when people and businesses leave communities, banks will not support investments, creating resource voids, where education, healthcare, employment, housing, and foodways become scarce.

The promise of prosperity and equality is still elusive to Black, Indigenous, and People of Color (BIPOC) living in Detroit. In this way, Detroit has long been a harbinger for urban America, reflecting the effects of the neoliberal agenda. The political landscape of the 1960s–1970s also fostered President Johnson's "War on Crime" and President Nixon's "War on Drugs," and these "wars" took place in the poorest urban centers of the United States (Alexander 2011; Alexander 2020; Thompson 2017). The "War on Crime" made way for the Detroit Police Department to create the "Stop the Robberies and Enjoy Safe Streets" (STRESS) Program—meant to "rein in Blacks" at the bequest of White voters (Thompson 2017). Black Americans were arrested and investigated at much higher rates than White Americans, a phenomenon that continues to be well documented across the United States.

Coleman Young, the city's first Black mayor in 1974, increased support of police rather than address the poverty caused by the "White Flight," which removed much of the tax base and weakened infrastructure. Supporting a crime-control model of criminal justice, Young oversaw the creation of twenty-three prisons while in office, and most of those incarcerated were from Detroit. Further making the marginalized invisible, the incarcerated also lost their right to vote. The effects of this are impactful when one considers that as of 2012 almost 230,000 children in Michigan had a parent who was incarcerated. Of these children, a disproportionately high number of them were from Detroit (Thompson 2017). The incarceration of Detroiters in other cities took away federal funding for roads, schools, and hospitals, again highlighting the persistence of structural violence as access to resources continued to erode.

From 2002 to 2013, there were 83,381 tax foreclosure cases reported in the city of Detroit, of which majority-Black neighborhoods were at ten times higher risk (Zahran et al. 2019). This contributed to the ongoing economic downturn, as increasing numbers of properties became "vacant." Researchers found that vacancy correlated with the number of Black American residents, unemployment rate, and food assistance recipients (Zahran et al. 2019). Rather than trying to work to help stabilize and protect the populace, tax foreclosures opened the door for desperate land grabs, evicting thousands of former homeowners and further devaluing property in the city with the deluge of vacancies and abandonments (Akers and Seymour 2019). This had a cascading effect, as the weakening of one's social system (e.g., housing) inevitably affects other cultural components (e.g., healthcare and labor), with correlations between vacancy, food insecurity, and unemployment.

The Great Recession of 2008 that was due to the subprime mortgage crisis led to Detroit filing for bankruptcy in July of 2013—the largest city in American history to ever do so. Consequently, Michigan's Republican Governor Rick Snyder appointed an Emergency Planner to take over financial responsibility of Detroit, overruling elected officials. The financial crisis in Detroit and *en masse* evictions led to creative attempts to "reinvent" the city. Currently, Detroiters are seven years deep into the fifty-year plan of "Detroit Future City" (DFC). The alleged politically neutral plan claims to reinvent Detroit as a green city, razing "vacant buildings" and developing retention ponds, greenways, and urban farms. At the same time, public services such as water and waste disposal will be *withdrawn* from some areas (Safransky 2014). Vacancies in Detroit have been described as a "new American Frontier" in need of cultivation (Safransky 2014). The ongoing neoliberal effort to gentrify and erase the inhabitants of Detroit in favor of privatization of public property continues despite the fact that 90,000 people, mostly BIPOC, still live—and die—in these "empty" areas. The progression of degraded, blighted, or "vacant" spaces embedded in existing communities has contributed to myriad impacts on residents.

Embodying Poverty: Arson, Access, and Allostatic Load for the Living

The interrelated effects of structural violence can be seen through the problem of "vacant" buildings (Zahran et al. 2019). An estimated 20 percent of homes in Detroit are abandoned or blighted, and with proliferation of "vacant buildings" there has been an increase in arsons—a last resort attempt to remove blight. The remnants of buildings pose economic, physical, and psychological dangers to communities. For example, as mentioned at the start of this chapter, a series of murder victims had been killed in an abandoned house owned by the city. The house remained standing over a year after the murders. In an interview with a local newspaper, a neighbor commented, "it's like they want this to keep happening" (LeDuff 2020), as the house, and many others like it, create a dangerous landscape of hunting ground for violent offenders. They also serve as a reminder that those living there go unseen by those with the power to intervene. Chronic stressors such as neighborhood safety may be commonly discussed in terms of psychological impacts, but also have real physiological responses when considering the HPA complex. Recurring stressors are believed to deplete the immune reserves to make individuals more susceptible to things such as the common cold and cause more frequent illness (Flinn 2008; Winburn et al. this volume).

Citizens of Detroit, by and large, have responded to the city's failure to respond through the observance of "Devil's Night" (i.e., the night before Halloween), when high rates of arson target neglected, vacant properties, attempting to rid neighborhoods of dangerous structures. Extending beyond Halloween, 300–600 buildings each month are currently burned by residents who otherwise have limited control of their environment (Zahran et al. 2019). In 2011, the Fire Commissioner of Detroit set a policy of "Let it Burn," where fire suppression would not be deployed for "abandoned" buildings. This policy had unintended consequences; when fires are not quickly extinguished, toxins are released into the air. Researchers used the data from "Devil's Night" in Detroit to measure additional toxins emitted citywide on those evenings. Zahran and colleagues (2019) linked the atmospheric levels of toxins measured with air quality monitors throughout the city and collected from the U.S. EPA's Air Quality System database. Although the policy may preserve scarce resources of the municipal fire departments and achieve clearing of landscapes, it also exposes inhabitants to hazardous gases, such as sulfur dioxide (SO_2), nitrogen dioxide (NO_2), and carbon monoxide (CO), and puts elderly residents with cardiopulmonary conditions at greater risk. The results demonstrated a significant correlation between these fires and air quality when looking at peak arson years (1980–1987) relative to non-peak years (1988–2013) (Zahran et al. 2019). Figure 8.1 shows the front steps of a house that had been burned to the ground by arson; decomposed and burned human remains were found among the debris. These unsafe living conditions are exacerbated not only by discriminatory practices, but also by the inability to access health insurance and healthcare.

When people lack adequate healthcare, preventive medicine also suffers. Mortality from "sentinel" causes of morbidity are those which are preventable by medical intervention or treatment. Between 1994 and 1996, Detroit was one of the top five cities in the United States with the highest Black/White ratio of death rates (per 100,000 per year) for individuals under sixty-five years for conditions that were treatable with medical attention (Polednak 2000). Further, the death rate for Black Americans from sentinel causes was at 20.5 per 100,000 per year compared to only 5.4 per 100,000 for White Americans (Polednak 2000). With decreased preventive medicine, disease severity and mortality inevitably increase. From 1973 to 1994, Black men in Detroit had higher rates of distant (i.e., advanced stage) prostate carcinoma compared to White men in Detroit, with Black men more than two times as likely to have distant carcinoma than White men, which ultimately increased the mortality rate because the pathology was not discovered soon enough

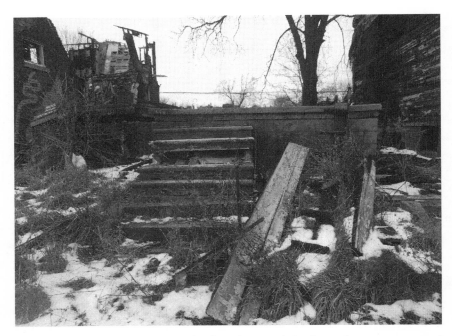

Figure 8.1   Burned house in Detroit where human skeletal remains were recovered.
Photograph by Megan K. Moore.

(Schwartz et al. 1996). Similar issues can be seen with Detroit women. Access to healthcare providers is limited due to the changing landscape, and women in middle-to-high-poverty regions of the city were more likely to have late-stage breast cancer diagnoses. Areas with fewer doctors' offices correlated to an increase in these late-stage diagnoses, showing a clear example of structural violence (Barry, Breen, and Barrett 2012).

While it is true that BIPOC are impacted by these factors at higher rates, it should be noted that the impacts of poverty, in a biological sense, are not limited to racialized groups. When looking at groups of people in Detroit, neighborhood poverty as a whole correlates to increased allostatic load, creating greater biological risk for those who have lower socioeconomic status. That correlation is independent of household income and demographic details—including race (Schulz et al. 2012). Poverty rates in Detroit are much higher than the national averages. In fact, between 35 and 38 percent of *all* residents in Detroit have annual reported incomes of less than $10,000, much lower than the national poverty rates for each group, which range between 6 and 15 percent (Geronimus et al. 2020). Interestingly, the allostatic load was just as high or higher for the poor Whites in Detroit as for the poor Blacks and Hispanics (Geronimus et al. 2020). This suggests that the effects of poverty reflect unseen heterogeneity in lived experiences, an important characteristic of the situationally specific poverty of Detroit. Grasping a sense of the documented struggles of the living, we ask how that translates into the missing and unidentified?

The Missing and Unidentified in Wayne County, MI

What do the missing persons and the bodies of the marginalized tell us when considering Crooks's (1998) biology of poverty or an osteology of structural violence? Do they reflect revitalization and prosperity or substandard living conditions with high allostatic loads? As forensic anthropologists serving Detroit during the last eight years, we have seen the effects of physical and structural violence among society as a whole and its effects on the human body through analysis of remains at the Wayne County M.E.O. To center our discussion on the violence made visible through the skeletal remains, we first consider the status of the missing and unidentified. Of Michigan's 3,992 missing persons, 2,955 (74%) of those are from Wayne County (H. Friedlander, Missing Persons Unit, Michigan State Police, personal communication, January 13, 2022). Concerning unidentified human remains, 265 of the 326 (81.3%) from Michigan are from the city of Detroit; 59.52 percent of the total unidentified cases are estimated to be BIPOC (www.namus.gov 2022) (table 8.1). Individuals of African ancestry make up 38.7 percent of the population of Detroit (www.census.gov 2020), yet they represent an estimated 54.69 percent of the forensic anthropology cases over the last eight years. From 2014 to 2021, we examined 141 forensic anthropology cases (excluding any cases involving non-human bones), the counts of 128 of these cases representing the adults are included in this preliminary analysis (see table 8.2). Like the unidentified individual at the start of this chapter who was found in a "vacant" building, the majority (73.4%) of the cases that we analyzed from 2014 to 2021 were also found in impoverished situations such

Table 8.1 The Number of Unidentified Remains in Wayne County, Michigan by "Racial" Classification Reported in www.NamUs.gov

Unidentified Persons Total and by "Racial" Classification	Total # of Cases in Wayne County
Total Unidentified Persons	265
Black	140
White	87
Hispanic/Latino	5
Uncertain	43

Note. Data reported to www.namus.gov as of January 10, 2022. There are 10 pending or circumstantial IDs not accounted for in the number of total unidentified persons.

Table 8.2 The Number and Frequencies of Adult Forensic Anthropology Cases by "Racial" Classification and/or Ancestry Estimation in Wayne County, Michigan

Sex and Ancestry	# of Cases	% of Cases	# of Unknowns	# of Identified	% Unknown ancestry specific	% Identified ancestry specific	% Unknown overall	% Identified overall
WF	16	12.5	3	13	18.75	81.25	7.14	15.12
WM	32	25.0	7	25	21.88	78.13	16.67	29.07
BF	24	18.75	9	15	37.5	62.5	21.43	17.44
BM	46	35.94	15	31	32.61	67.39	35.71	36.05
HF	1	0.78	0	1	0	100	0	1.16
HM	1	1.56	1	1	50	50	2.38	1.16
?	7	5.47	7	0	100	0	16.67	0

Note. Data based on adult forensic anthropology cases from 2014 to 2021.

as in abandoned houses or buildings or in empty lots beside vacant dwellings. Another 15.6 percent have been recovered from homeless encampments or wooded areas.

Structural violence and physical violence are not mutually exclusive. This can be seen in the widely recognized disproportionately high rates of missing and murdered Indigenous women (MMIW) in the United States and Canada when compared to rates of missing for the general population (Kim 2014; Kim 2018). Structural violence contributes to the physical violence vis-à-vis absence of a coordinated systemic response, low prioritization in case load, deterrence from reporting, and other policies, practices, and beliefs that create barriers (Kaplan et al. this volume; Bird and Bird this volume). A similar relationship between structural and physical violence can also be seen among the cases of Detroit. For example, the medical examiners ruled homicide in 32 percent of the adult cases, with perimortem blunt force trauma in fourteen cases (10.9%), perimortem high velocity projectile trauma in fifteen cases (14.1%), perimortem sharp force trauma in six cases, and strangulation in two cases. When considering how poverty shrouds victims in invisibility, this sometimes can have quite a literal interpretation, as eight of the adult homicide victims were found discarded in some way: two decedents were found in garbage cans, one was found in a 50-gallon drum, one was found dismembered in a duffle bag, one was dismembered and hidden in two separate storage bins, and three were wrapped in a sheet, garbage bag, or plastic tarp. Of the six sharp force trauma cases, three of those were cases of dismemberment. There were signs of healed gunshot trauma in five individuals, representing the long-term physical violence to which many of the Detroit residents are exposed. Watkins (2012) similarly found significantly higher rates of healed fractures and evidence of interpersonal violence in individuals from the Cobb Skeletal Collection who had lived and died in an almshouse in Washington, D.C. compared to those individuals from the general population from the same skeletal collection. Considering the historical backdrop and positionality of the living, we interrogate our casework further and the narratives embedded within the remains.

PATHOLOGIES OF POVERTY—A BRIEF OVERVIEW OF CASEWORK

Farmer (1999) describes the "pathologies of power" made apparent when examining health insecurity. Looking at structural violence through a public health lens, he discusses how different groups within a culture experience differential access to healthcare and resources that support physical and mental well-being. Using a similar approach, we examine pathologies of poverty to understand how the disparate access to health and shelter, labor, and physical trauma can manifest skeletally and contribute to structural violence and marginalization. Each of the following subsections challenges the forensic anthropologist to interrogate the highlighted aspect of marginalization and how skeletal analyses can evidence the lived experiences of individuals. While statistical analyses of pathologies (e.g., controlling for age and other variables) is beyond the scope of the current chapter, raw frequencies are presented to emphasize the skeletal data that are seen in the Wayne County forensic anthropology casework. These case examples paint a picture of limited access to resources and epitomize the reality of living in "vacant" or invisible spaces, both literally and metaphorically.

Access to Shelter and Exposure to the Elements—Postmortem Evidence

We commonly encounter mummified human remains in the Detroit and Wayne County area. Mummification occurs naturally when remains are stored in a dry location, such as inside a building. The process of mummification can begin as early as three weeks after death but is facilitated when the remains are wrapped in cloth, especially cotton (Dautartas 2009; White 2013). For a body to become fully mummified, at least several months have elapsed since death. Nearly one-third of the adult remains (n=38) from the forensic anthropology cases that we analyzed exhibit extensive desiccation of soft tissues. When contextualizing these remains, many have been recovered from vacant houses, vacant lots, and homeless encampments, as well as deaths at legal residences that had passed unnoticed for extended periods of time. Individuals who live in these abandoned and "vacant" homes are invisible in life; not being found for several months after death is a continuation of this invisibility and marginalization well into the postmortem interval.

Contributing to mummification, we find individuals wrapped in several layers of clothing and blankets as they had lived in spaces with no access to heating. January is typically the coldest month of the year in Detroit with an average high temperature of 29.3°F (−1.5°C) (Weather-Atlas 2021). One individual was found below the highway underpass inside a sleeping bag; one was found in a sleeping bag in a vacant garage; several others were wrapped in blankets inside vacant houses and buildings—including crawl spaces. Another was found in the backseat of a car. Many of these individuals were found bundled in several layers of clothing. Three individuals exhibited evidence of prior amputations, two of which had medical documentation of frostbite necessitating the amputation. One of these individuals exhibited an active infectious process of the soft tissues of the ankles and feet, and he used newspapers and sugar packets to bandage his injuries (figure 8.2). When

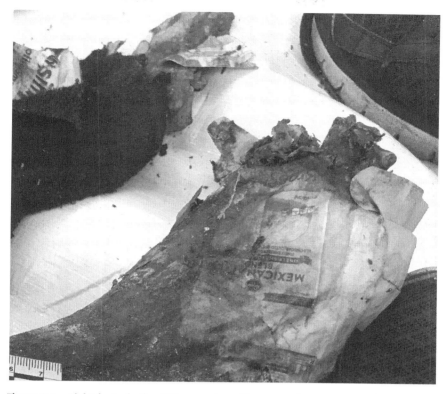

Figure 8.2   Right foot of a frostbite amputee with scraps of newspaper and sugar packets used as bandages. Photograph by Megan K. Moore.

considering a pathological aspect to the biology of poverty, skeletal indicators of exposure highlight the lived realities of those without access to shelter, even in the coldest months of urban Michigan, and limited access to medical care and resources to treat the cold-related injuries.

Access to Dental Care and Nutrition—Postmortem Evidence

One privilege typically associated with healthcare of wealthier developed nations is access to dental care, though this is not the case for all U.S. residents. The relationship between marginalization, oral pathology, and other pathology is discussed by other authors in this volume (Soler, Beatrice, and Martínez this volume; Winburn et al. this volume). A previous study by Nriagu and colleagues (2006) revealed that of Detroit's low-income adult residents 95.5 percent had evidence of clinical caries and 80 percent had carious lesions that progressed through the enamel and into the dentin. The average number of teeth lost in the living sample was 3.4 teeth per individual, with thirty carious lesions on average (Nriagu et al. 2006). Our casework reflects the same poor dental health, with the antemortem tooth loss for this forensic anthropology sample even more dire. We found the average number of antemortem absent teeth per person to be 9.2 (S.D. 10.45), with a median antemortem tooth loss of 4. The mean age of the identified decedents from our casework is 44.8 years (S.D. 17.05). Antemortem tooth loss is a complicated variable, as mentioned earlier by Soler and colleagues (this volume). For our preliminary analysis, the average antemortem tooth loss excludes possible third molar extractions or congenital absence for those individuals in which all other teeth were present. Additionally, only the counts of antemortem tooth loss of the maxillae are reported for two cases with edentulism, as the mandible was not recovered; thus, our calculation provides a conservative estimate of overall antemortem tooth loss in this particular sample. Figures 8.3a and 8.3b exhibit the more severe examples of poor dental health observed from the forensic anthropology cases.

Other pathological conditions related to dental health reveal nutritional deficiencies for the decedents in our sample. Scurvy is a vitamin C-deficiency disease that is historically associated with long periods of sea travel, and it can impact dental health, osteoblast function, and healing (Callus, Verra, and Ferry 2018). Modern-day cases still occur and are higher in developing nations associated with malnutrition, sometimes reaching epidemic levels in refugee camps, though rarely in the Global North (Wijkmans and Talsma 2016). The modern causes of scurvy can be related to poor diet, which occurs more frequently in adult males who live alone and/or in individuals living in poverty in the United States (Connelly, Becker, and McDonald 1982; Wang and Still 2007; Wijkmans and Talsma 2016). In at least three forensic anthropology cases from Detroit, we see evidence of lesions that are diagnostic of adult scurvy, with another four individuals having more mild skeletal manifestations that are suggestive. The anterior facial skeleton of Case 0002 shows bilateral fine cortical porosity (pin- to pen-point, sized<1mm) of the

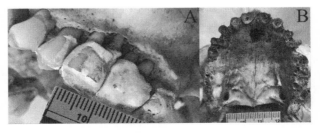

Figure 8.3 A) Severe calculus of the left maxillary dentition indicating no access to dental care. B) Inferior view of maxillae of adult male with carious destruction of all remaining crowns. Credit for all photographs: Megan K. Moore.

anterior right and left maxillae, inferior to the nasal aperture, and along the alveolar margin, which are diagnostic for adult scurvy (Ortner 2003, Snoddy et al. 2018). Figure 8.4 shows the inferior aspect of the cranium with bilateral fine cortical porosity (pin- to pen-point, <1mm in diameter) of the palatine processes and posterior maxillae, basilar portion of the occipital bone, and greater wings and pterygoid fossae of the sphenoid bone, the specific distribution of the porosity for which is also diagnostic of scurvy. Pathological presentations like this are diagnostic of scurvy, but natural variation, other nutritional deficiencies, trauma, and localized infection cannot be ruled out (Ortner 2003; Snoddy et al. 2018). Alternatively, a differential diagnosis of anemia or untreated infection tells a similar story of poverty and homelessness through the lack of access to proper nutrition, medical care, clean drinking water, and personal hygiene materials.

Severe presentation of rheumatoid arthritis was also observed in Case 0003. This pathology is not correlated with activity and appears to have an environmental component, but there is clearly a genetic link (Ortner 2003). Figure 8.5 shows the example of severe rheumatoid arthritis of the wrist and hand for Case 0003 who was found in a vacant residence. The severity of the condition in this case suggested that the individual was not being medically treated for the condition.

Frequently, the individuals in this sample exhibit skeletal and dental pathologies consistent with restricted access to medical care, dental care, and show signs of malnutrition—all of which are physical markers of poverty and lack of access to necessary resources (Soler, Beatrice, and Martínez this volume; Winburn et al. this volume). The evidence of pathology in the adult skeletal remains must be considered in association with the contextual evidence of poverty and the locations from where the remains are found—often in vacant buildings.

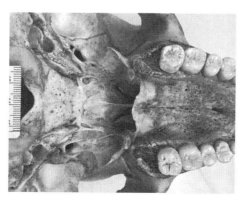

Figure 8.4   Pinpoint porosity along the palatine processes, basilar portion, and greater wings of sphenoid as evidence of malnutrition diagnostic as scurvy. Photograph by Megan K. Moore.

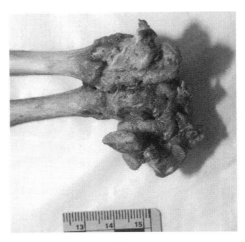

Figure 8.5 Severe ankylosing of the wrist due rheumatoid arthritis. Photograph by Jaymelee J. Kim.

In addition to being found in vacant residences, human remains have been found in vacated funeral homes—specifically those of fetuses and neonates.

Access to Mortuary Practices and Infant Mortality—Postmortem Evidence

On October 13, 2018, eleven fetuses/neonates were discovered hidden in a crawl space of a recently shuttered funeral home. This led to the discovery of multiple funeral homes and cemeteries improperly handling the remains of fetuses and infants, as well as adult remains. The Wayne County M.E.O. received the cases in one large cardboard box. Each infant was packaged just as uniquely as were the delicate remains wrapped within. Many of the desiccated neonates had hospital tags tied around their ankles with the first name listed as "Baby Girl" or "Baby Boy." One had a diaper and several had the umbilical cord clamps still attached. One had an IV attached as evidence of life-saving attempts. All but one infant had some form of hospital documentation that indicated the child was stillborn. The estimated ages-at-death ranged from an eighteen-week-old fetus to an approximately one-week old neonate based on the length of the femur and humerus as measured from radiographs.

These remains were not repatriated to their parents or given a proper burial, leading to further traumatization of families as they learned of the discovery in the news and from law enforcement personnel. While beyond the scope of this chapter, the infant remains could potentially be described as victims of necroviolence, as described by Reineke (2019) and De León

(2015). Building upon seminal works of scholars such as Verdery (1999) and Das and Poole (2004) and "the continuum of violence," De León framed necroviolence (2015, 69) as the "violence performed and produced through the specific treatment of corpses that is perceived to be offensive, sacrilegious, or inhumane." Other authors in this volume discuss the mistreatment of the dead as a continuation of structural violence (Bird and Bird this volume; Nystrom 2014; Kaplan et al. this volume; Winburn et al. this volume). The mistreatment of infant remains also draws attention to the high crude infant mortality of Black women in Detroit, which is more than twice that for their White counterparts (14.0 vs. 5.9 deaths per 1,000 live births) (Wallace et al. 2019). From 2010 to 2013, 72 percent of 845 infant deaths were born to Black women and "the risk of infant mortality was greater in areas of concentrated deprivation relative to areas of concentrated privilege. Joint racial and socioeconomic segregation contributes to the persistent racial inequity in infant mortality" (Wallace et al. 2019, 208; Sealy-Jefferson, Mustafaa, and Misra 2019; Zuberi et al. 2016). Some speculated that the infant remains found hidden at the funeral home in Detroit represented hoarding or evidence of an unsanctioned abortion enterprise, but the reason is still unclear. More likely, the families did not have the money to pay for infant funerals—unprepared for this tragic birth outcome.

It is a felony in the state of Michigan for a funeral home to retain human remains beyond 180 days without final disposition (Michigan Penal Code: MCL 750.160c(2)(b)). It could have been due to the lack of resources afforded to family members with stillborn infants; however, one family claimed that they returned for the infant, but funeral home employees told them the remains had been discarded (Selk 2018). Regardless, the violence against the neonates and their parents persisted, as families were unable to choose the mortuary rites for their deceased.

The funeral home revelation led to the discovery of sixty-three fetuses/neonates found at another funeral home, with the possibility of more yet to be discovered (Selk 2018). Evidence later emerged, and a lawsuit followed, that alleged that one funeral home had billed Medicaid for funeral expenses that were never completed. Both funeral homes have since been closed (Selk 2018). Nonetheless, these cases provide evidence of invisible violence that further traumatize families (De León 2015; Reineke 2019) and serve as a reflection of lesser-known struggles facing the community.

Access to Healthcare and Drug Intervention, The Opioid Crisis—Postmortem Evidence

The United States has faced an opioid crisis which is only recently being addressed through legal proceedings holding the pharmaceutical industry accountable (Sherman 2020). With limited access to mental and physical healthcare, Wayne County also experienced the opioid epidemic that contributed to mortality, especially after carfentanil was released into the global distribution. Carfentanil is a synthetic opioid which serves as an elephant tranquilizer, an estimated 10,000 times more potent than morphine, with chronic pain sufferers becoming victims of the black-market manufacture of opioids and their addiction that was initially started by the American medical system (King et al. 2019). This led to a spike in deaths at the Wayne County M.E.O. in 2016, with Detroit at the center of the epidemic from 2015 to 2017.

Many of the cases of overdose witnessed at the Wayne County M.E.O. are of those who suffered from chronic pain, which can lead to addiction and self-prescription (Andronowski and Depp this volume). One individual had documentation of two serious accidents in his youth. He had a healed fracture of the humerus and an avulsion fracture of the ischium that never fused likely causing severe pain while walking. He also lost his left eye and had reconstructive surgery to his face. With a history of drug abuse, he disappeared shortly after being released from the hospital at the age of fifty-three. Evidence at the scene suggests he overdosed soon thereafter, and his skeletal remains were found undisturbed in a homeless encampment in SW Detroit.

In another case, a thirty-eight-year-old mother of five children was found located on the floor of a vacant house in what appeared to be a partially seated position in a state of advanced decomposition. Syringes were found closely associated at the scene according to the case report summary completed by the Medical Examiner Investigator. In her medical record, it was documented that she suffered from chondrosarcoma and had a craniotomy with orthopedic plates and surgical removal of most of her left maxilla. The case report summary briefly explained how she had been addicted to pain pills and had been arrested multiple times on drug possession charges. When formal medical institutions failed to provide the needed treatments for individuals such as these, they turned to drug use.

CONCLUDING REMARKS

Mass deaths affiliated with warfare, human rights violations, or disaster and refugee diaspora carry with them an expectation that forensic analyses will evidence individuals' suffering and prevent governments and leaders from masking or revising history. Domestic casework in the United States, outside of these contexts, also assumes reconstruction of trauma and disease; however, there is no expectation to document evidence of experiences of mass violence, let alone forms of structural violence. While no court awaits evidence of policies, practices, and beliefs that deny access to resources, that is the evidence forensic anthropologists may be positioned to provide, if not for the courts, then for the historical record, for both policymakers and service providers.

When pushing the field of forensic anthropology forward, we interrogate the humanitarian aspect of individual case analysis and the ability to contextualize it in broader sociocultural dynamics, particularly in countries of the Global North. To thoroughly understand the demographics, trauma, and pathology of the deceased, we respond to Crooks's challenge and build on emerging work, particularly of those working in the U.S. borderlands or in African American and residential school cemeteries (Beatrice and Soler 2016; Cress 2018; Goad 2020; Kim 2014; King 2010; Reineke 2019; Soler and Beatrice 2018; Soler et al. 2019; Spradley et al. 2019). Going a step further, we demonstrate that forensic anthropology can illuminate an osteology of structural violence as part of biology of poverty by using a more holistic approach to investigate cases within the broader sociopolitical and sociohistorical context.

The biology of poverty that we observed based on this forensic anthropology sample from Detroit exhibited evidence of limited access to food, shelter, healthcare, medications, and dental care. Many of the bodies exhibited evidence of physical labor in an economically unstable community as vacant spaces and homelessness proliferate. Increasing rates of homelessness accompany economic decline with a policy of eviction by the state for delinquent taxes. Many of the persons who died due to the harsh winters did not die entirely from natural causes. Socio-political forces rendered them invisible and placed them in a state of precarity as they experienced the effects of structural violence. Through review of historical dynamics of Detroit, evictions and the role of "vacant" buildings, health status of the living, and contemporary casework, we present the skeletal impacts of structural violence and how poverty is embodied in the remains, deposition, and care of the dead. Just as forensic anthropologists commit to evidencing the overt violence of homicide and warfare, we also bear witness to the insidious and longstanding structural violence experienced by marginalized groups through interrogating modern America's biology of poverty. We conclude with a call for forensic anthropologists to engage with a holistic approach to casework and violence. As the forensic investigator, we attempt to minimize bias, but also recognize that, as with all disciplines, to fail to recognize biases and positionality would be in error, and we know that our actions can contribute to ongoing narratives of erasure and marginalization. Using our skills, we can attempt to minimize violence that can persist even after death and accurately document the physical and structural violence experienced in life. We are some of the last people to witness and to document these abuses. With that comes an obligation and responsibility to reveal, rather than obscure systems of power and oppression.

The following words paraphrased from our friend and fellow anthropologist, Dr. Elizabeth DiGangi resonate here:

Documentation of the violence will hopefully prevent others from being hurt. Not everyone can do the work we do. It is difficult, but it is very important work.

If not us, then who?

NOTE

1. Acknowledgments: A special recognition to the individuals from the cases described herein and to the many missing and unidentified individuals and their families. Dr. Carl Schmidt, Chief Medical Examiner, Wayne County, MI and all the pathologists, autopsy technicians, and the medical examiner investigators. Sgt. Shannon Jones, Detroit Police; Lt. Sarah Krebs, Hanna Friedlander, Sgt. Dave Yount, cadaver dogs Lightning, Fil, Chappy, and Jameson, of the Michigan State Police. Dr. Elizabeth DiGangi was gracious to provide feedback on a draft of this manuscript, as well as to serve as a close friend and confidant. Our students who helped in the field, in the morgue, and in the classroom have helped inspire this work. Finally, thank you to the reviewers and editors of this volume for their insightful comments.

REFERENCES

Akers, Joshua and Eric Seymour. 2019. "The eviction machine: Neighborhood instability and blight in Detroit's neighborhoods." Poverty Solutions at the University of Michigan. Working Paper Series #5-19, July 2019. https://poverty.umich.edu/files/2019/08/Akers-et-al-Eviction-Machine-Revised-August-12.pdf.

Alexander, Michelle. 2011. "The new Jim Crow." *Ohio St. J. Crim. L.* 9: 7.

———. 2020. *The New Jim Crow: Mass Incarceration in the Age of Colorblindness.* The New Press.

Barry, Janis, Nancy Breen, and Michael Barrett. 2012. "Significance of increasing poverty levels for determining late-stage breast cancer diagnosis in 1990 and 2000." *Journal of Urban Health* 89, no. 4: 614–27.

Beatrice, Jared S., and Angela Soler. 2016. "Skeletal indicators of stress: A component of the biocultural profile of undocumented migrants in southern Arizona." *Journal of Forensic Sciences* 61, no. 5: 1164–72.

Beatrice, Jared S., Angela Soler, Robin C. Reineke, and Daniel E. Martínez. 2021. "Skeletal evidence of structural violence among undocumented migrants from Mexico and Central America." *American Journal of Physical Anthropology* 176, no. 4: 584–605.

Bethard, Jonathan D. and Elizabeth DiGangi. 2020. "Letter to the editor—Moving beyond a Lost Cause: Forensic anthropology and ancestry estimates in the United States." *Journal of Forensic Sciences* 65, no. 5: 1791–2.

Callus, Claire Ann, Samantha Vella, and Peter Ferry. 2018. "Scurvy is back." *Nutrition and Metabolic Insights* 11: 1178638818809097.

Census.gov. n.d. "Quick facts." Accessed March 1, 2020. https://www.census.gov/quickfacts/waynecountymichigan.

Centers for Disease Control and Prevention. 1997. "Urban community intervention to prevent Halloween arson – Detroit, Michigan, 1985–1996." *MMWR Wkly* 46, no. 14: 299–304. https://wonder.cdc.gov/wonder/prevguid/m0047208/m0047208.asp.

———. 2017a. Trends in infant mortality in the United States, 2005–2014. NCHS Data Brief 279. https://www.cdc.gov/nchs/products/databriefs/db279.htm#:~:text=Over%20the%20past%20decade%2C%20the,mortality%20(4%2C5).

———. 2017b. Assessing Access to Water and Sanitation. Global Water, Sanitation, and Hygiene. https://www.cdc.gov/healthywater/global/assessing.html.

Connelly, Thomas J., Andera Becker, and John W. McDonald. 1982. "Bachelor scurvy." *International Journal of Dermatology* 21, no. 4: 209–10.

Cress, Joseph. 2018. "Forensic anthropologist discusses process of finding remains of three Carlisle Indian School students." *The Sentinel*. https://cumberlink.com/news/local/forensic-anthropologist-discusses-process-of-finding-remains-of-three-carlisle-indian-school-students/article_4515f4f4-1102-5f3e-963d-ac202e94545e.html.

Crooks, Deborah L. 1995. "American children at risk: Poverty and its consequences for children's health, growth, and school achievement." *American Journal of Physical Anthropology* 38, no. S21: 57–86.

Das, Veena, and Deborah Poole, eds. 2004. *Anthropology in the Margins of the State*. Santa Fe: School of American Research Press.

Data Driven Detroit. *State of the child: 2010*. Detroit, Michigan. https://sdc.datadrivendetroit.org/.

———. Detroit residential parcel survey of 2009 [Dataset and codebook]. 2010. Retrieved from http://portal.datadrivendetroit.org/.

Dautartas, Angela M. 2009. "The effect of various coverings on the rate of human decomposition." Unpublished Master's Thesis. University of Tennessee, Knoxville.

Detroit News, The. "Suspected Detroit serial killer to be tried in four slayings." 2020. https://www.detroitnews.com/story/news/local/detroit-city/2020/08/13/suspected-detroit-serial-killer-tried-4-slayings/3370771001/.

De León, Jason. 2015. "Necroviolence." In *The Land of Open Graves: Living and Dying on the Migrant Trail*, 62–85. University of California Press.

DiGangi, Elizabeth A., and Jonathan D. Bethard. 2021. "Uncloaking a Lost Cause: Decolonizing ancestry estimation in the United States." *American Journal of Physical Anthropology*. 175, no. 2: 422–36. https://doi.org/10.1002/ajpa.24212.

Eisinger, Peter. 2014. "Is Detroit dead?" *Journal of Urban Affairs* 36, no. 1: 1–12.

Farmer, Paul. 1999. "Pathologies of power: Rethinking health and human rights." *American Journal of Public Health* 89, no. 10: 1486–96.

———. 2003. "Pathologies of power: Health, human rights, and the new war on the poor." *North American Dialogue* 6, no. 1: 1–4.

Farmer, Paul E., Bruce Nizeye, Sara Stulac, and Salmaan Keshavjee. 2006. "Structural violence and clinical medicine." *PLoS Med* 3, no. 10: e449.

Flinn, Mark V. 2008. "Why words can hurt us: Social relationships, stress, and health." *Evolutionary Medicine and Health* 13: 247–58.

Garland, Carey J., and Laurie J. Reitsema. 2019. "Colonialism and structural violence: Implications for childhood physiological stress and mortality risk." *American Journal of Physical Anthropology* 168: 82–83.

Geronimus, Arline T., Jay A. Pearson, Erin Linnenbringer, Alexa K. Eisenberg, Carmen Stokes, Landon D. Hughes, and Amy J. Schulz. 2020. "Weathering in Detroit: Place, race, ethnicity, and poverty as conceptually fluctuating social constructs shaping variation in allostatic load." *The Milbank Quarterly* 98, no. 4: 1171–218.

Goad, Gennifer. 2020. "Expanding humanitarian forensic action: An approach to US cold cases." *Forensic Anthropology* 3, no. 1: 50–59.

Gravelee, Clarence C. 2009. "How race becomes biology: Embodiment of social inequality." *American Journal of Physical Anthropology* 139: 47–57.

Juster, Robert-Paul, Bruce S. McEwen, and Sonia J. Lupien. 2010. "Allostatic load biomarkers of chronic stress and impact on health and cognition." *Neuroscience & Biobehavioral Reviews* 35, no. 1: 2–16.

Kim, Jaymelee J. 2014. "They made us unrecognizable to each other: Human rights, truth, and reconciliation in Canada." Unpublished PhD dissertation, University of Tennessee, Knoxville, Tennessee.

———. 2018. "Perspectives from the ground: Colonial bureaucratic violence, identity, and transitional justice in Canada." *Conflict and Society* 4, no. 1: 116–34.

Kim, Jaymelee J., and Tricia Redeker Hepner. 2019. "Of justice and the grave: The role of the dead in post-conflict Uganda." *International Criminal Law Review* 19, no. 5: 819–43.

Kim, Jaymelee J., and Adam Rosenblatt. In Press. "Whose Humanitarianism? Whose Forensic Anthropology?" In *Anthropology of Violent Death: Theoretical Foundations for Forensic Humanitarian Action*. edited by Robert C. Parra and Douglas H. Ubelaker, Wiley: Hoboken, NJ.

Kimmerle, Erin H., and José Pablo Baraybar. 2008. *Skeletal Trauma: Identification of Injuries Resulting from Human Rights Abuse and Armed Conflict*. CRC Press.

King, Andrew, Daniel Foley, Cynthia Afrken, Cynthia Aaron, Lokman Sung, and Leigh Hlavaty. 2019. "Carfentanil-associated mortality in Wayne county, Michigan, 2015–2017." *American Journal of Public Health* 109, no. 2: 300–2.

King, Charlotte. 2010. "Separated by death and color: The African American cemetery of New Philadelphia, Illinois." *Historical Archaeology* 44, no. 1: 125–37.

Klaus, Haagen D. 2012. "The bioarchaeology of structural violence: A theoretical model and a case study." In *The Bioarchaeology of violence*, edited by Debra L. Martin, Ryan P. Harrod, and Ventura R. Pérez, 29–62. Gainesville, Tallahassee, Tampa, Boca Raton, Pensacola, Orlando, Miami, Jacksonville, Ft. Myers, Sarasota: University Press of Florida.

Knudson, Kelly J., and Christopher M. Stojanowski. 2008. "New directions in bioarchaeology: Recent contributions to the study of human social identities." *Journal of Archaeological Research* 16, no. 4: 397–432.

LeDuff, Charlie. 2020. "LeDuff: Detroit serial killer house still stands a year later in the land of the lost." *Deadline Detroit*. July 30, 2020. https://www.deadlinedetroit .com/articles/25872/leduff_detroit_serial_killer_house_still_stands_a_year_later _in_the_land_of_the_lost.

Martínez, Daniel E., Robin Reineke, Raquel Rubio-Goldsmith, and Bruce O. Parks. 2014. "Structural violence and migrant deaths in southern Arizona: Data from the Pima County Office of the Medical Examiner, 1990–2013." *Journal on Migration and Human Security* 2, no. 4: 257–86.

Mathena-Allen, Sarah, and Molly K. Zuckerman. 2020. "Embodying industrialization: Inequality, structural violence, disease, and stress in working-class and poor British women." In *The Bioarchaeology of Structural Violence*, edited by Lori A. Tremblay and Sarah C. Reedy, 53–79. Cham: Springer.

McClure, Elizabeth, Lydia Feinstein, Evette Cordoba, Christian Douglas, Michael Emch, Whitney Robinson, Sandro Galea, and Allison E. Aiello. 2019. "The legacy of redlining in the effect of foreclosures on Detroit residents' self-rated health." *Health & Place* 55: 9–19.

McEwen, Bruce S. 2003. "Mood disorders and allostatic load." *Biological Psychiatry* 54, no. 3: 200–207.

Meyers, Todd, and Nancy Rose Hunt. 2014. "The other global south." *The Lancet* 384, no. 9958: 1921–2.

Michigan Penal Code: MCL 750.160c(2)(b), accessed March 1, 2021. https://www .michigan.gov/documents/lara/Bulletin_-_Embalming_and_Final_Disposition _626268_7.pdf.

Moore, Megan. 2016. "The osteology of poverty in Detroit: Forensic anthropology case reports from 2014." *Michigan Academician* 43, no. 1–2: 183–347.

National Missing and Unidentified Persons System (NamUs). n.d. www.namus.gov. Accessed March 1, 2021.

Nriagu, Jerome, Brian Burt, Aaron Linder, Amid Ismail, and Woosung Sohn. 2006. "Lead levels in blood and saliva in a low-income population of Detroit, Michigan." *International Journal of Hygiene and Environmental Health* 209, no. 2: 109–21.

Nystrom, Kenneth C. 2014. "The bioarchaeology of structural violence and dissection in the 19th-century United States." *American Anthropologist* 116: 765–79.

Ortner, Donald. 2003. *Identification of Pathological Conditions in Human Skeletal Remains*. 2nd ed. Amsterdam: Academic Press.

Plecher, H. 2020. "Mexico: Infant mortality rate from 2009 to 2019." *Statista*. https:// www.statista.com/statistics/807025/infant-mortality-in-mexico/.

Polednak, Anthony P. 2000. "Black-white differences in sentinel causes of death: Counties in large metropolitan areas." *Journal of Urban Health* 77, no. 3: 501–7.

Reineke, Robin. 2019. "Necroviolence and postmortem care along the US-México border." In *The Border and Its Bodies: The Embodiment of Risk Along the*

US-México Line, edited by Thomas E. Sheridan and Randall H. McGuire, 144–72. University of Arizona Press.

Reveal News. 2020. From the center of investigative reporting. https://revealnews.org/episodes/the-lost-homes-of-detroit/, accessed January 11, 2020.

Rosenblatt, Adam. 2015. *Digging for the Disappeared*. Stanford University Press.

———. 2019. "The danger of a single story about forensic humanitarianism." *Journal of Forensic and Legal Medicine* 61: 75–7.

Rylko-Bauer, Barbara, and Paul Farmer. 2016. "Structural violence, poverty, and social suffering." *The Oxford Handbook of the Social Science of Poverty*: 47–74.

Safransky, Sara. 2014. "Greening the urban frontier: Race, property, and resettlement in Detroit." *Geoforum* 56: 237–248.

Schulz, Amy J., Graciela Mentz, Laurie Lachance, Jonetta Johnson, Causandra Gaines, and Barbara A. Israel. 2012. "Associations between socioeconomic status and allostatic load: Effects of neighborhood poverty and tests of mediating pathways." *American Journal of Public Health* 102, no. 9: 1706–14.

Schwartz, Kendra L., Richard K. Severson, James G. Gurney, and James E. Montie. 1996. "Trends in the stage specific incidence of prostate carcinoma in the Detroit metropolitan area: 1973–1994." *Cancer: Interdisciplinary International Journal of the American Cancer Society* 78, no. 6: 1260–6.

Sealy-Jefferson, Shawnita, Faheemah N. Mustafaa, and Dan P. Misra. 2019. "Early-life neighborhood context, perceived stress, and preterm birth in African American Women." *SSM - Population Health* 7: 100362.

Selk, Avi. 2018. "Dozens more infant corpses found as Detroit police widen investigation of funeral homes." *Washington Post*, October 21, 2018 at 9:05 a.m. EDT. https://www.washingtonpost.com/nation/2018/10/20/dozens-more-infant-corpses-found-detroit-police-widens-investigation-funeral-homes/. Accessed online March 2, 2021.

Sherman, Natalie. 2020. "Purdue Pharma to plead guilty in $8bn opioid settlement." *BBC News Business Reporter*. New York, Published 21 October 2020. https://www.bbc.com/news/business-54636002.

Snoddy, Anne Marie E., Hallie R. Buckley, Gail E. Elliott, Vivien G. Standen, Bernardo T. Arriaza, and Siân E. Halcrow. 2018. "Macroscopic features of scurvy in human skeletal remains: A literature synthesis and diagnostic guide." *American Journal of Physical Anthropology* 167, no. 4: 876–95.

Soler, Angela, and Jared S. Beatrice. 2018. "Expanding the role of forensic anthropology in a humanitarian crisis: An example from the USA-Mexico border." In *Sociopolitics of Migrant Death and Repatriation*, edited by Krista E. Latham and Alyson J. O'Daniel, 115–128. Cham: Springer.

Soler, Angela, Robin Reineke, Jared Beatrice, and Bruce E. Anderson. 2019. "Etched in bone: Embodied suffering in the remains of undocumented migrants." In *The Border and Its Bodies: The Embodiment of Risk Along the US-México Line*, edited by Thomas E. Sheridan and Randall H. McGuire, 173–207. University of Arizona Press.

Spradley, M. Katherine, Nicholas P. Herrmann, Courtney B. Siegert, and Chloe P. McDaneld. 2019. "Identifying migrant remains in South Texas: Policy and practice." *Forensic Sciences Research* 4, no. 1: 60–68.

Stubblefield, Phoebe R. 2021. "Don't let your world be too small: The relevance of identity and skeletal populations." Webinar, *Blinded by the White: Forensic Anthropology and Ancestry Estimation*. February 19, 2021. Sponsored by Binghamton University, Davidson College, and Louisiana State University.

Thompson, Heather Ann. 2017. *Whose Detroit?: Politics, Labor, and Race in a Modern American City*. Cornell University Press.

Tremblay, Lori A., and Sarah C. Reedy, eds. 2020. *The Bioarchaeology of Structural Violence: A Theoretical Framework for Industrial Era Inequality*. Springer Nature.

UN News. "In Detroit, city-backed water shut-offs 'contrary to human rights,' say UN experts." October 20, 2014. https://news.un.org/en/story/2014/10/481542-detroit-city-backed-water-shut-offs-contrary-human-rights-say-un-experts.

Verdery, Katherine. 1999. *The Political Lives of Dead Bodies: Reburial and Postsocialist Change*. Columbia University Press.

Wagner, Sarah. 2008. *To Know Where He Lies: DNA Technology and the Search for Srebrenica's Missing*. University of California Press.

Wallace, Maeve E., Joia Crear-Perry, Carmen Green, Erica Felker-Kantor, and Katherine Theall. 2019. "Privilege and deprivation in Detroit: Infant mortality and the Index of Concentration at the extremes." *International Journal of Epidemiology* 48, no. 1: 207–16.

Wang, Alan H., and Christopher Still. 2007. "Old world meets modern: A case report of scurvy." *Nutrition in Clinical Practice: Official publication of the American Society for Parenteral and Enteral Nutrition* 22, no. 4: 445–8.

Watkins, Rachel. 2012. "Variation in health and socioeconomic status within the W. Montague Cobb skeletal collection: Degenerative joint disease, trauma and cause of death." *International Journal of Osteoarchaeology* 22, no. 1: 22–44. https://doi.org/10.1002/oa.1178

Weather-Atlas. 2021. https://www.weather-us.com/en/michigan-usa/detroit-climate, accessed on March 1, 2021.

White, Teresa. 2013. A. *Avian scavenging, mummification, and variable micro-environments as factors affecting the decomposition process in western Montana*. Unpublished Master's Thesis, University of Montana, Missoula.

Wijkmans, Rian AA, and Koen Talsma. 2016. "Modern scurvy." *Journal of Surgical Case Reports* 2016, no. 1: rjv168.

Williams, Brett. 1992. "Poverty among African Americans in the Urban United States." *Human Organization* 51, no. 2: 164–74.

Wolputte, Steven Van. 2004. "Hang on to Your Self: Of bodies, embodiment, and selves." *Annual Review of Anthropology* 33: 251–69.

Zahran, Sammy, Terrence Iverson, Shawn P. McElmurry, Stephan Weiler, and Ryan Levitt. 2019. "Hidden Costs of Blight and Arson in Detroit: Evidence from a Natural Experiment in Devil's Night." *Ecological Economics* 157: 266–77.

Zuberi, Anita, Waverly Duck, Bob Gradeck, and Richard Hopkinson. 2016. "Neighborhoods, race, and health: Examining the relationship between neighborhood distress and birth outcomes in Pittsburgh." *Journal of Urban Affairs* 38, no. 4: 546–63.

Chapter 9

A Social Autopsy of Honolulu, Hawai'i

Forensic Anthropology Case Files as an Archive of Marginalization

Jennifer F. Byrnes, William R. Belcher, and Katharine C. Woollen

INTRODUCTION

Although forensic anthropologists commonly publish case studies (e.g., Garvin and Langley 2020), few have examined the mortality demographics of their case files.[1] Nevertheless, when published, these studies have provided synchronic, diachronic, and geographic insights into medicolegal mortality trends at the local, regional, and national scale (e.g., Grisbaum and Ubelaker 2001; Kimmerle, Falsetti, and Ross 2010). For example, decedents identified as "White" males comprise the most common demographic groups in forensic anthropology casework throughout North America (e.g., Hughes, Juarez, and Yim 2021; Kimmerle, Falsetti, and Ross 2010). However, as Hughes, Juarez, and Yim (2021) aptly note, Whites are underrepresented in forensic anthropology casework relative to the overall population in the United States. Hughes, Juarez, and Yim (2021) also report the most common forensic anthropology case age cohorts in the national Forensic Anthropology Database for Assessing Methods Accuracy (FADAMA) to be young adults (twenty to thirty-four years), followed closely by old adults (fifty-nine years median). This bimodal age distribution can be attributed to the relatively high homicide rate of younger adults and the typical life expectancy of older adults. Their findings from this nationwide database allow their results to be extrapolatable to the U.S. context at large. However, whether these patterns are consistent and predictable in various regional settings has remained hitherto unexplored.

We therefore examined forensic anthropology casework from the City and County of Honolulu,[2] Department of the Medical Examiner, to illustrate the importance of retrospective archival analysis for public health policy.

Forensic anthropology cases are not a representative sample of the living population. Rather, due to what might be called a forensic anthropological paradox (cf. Wood et al. 1992), a non-random subset of people is likely to have their remains examined through forensic anthropology casework. A smaller, again, non-random, proportion of these cases are likely to be identified, the remainder becoming cold cases (Goad 2020). We used Klinenberg's (2002) social autopsy method to model how the social and political conditions in Hawai'i shaped the demographic profile of forensic anthropology casework. In his social autopsy of the 1995 Chicago heat wave, Klinenberg found that of the more than 485 Chicago residents who died of heat-related causes, most were elderly and/or African American, and/or lived in low-income, and/ or violent neighborhoods of the city. Significantly, many of these individuals died alone due to the marginalized places they occupied in their community social networks. Subsequently, researchers have usefully applied the social autopsy framework in the fields of public health (e.g., Streinzer 2021), sociology (e.g., Timmermans and Prickett 2021), and to a lesser extent medical anthropology (Mulligan and Weil 2022) and forensic archaeology (Ferrándiz 2011, 2013). We wanted to know what insights a social autopsy of Honolulu forensic anthropology casework would reveal.

Social autopsy has been well received by many social scientists, perhaps because it offers a replicable method useful for investigating phenomena of perennial interest. As Timmermans and Prickett (2021, 2) pointed out, many early social scientists were interested in the conditions surrounding death of the underprivileged (i.e., Du Bois 1906, Durkheim 1979, Engels 1969). More recently, the theory of structural violence (Galtung 1969) has helped researchers conceptualize how social institutions, economic divides, and policies selectively increase morbidity and mortality rates among marginalized people, producing what Paul Farmer (2001, 5) referred to as a "biological reflection of social fault lines." Implementing social autopsy as a methodology allows social scientists to systematically examine and further understand the conditions and/or circumstances that result(ed) in excess death rates for various groups (e.g., populations, communities, neighborhoods, organizations, and so on). Social autopsy typically starts with the examination of death patterns among contemporary groups, then probes these phenomena and the causality of past social, economic, and political policies that resulted in the perpetuation of these deaths over time. The social autopsy method expands these arenas of long-standing and evergreen social inquiry to highlight how individuals who fall through these social fissures and suffer with a poor quality of life also die needlessly isolated deaths, making it possible for at-risk individuals' deaths to go unnoticed and become overlooked—becoming what Jenny Edkins terms "unmissed" persons (2011). When marginalized people die alone in the United States, the forensic anthropologist is often called upon to make an identification.

On the island of O'ahu, where our analysis is focused, prevailing patterns of inequality and discrimination stem from the Euroamerican colonization of the Hawaiian Islands, including the entwined pressures of military occupation and capitalist exploitation that intensified throughout the nineteenth and twentieth centuries and that continues today. These historical traumas have created a variety of persistent and worsening social fault lines, including a high cost of living, a lack of affordable housing (February 2016), and low median incomes (U.S. Department of Housing and Urban Development [HUD]). This confluence of social problems has led to high rates of houselessness. While houselessness has been identified as a public health issue for some time, investigating why some bodies of deceased houseless people are more likely to reach an unidentifiable postmortem state than others has not yet been addressed.

Overview of Terms and Concepts

In specific governmental contexts, we use the generic and widely accepted term "homeless" or "homelessness" following the U.S. Department of Housing and Urban Development (HUD's Definition of Homelessness: Resources and Guidance—HUD Exchange) to include individuals that are living "on the streets," in transitional housing, or in emergency shelters. However, in Hawai'i and other sociocultural contexts, the terms "houseless" or "unhoused" are used to separate the concepts of "home" and "house," as they are inherently different. Home does not necessarily require a physical structure of four walls and a roof (Mallett 2004) but is where domestic tasks or practices occur ultimately creating a place of security and comfort for an individual as well as producing a sense of identity (Hopwood 2020). Thus, houseless communities are not without a home, but are without the traditional idea of a physical house structure. Houseless communities are just that—they can be made up of nuclear and extended families with actual and fictive kin relations but do not reside in traditional permanent housing (Groot and Hodgetts 2012). Instead, shelters in these communities can be made of motor vehicles, tents, tarps, among others. Use of the term *homeless/homelessness* can be offensive and does not recognize the nuances of this specific Hawaiian context as well as other numerous cultural or socioeconomic contexts (Julien-Chinn and Park 2021).

This chapter uses aspects of ancestry or geographic origin, and we acknowledge that these terms may imply meaning that is beyond pure individual identification. Several of our colleagues have powerfully critiqued mainstream forensic anthropology practices that claim to morphologically identify the genetic ancestry of decedents (e.g., Bethard and DiGangi 2020; DiGangi and Bethard 2021; Stull et al. 2021; Ross and Williams 2021). Nevertheless, assigning ancestry remains standard practice in the creation of the biological profile to build evidence towards a personal identification because it relates to self- and peer-identified racial categories. We will not repeat here the oft-cited arguments on the use of "race" and the implications of its use in forensic anthropology, as that is beyond the scope of this chapter, but we accept the critique that the procedures employed tend to bias against the identification of Black, Indigenous, and People of Color (BIPOC).

A Social Autopsy of Hawai'i—The External Examination

As one might expect in a colonial context, minority and marginalized groups, especially Indigenous people, are disproportionately engulfed by the social fissures outlined above. For example, the Indigenous people of Hawai'i historically suffered the ravages of introduced diseases and currently have higher morbidity rates and shorter life expectancies than other ethnic groups in Hawai'i (Johnson et al. 2004). Compared to other demographic groups, Native Hawaiians (or *kānaka 'ōiwi, kānaka maoli,* and *Hawai'i maoli*) also tend to have relatively low incomes (Naya 2007) and high rates of incarceration (Taschner 2021). In contrast, Whites (or *haoles*) tend to occupy privileged socioeconomic positions in contemporary Hawai'i. Originally, the term *haole* referred to foreigners in general but has come to be associated with individuals of European descent (Pukui and Elbert 1986).

In addition to Native Hawaiians and whites, modern Hawai'i is ethnically diverse, and again this is a consequence of historical events and processes. For example, in 1850, plantation owners began to recruit large numbers of indentured laborers from abroad. The first indentured servants came from China, but later groups hailed from a multitude of countries, including Japan (1860s), Portugal (1870s), and Korea (1903) (Buck 1993, 74; Daws 1968, 303–306). In a classic divide and conquer strategy, the plantation owners intentionally pitted ethnic groups against each other (Takaki 1984), contributing to ethnic tensions that persist today (Rosa 2018). Additionally, the modern population also includes individuals from various Polynesian, Melanesian, and Micronesian island groups that have relocated to the State of Hawai'i for employment, healthcare, and family. Nevertheless, in the crucible of oppression, a new Local ethnic identity was forged.

To be Local in Hawai'i implies membership to a community by virtue of a shared history and culture. "Locals," as Rosa framed it, "are the descendants of specific immigrant groups—mostly from east Asia, the Philippines,

Portugal, and Puerto Rico—who were recruited as plantation laborers from the mid-nineteenth century to the mid-twentieth century" (2018, 79). However, local identity is more complicated than ancestry and reflects a shared regional or island culture. According to Spickard (2018, 181), "'local' denotes people who are part of the fabric of life in Hawai'i." Implicitly, local is a social identity, rather than an individual one. Thus, "you are local when local people see you as one of themselves and not an outsider" (Spickard 2018, 184). Being integrated into the community's social fabric means that Local people, even poor and otherwise marginalized people, are likely to have access to informal support networks and, significantly for the purposes of this study, are less likely to die alone and become an unmissed person (Edkins 2011). We want to emphasize that as long as individuals are participating in a local culture, they can be considered as locals, regardless of ancestry. Thus, we may find Locals of Japanese, White European, Portuguese, Korean, and other areas of geographic origin or ancestry.

Excellent examples of how marginalized Local people form robust informal support networks are the houseless camps located primarily on the western side of the island of O'ahu, especially Pu'uhonua 'O Wai'anae (Mello 2017) and Pu'uhonua Mākua (Niheu 2014). Far from evolving to describe modern conditions leading to houselessness, "pu'uhonua" is a Native Hawaiian term for "sanctuary" or "refuge." As Niheu explained, "[i]n traditional times there were many pu'uhonua, commonly known as 'places of refuge,' where those who violated the strict kapu, or laws, could flee and find sanctuary, even from penalties requiring death" (2014, 165). As such, conveying the title of pu'uhonua upon the western O'ahu camps and acknowledging that they are continuing this tradition of pu'uhonua has great significance. As Niheu (2014) eludes the past "places of refuge" provided a safe haven for those that broke "kapu," usually against the royalty or *ali'i* [chiefs]. Usually, the offenders were commoners and women, the disadvantaged from our modern cultural lens. The offenders could offer prayer to the gods to ask for a second chance and avoid execution (National Park Service 2018). In essence, today's houseless communities provide modern sanctuary for anyone willing to join them, mostly including people of at least part Native Hawaiian descent. In these communities, whites are significantly underrepresented relative to their overall population, while Native Hawaiians and other BIPOC are overrepresented.

The underrepresentation of Whites in these Indigenous-inspired houseless communities is partially attributable to the privileged socioeconomic position that most Whites occupy and, as a result, their underrepresentation in the houseless community in general (table 9.1). However, in addition to economic variables, social factors must be considered. Spickard aptly noted, "it is more difficult for

Table 9.1 **"Social Race" categories from 2020 for the City and County of Honolulu general population compared to the houseless population***

"Social Race" Category	City and County of Honolulu as a Whole		City and County of Honolulu Sheltered and Unsheltered "Houseless" Combined	
	Population	%	Population	%
Asian	436,853	43.0	378	8.5
Two or more	248,686	24.5	1,100	24.7
White	188,462	18.5	712	16.0
Native Hawaiian/Pacific Islander	102,099	10.0	1,383	31.1
Black/African American	20,723	2.0	212	4.8
Other	17,407	1.7	102	2.3
American Indian/Alaska Native	2,278	0.2	36	0.8
Unknown/Refused	NA	NA	525	11.8
TOTAL	1,016,508	100	4,448	100

*Sources: Data from U.S. Census Bureau's American Community Survey (2020); Partners in Care/Oahu's Continuum of Care (2020).

a White person to be accorded local status than it is for a person of color" (2018, 181). A White person can generally only manifest a Local identity "if their worldview, social connections, and loyalties are local," and if other Locals accept them as Local (Spickard 2018, 181). Because most Whites occupy relatively privileged social positions, the average White person is likely to die in the presence of someone or be found shortly after death. However, in addition to lacking economic privilege, houseless whites might also lack a sense of belonging to the local community. This is a recipe for a lonely death, leading to an unidentifiable postmortem state and contributing to the growing missing persons mass disaster (Ritters 2007).

Based on our social autopsy and the socioeconomic context and history outlined above, we generated a simple hypothesis and prediction. We hypothesize that houseless Whites will die alone and not be found, or become an unmissed person, at higher rates than other ethnic groups on Oʻahu. We predicted that, if this were true, then houseless Whites would be overrepresented in forensic anthropology casework on the island of Oʻahu.

METHODS AND MATERIALS

Our sample consisted of fifty-one years (1967–2018) of case work from the City and County of Honolulu, Department of the Medical Examiner, which we arbitrarily divided into two categories: pre-2004 (n=21) and post-2004 (n=30). The rationale for this division was twofold. First, after 2004, the forensic anthropology literature increased voluminously. Second, in Honolulu, the annual caseload that required forensic anthropology consults increased significantly after 2004, from an average of 0.57 cases per year between 1967 and 2004 to an average of 2.1 cases per year thereafter.

The cases were coded for biological profile findings such as skeletal sex, age-at-death, ancestry, and trauma. The cases were further coded based on the Medical Examiner's conclusions of manner of death, as well as personal identification status. If an identification was reached, then information was gathered in-so-far-as-possible into the decedent's residency and/or house-lessness status, mental illness(es), and drug abuse/use history based on the Investigator's report. For those who remained unidentified at the time of this chapter's writing, the biological profile determination of sex and estimation of ancestry were used. For age-at-death of the unidentified, the mean of the upper and lower age range provided in the forensic anthropology report was used as a point estimate. These point estimates were used alongside the known age-at-death of identified cases to calculate the overall mean age for the fifty-one cases. Cases were also grouped by decade of age-at-death using either their known age-at-death for identified cases or the mean point estimate for those who remain unidentified (e.g., the first decade of life is 0–9 years).

Forensic anthropological ancestry estimation methods and conceptualization have dramatically changed over our sample's time frame (i.e., 1967–2018), and this was reflected in the skeletal ancestry or "race" reported by forensic anthropologists in their casework. Reports primarily included results as one of the "big three" ancestry categories: "Caucasoid," "Mongoloid," and "Negroid." These ancestry categorizations are an artifact of the agency that performed the casework, that is, the Defense POW/MIA Accounting Agency (DPAA) or formerly the Joint POW/MIA Accounting Command (JPAC), as well as the time period the casework was performed. The DPAA's Forensic Anthropology Report Standard Operating Procedures (DPAA SOP 3.4 *Skeletal Analysis*) called for the analyst to use these "big three" categories for "race" or ancestry up until 2013 when they semantically shifted to "European," "Asian," and "African." By mid-2015, the DPAA stopped performing casework for the Honolulu Medical Examiner's Office due to a legal opinion which banned the Department of Defense from assisting with police investigations, in accordance with the *Posse Comitatus* Act of 1878. Other anthropologists who performed Honolulu County casework were either former employees of the DPAA and/or were using the methods they were familiar with at the time they received their training (e.g., Bass 1971, 1986, 1994, 1996, 2005). However, there were a handful of reports that used the terms "Asian," "Hispanic," "White," "Pacific Islander," and "European." Thus, to standardize different analysts' case reports, we chose to group ancestral terms into "European" (i.e., "Caucasoid," "White," and "European") and "non-European'' for the purposes of this study.

To provide a snapshot of the houselessness trends on Oʻahu, we analyzed demographic data from the U.S. Census Bureau and the local non-profit Partners in Care. The forensic case file data were tested for statistical significance, where appropriate. Chi-squared analyses, Fisher's Exact Test, and Independent T-tests were run using SPSS version 26.

RESULTS

Of the fifty-one forensic anthropology cases from Oʻahu, twenty-six (51%) were positively identified, and twenty-five remain unidentified (49%). Analyzing those who have been positively identified across time using a two-tailed chi-square test displayed a statistical difference in pre-2004 versus post-2004 cases (χ^2 [1, N=51]=10.546, **p=0.001**). Prior to 2004, only five out of twenty-one cases were positively identified (24%), with the majority remaining unidentified (76%). Counter to this, from 2004 onward, twenty-one out of thirty cases (70%) were positively identified. The sex ratios of male to female were consistent over time, hovering around 70:30 in male: female ratio.

The overall age-at-death mean was 44.3 years. The pre-2004 age-at-death mean was 37.85 years (SD=16 years), while the post-2004 mean was 52.07 years (SD=12.27 years). A two-tailed independent T-test at a 95% CI was conducted on these two time periods by age-at-death, which revealed a significant difference between the age-at-death means (t[43]=-3.371, **p=0.002**). The male age-at-death mean was 48.36 years (SD=14.32 years) while the female age-at-death mean was 39.77 years (SD=17.61 years); however, they were not statistically different using a two-tailed independent T-test at a 95% CI (t[43]=1.674, p=0.101). The age-at-death distribution is displayed in figure 9.1, which indicates the sixth decade of life was the most frequent (27%).

When comparing those who have been identified by ancestry, there was no statistical difference for those of European ancestry over time based on identification status using a two-tailed Fisher's Exact Test (1, N=21, p=0.354). A two-tailed chi-square test showed a significant difference for those of non-European ancestry over time based on identification status (χ^2 [1, N=26]=15.367, **p<0.001**), in which more were identified in the post-2004 period than the pre-2004 period (figure 9.2). Overall, there were more individuals of European ancestry with twenty-one out of fifty-one individuals (41%). Of the twenty-one individuals of European ancestry, fifteen individuals (71%) were in the post-2004 period and six (29%) in the pre-2004 period.

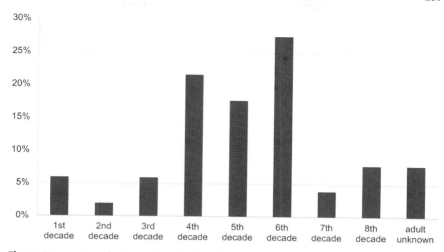

Figure 9.1   Age-at-death by decade. Credit: Jennifer F. Byrnes.

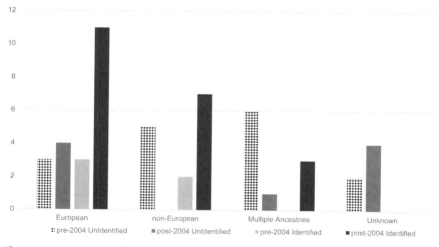

Figure 9.2   Ancestry distribution by time period and identification status. Credit: Jennifer F. Byrnes.

A two-tailed chi-square test showed no significant difference in identification status between individuals of European and non-European ancestry (χ^2 [1, N=45]=1.275, p=0.259) when those of unknown ancestry were removed from the analysis.

Approximately a quarter of individuals had antemortem trauma (28%; n=14), ranging from healed fractured toes to noses (table 9.2). Two (14%) were female while twelve (86%) were male. There were no significant differences for antemortem trauma between the time periods (χ^2 [1, N=43]=0.973,

Table 9.2 Time period, identification status, demographics, manner of death, trauma, housed status, mental illness, and substance abuse status. Cases with no identification were based on the forensic anthropology reports for demographics, while cases with an identification were based on the individual's personal identification from the investigator's report for sex, age, and ancestry

Date	ID?	Sex	Age (years)	Ancestry	Manner of Death	Trauma	Housed or houseless?	Mental Illness?	Substance abuse?
Pre-2004	No	Male	22–31	Unknown	Undetermined	None	N/A	N/A	N/A
Pre-2004	No	Male	28–35	Asian or mixed Asian	Homicide	None	N/A	N/A	N/A
Pre-2004	No	Male	50–55	White	Undetermined	Ante: right arm and clavicle; Peri: spinous processes of L4 and L5	N/A	N/A	N/A
Pre-2004	No	Female	19–22	Mongoloid	Undetermined	None	N/A	N/A	N/A
Pre-2004	No	Male	35–45	Caucasoid with probable Mongoloid admixture	Undetermined	none	N/A	N/A	N/A
Pre-2004	No	Male	45+, likely 50+	Mongoloid, with possible admixture	Undetermined	Ante: right fibula, three right ribs, two left ribs, with possible additional left rib and right frontal (superior orbit)	Likely houseless based on circumstances at death scene	N/A	N/A

Pre-2004	No	Male	25–35	Probably Mongoloid, possible with some Caucasoid admixture	Undetermined	none	N/A	N/A	N/A
Pre-2004	No	Female	40+	Caucasoid with possible admixture	Undetermined	none	Likely houseless based on circumstances at death scene	N/A	N/A
Pre-2004	No	Female	30–40	Mongoloid	Not Noted (coded as undetermined)	none	N/A	N/A	N/A
Pre-2004	No	Male	>22	Indeterminate	N/A (coded as undetermined)	none	N/A	N/A	N/A
Pre-2004	Yes	Male	61	Portuguese	Natural	none	Houseless	None noted	None noted
Pre-2004	No	Male	50+	Caucasoid	Not noted (coded as undetermined)	none	N/A	N/A	N/A
Pre-2004	No	Female	7.5–10	Mongoloid	Undetermined	none	N/A	N/A	N/A
Pre-2004	Yes*	Female	40	Korean	Undetermined or Suicide	none	Housed	Yes	None noted
Pre-2004	Yes*	Female	32	Chinese	Accident	none	Housed	None noted	None noted
Pre-2004	Yes	Male	28	Caucasian	Undetermined	none	Housed	None noted	None noted

(continued)

Table 9.2 Continued

Date	ID?	Sex	Age (years)	Ancestry	Manner of Death	Trauma	Housed or houseless?	Mental Illness?	Substance abuse?
Pre-2004	Yes	Male	75	Portuguese	undetermined	Ante: 2nd, 3rd, 4th, and 5th left ribs; 10th and 11th right ribs; right femur; left tibia; cranium had suffered effects of at least 2 surgeries. Peri: mandible, 8th right rib	Housed	Yes	None noted
Pre-2004	No	Male	25–45	Caucasoid, Mongoloid, or Hispanic	Undetermined	Ante: fibula, femur	N/A	N/A	N/A
Pre-2004	No	Male	Adult	Caucasoid	Undetermined	none	N/A	N/A	N/A
Pre-2004	Yes*	Male	49	Chinese	Undetermined	Ante: broken arm	N/A	N/A	N/A
Pre-2004	No	Male	13–16	Mongoloid	Undetermined	none	N/A	N/A	N/A
Post-2004	No	Male	34–62	Probable Caucasoid	Undetermined	Peri: T1	N/A	N/A	N/A
Post-2004	Yes*	Female	38	Chinese	Undetermined	none	Housed	Yes	None noted
post-2004	Yes	Male	53	Part Hawaiian, Japanese, Portuguese	Accident	Ante: nose. Peri: skull, vertebrae, tibiae, fibula.	Houseless	None noted	Yes
Post-2004	Yes	Male	55	Caucasoid	undetermined	Ante: skull, ribs, sternum	Houseless	Yes	None noted
Post-2004	Yes	Female	79	Filipino	undetermined	Ante: clavicle, ribs. T6, T7	Housed	Yes	None noted

Post-2004	Yes	Male	58	Hawaiian, Filipino, Caucasoid	Undetermined	Ante: clavicle, nose.	Houseless	Yes	None noted
Post-2004	Yes	Male	78	Caucasoid	Undetermined	None noted	Housed	None mentioned	None noted
Post-2004	No	Male	40-57	Caucasoid	Homicide	Peri: Gunshot wound	N/A	N/A	N/A
Post-2004	Yes	Male	72	Portuguese	Undetermined	none	Housed	None noted	None noted
Post-2004	Yes*	Male	51	Vietnamese	undetermined	Peri: scapula, ribs, L3. (BFT, fall?)	Housed	Yes	None noted
Post-2004	Yes	Male	45	Portuguese/German/Filipino	Undetermined	none	Housed	None noted	Yes
Post-2004	Yes	Male	34	Caucasian	Undetermined	N/A	Houseless	Yes	None noted
Post-2004	Yes	Male	38	Caucasian	Suicide	N/A	Houseless	Yes	None noted
Post-2004	No	Male	55+	Caucasoid	undetermined	Ante: nose, facial bones, ribs	Likely houseless based on circumstances at death scene	N/A	N/A
Post-2004	Yes	Male	47	Korean	Suicide	Peri: Gunshot wound	Housed	Yes	None noted
Post-2004	Yes	Male	49	Caucasian	Suicide	Peri: Gunshot wound	Housed	Yes	Yes
Post-2004	No	Unknown	Young child	N/A	Not noted (coded as undetermined)	N/A	N/A	N/A	N/A
Post-2004	Yes*	Female	53	Korean	Undetermined	none	Houseless	Yes	None noted

(continued)

Jennifer F. Byrnes et al.

Table 9.2 Continued

Date	ID?	Sex	Age (years)	Ancestry	Manner of Death	Trauma	Housed or houseless?	Mental Illness?	Substance abuse?
Post-2004	No	Unknown	Unknown	Unknown	N/A	N/A	N/A	N/A	N/A
Post-2004	No	Unknown	4.4–5.6	Indeterminate	Undetermined	None	N/A	N/A	N/A
Post-2004	Yes	Female	56	Japanese	Undetermined	None	Housed	Yes	None noted
Post-2004	Yes	Male	61	Caucasian	Undetermined	N/A	Houseless	Yes	None noted
Post-2004	Yes	Male	33	Caucasian	Suicide	None	Housed	N/A	N/A
Post-2004	Yes	Female	36	Chinese/Mongolian/Irish	Suicide	None	Housed	Yes	None noted
Post-2004	No	Male	N/A	N/A	Undetermined	None	N/A	N/A	N/A
Post-2004	No	Male	40–72	Asian and/or European	Undetermined	Ante: nose, left radius, left toe, right side of crania, maxilla PM. Peri: S5-6.	Likely houseless based on circumstances at death scene	N/A	N/A
Post-2004	Yes	Female	39	Filipino	Homicide	Ante: T7. Peri: mandible, multiple upper vertebrae, manubrium	Housed	None	None
Post-2004	Yes*	Male	50	Caucasian	Undetermined	Ante: nose, tibiae, right fibula	Houseless	None noted	Yes
Post-2004	No	Male	45–70	European	Undetermined	Ante: mandible, hyoid, ribs, nose, right and left hands	Likely houseless based on circumstances at death scene	N/A	N/A
Post-2004	Yes	Male	45–65	European	Undetermined	None	Houseless	None noted	Yes

*circumstantial or tentative identification

p=0.324) or identification status (χ^2 [1, N=43]=0.102, p=0.750). Ten individuals (20%) were reported as having perimortem trauma, one of which was a female, and the rest were males. Three cases involved gunshot wounds, of which two were deemed suicides and one a homicide. Seven cases displayed blunt force trauma of the thorax, of which three individuals also displayed blunt force trauma of the skull and one individual also had blunt force trauma of the leg bones. The only blunt force trauma case that was determined to be a homicide was that of the sole female case, with perimortem trauma to the mandible and upper thorax. Of the other six cases with blunt force trauma, one was an accident and five were undetermined for manner of death. Overall, most cases were classified as undetermined for manner of death (n=39; 76%), with the next most common as suicide (n=5; 10%) and homicide (n=4; 8%). There were two accidental deaths (4%) and one natural death (2%).

Of the twenty-six identified decedents, ten (39%) were known to be houseless at the time of their death (table 9.2). Of the twenty-five unidentified, five individuals (20%) were likely to be houseless based on the circumstances in which their remains were found. Of the nine individuals who were houseless and identified, almost all had a history of either mental illness, drug abuse, or both (n=8; 89%). One individual who was houseless and identified had no accompanying medical or historical data, and thus they were excluded. Of the fourteen individuals who were not houseless and identified, ten (71%) individuals had either a documented mental illness, mental degenerative disease, and/or a history of drug abuse. Two individuals did not have enough information to categorize mental illness or drug use status, and thus they were excluded.

Table 9.1 displays the 2020 general population for O'ahu to a Point in Time (PIT) census of houseless populations conducted on January 28, 2020. Salient points of comparison from O'ahu general population versus the houseless population are that Native Hawaiians and Other Pacific Islanders were overrepresented by 210 percent in houseless population. In other words, they were 2.1 times more likely to be represented in the PIT count compared to the general population. Additionally, Blacks or African Americans were 67 percent overrepresented in the PIT count. Whites were 24 percent less likely to be represented in houseless populations, with individuals of Asian ancestry 81 percent less likely to be in the houseless PIT count compared to the general population.

DISCUSSION

A Social Autopsy of Hawai'i - The Internal Examination

In this study, we conducted a social autopsy of Honolulu, Hawai'i. Our specific interest was in using this method to model who was most likely to have their remains examined by a forensic anthropologist. By building a robust sociohistorical context, we identified the houseless community to be one of the most marginalized and vulnerable groups in Honolulu (e.g., Gray 2020). Non-Whites were typically more marginalized than Whites, leading to an over-representation of the former group among the houseless and an under-representation of the latter (HUD 2019). We also noted that non-Whites in Hawai'i were more likely to identify as Local than Whites. We then hypothesized that, because Local identity connotes a position within the social fabric of Honolulu, non-White houseless people in Honolulu were less likely to die alone and not be found than White houseless people. We predicted that, if our hypothesis were true, houseless Whites would be disproportionately represented in the forensic anthropology case files.

Contrary to other regions in the United States (e.g., Hughes, Juarez, and Yim 2021; Kimmerle, Falsetti, and Ross 2010) and consistent with our hypotheses, our results indicated that individuals identified as middle-aged and White were disproportionately overrepresented in O'ahu forensic anthropology case files, relative to the overall population of Honolulu. We suggest that this anomalously low age-at-death would be consistent with a primarily houseless and marginalized population. Nationally, houseless people tend to die before their housed counterparts due to a variety of physical and mental health issues related to stress, addiction, and Post-Traumatic Stress Disorder (PTSD) (e.g., North, Smith, and Spitznagel 1994; Rosenheck et al. 1997). According to an analysis by the City and County of Honolulu Office of the Medical Examiner, for the 373 people considered "homeless/houseless" at the time of their deaths, between 2014 and 2018, the average age-at-death was about 53 years. In contrast, the life expectancy of the general population of the island of O'ahu was more than eighty years (City and County of Honolulu 2019). Contextualization of these results required additional historical and sociological information.

We suggest that the number of identifications made post-2004 is due to the progress of the forensic sciences, as well as advancements in DNA technology, testing, and availability. The City and County of Honolulu Department of the Medical Examiner only recently collected and sent cold case samples to the Center for Human Identification (CHI) at the University of North Texas for DNA sequencing in 2019 (personal communication). Prior to the efforts from the National Institute of Justice funding cold case identification efforts such as National Missing and Unidentified Persons System (NamUs), medical examiner and coroners offices had to fund DNA sequencing and other identification efforts. National databases such as NamUs, which allow offices across the country to input missing person and unidentified case data, did not exist prior to 2007 (National Institute of Justice n.d.). Since many medical examiner and coroners offices are historically underfunded, this led to 1) no samples being taken for DNA sequencing, or 2) mismanagement of the sampling (Committee on Identifying the Needs of the Forensic Sciences Community 2009). Thus, the pre-2004 cases, which are primarily unidentified, are the result of this confluence of factors. Hopefully with the renewed efforts of sampling cold cases, there may be new identifications made.

This study demonstrates that even extremely marginalized houseless people can ameliorate the final insult of postmortem anonymization through effective social interactions. In addition to improving their quality of life, Indigenous-inspired and ethnically diverse Hawaiian houseless communities reduce the likelihood of dying alone and not being found. These houseless communities are composed of people who Haraway (2016, 4) might call "oddkin"—groups that come together "in unexpected collaborations and combinations." Given their cultural dispositions and Local identities, Native Hawaiians and Asians might have better social support networks and be better at making oddkin than houseless Whites. As McDonell theorized (2014), this makes the Local subgroup more resilient to daily risks involved with being unhoused.

An additional possibility is that Locals have had more time to acquire these social support networks within their houseless communities as compared to non-local Whites. Native Hawaiians are more likely to directly experience the growing shortage of affordable housing and the economic burden of living in Hawaiʻi earlier in life, potentially leading to poverty and houselessness at an earlier age (McDonell 2014, 31). It can come as quite a shock to mainlanders who move to Hawaiʻi that their middle-class lifestyle is what many would consider a life of poverty, where individuals are living paycheck to paycheck with little expendable income (Leong 1997, 216). Furthermore, it is possible that houseless, non-local Whites become "stuck." Trips to the mainland are increasingly expensive, with many unable to afford air travel once they are in Hawaiʻi. Thus, it is reasonable to consider that Native Hawaiians and Asians are better at making oddkin due to potential long-term houselessness, whereas non-local Whites lack the time to create meaningful oddkin networks (Leong 1997; Rohrer 2008).

As Klinenberg (2002) discussed, marginalized neighborhood residents often keep close tabs on one another to reduce their vulnerability to violence and other broader social problems. The sense of community that develops in these marginalized neighborhoods also allows individuals to gauge who can and cannot be trusted. When individuals do not develop a sense of community, or are viewed as outsiders that cannot be trusted, those individuals fall through the cracks in society. Klinenberg (2002, 45) suggested that individuals that live in isolation were more likely "to be depressed, impoverished, fearful of crime, and removed from proximate sources of support." Houseless white males in Hawai'i seem to have fallen through those cracks and become isolated from the larger community at higher rates than non-Whites.

While the factors contributing to houselessness are well known, such as poverty, lack of affordable housing, mental illness, substance abuse, and domestic violence (Fitzpatrick 2005), understanding that there are structural and individual forces leading to a path to houselessness can help frame the current situation. As well, once someone has experienced houselessness, it is more likely they will experience it again in the future due to the inadequate social support networks in place, leading to intermittent or houselessness recidivism (Shinn et al. 2017). Anti-houseless legislation and the general apathy from housed voters leads to policies that further stigmatize houseless individuals, treating houseless individuals as non-citizens, literally pushing them to the margins physically and socially, making them invisible (Mitchell 2003; Somerville 1992). The criminalization of houseless individuals is a problem across the nation (National Law Center on Homelessness & Poverty 2019), but in Hawai'i unhoused people are advocating for a novel solution which should be supported: build a new community from scratch (Terrell 2021). Since many have co-occurring issues contributing to their houseless status, such as having both mental illness and substance abuse, public health measures and outreach should be targeting programs that are capable of addressing these. While we are not experts in public policy, we feel that our findings are imperative to help push more progressive public services forward, as we show that not only are houseless individuals experiencing increased morbidity and lower life expectancy, but they are also at risk of losing their identity in the postmortem interval altogether, permanently disappearing them or making them invisible as "unmissed" persons (Edkins 2011). Lastly, the intersectionality of their social identities creates unique sets of vulnerabilities (Crenshaw 1989, 1991). In this instance, identifying as a White middle-aged male who is houseless, and has mental impairment/illness a substance addiction creates a social identity that structurally and individually is vulnerable to dying alone and experiencing postmortem identity erasure.

CONCLUSION

The results of this local-level examination of sociocultural trends provide us with more information on who may be at a differential risk of becoming a forensic anthropology case on the island of O'ahu. Our case study represents a unique socioeconomic situation, where houselessness reached epidemic proportions with Whites experiencing greater difficulties in becoming integrated into Local social support networks. This led to the hypothesis that houseless whites would be overrepresented in the forensic anthropology case files. We do not expect that other researchers would find similar patterns in other regions of the United States since Hawai'i is a majority minority state with most of the population comprising traditionally recognized racial/ethnic minority groups in the United States. Nevertheless, this chapter emphasizes that more attention from public administration officials is needed to address the systemic postmortem erasure of identity experienced by those who are houseless or are otherwise marginalized people. Although forensic anthropologists tend to approach their work on an individual, case-by-case basis, we might be missing the forest for the trees. By stepping back and viewing our casework patterning, forensic anthropologists can help to inform both the public and policymakers about the inequalities that communities experience, including the indignity of postmortem identity erasure. As we demonstrate here, aggregate forensic anthropology casefiles can function as an archive of marginalization. People experiencing houselessness are at risk of a multitude of injustices in life, and they also face injustice in death by the loss of their personal identity and untold narratives.

NOTES

1. Acknowledgments: This chapter is based on a poster by Jennifer Byrnes, William Belcher, and Christy Mello, presented at the 2019 Annual American Academy of Forensic Sciences Annual Scientific Conference in Baltimore, Maryland. We would like to thank the City & County of Honolulu Office of the Medical Examiner, specifically Charlotte Carter and Susan Faulk. As well, the Defense POW/MIA Accounting Agency (Joint Base Pearl Harbor-Hickam), specifically Mr. Vince Sava, who helped track down some of the case work and Ms. Tina Schmidt who created the case work spreadsheet/database. Lastly, we'd like to acknowledge Roxayn Povidas who assisted in compiling the raw data from the case files, Liam Johnson for reviewing a version of this draft, David Ingleman for his thoughtful suggestions on Hawaiian colonial history, and the two anonymous reviewers for their insightful and constructive comments.

2. Each island is organized as a county within the State of Hawai'i; thus, the City and County of Honolulu is synonymous with the island of O'ahu and will be used interchangeably in this chapter.

REFERENCES

Bass, William. 1971, 1986, 1994, 1996, 2005. *Human Osteology: A Laboratory and Field Manual of the Human Skeleton*. Missouri Archeological Society, Columbia, MO.

Bethard, Jonathan D., and Elizabeth A. DiGangi. 2020. "Letter to the Editor—Moving Beyond a Lost Cause: Forensic Anthropology and Ancestry Estimates in the United States." *Journal of Forensic Sciences* 65, no. 5: 1791–92. https://doi.org/10.1111/1556-4029.14513

Buck, Elizabeth. 1993. *Paradise Remade: The Politics of Culture and History of Hawai'i*. Philadelphia, PA: Temple University Press.

C. Peraro Consulting, LLC. (2020, January). *State of Hawai'i Homeless Point-in-Time Count (PIT)*. Partners in Care. Retrieved July 15, 2021. https://www.partnersincareoahu.org/pit-reports

City and County of Honolulu. 2019. "2019 Homeless Deaths Demonstrate Need to House Vulnerable Population." Press Release Department of Customer Services. Last Updated: June 13, 2019, Accessed November 24, 2021. https://www.honolulu.gov/cms-csd-menu/site-csd-sitearticles/1257-site-csd-news-2019-cat/35185-06-05-19-homeless-deaths-demonstrate-need-to-house-vulnerable-population.html

Committee on Identifying the Needs of the Forensic Sciences Community. 2009. *Strengthening Forensic Science in the United States: A Path Forward*. Washington, DC: The National Academies Press.

Crenshaw, Kimberlé W. 1989. "Demarginalizing the Intersection of Race and Sex: A Black Feminist Critique of Antidiscrimination Doctrine, Feminist Theory and Antiracist Politics." *University of Chicago Legal Forum*: 139–67.

———. 1991. "Mapping the Margins: Intersectionality, Identity Politics, and Violence against Women of Color." *Stanford Law Review* 43, no. 6: 1241–99.

Daws, Gavan. 1968. *Shoal of Time: A History of the Hawaiian Islands*. Honolulu, HI: University of Hawai'i Press.

Department of Housing and Urban Development (HUD). Accessed November 14, 2021. https://www.huduser.gov/portal/datasets/il.html#2019

DiGangi, Elizabeth A., and Jonathan D. Bethard. 2021. "Uncloaking a Lost Cause: Decolonizing Ancestry Estimation in the United States." *American Journal of Physical Anthropology* 175, no. 2: 422–36. https://doi.org/10.1002/ajpa.24212

Du Bois, W.E.B. 1906. *The Health and Physique of the Negro American. Report of a Social Study Made under the Direction of Atlanta University*. Together with the Proceedings of the Eleventh Conference for the Study of the Negro Problems, Held at Atlanta University, on May the 29th, 1906. Atlanta, GA: Atlanta University Press.

Durkheim, Émile. 1979 (1897). *Suicide: A Study in Sociology*. Trans. John A. Spaulding. New York: The Free Press.

Edkins, Jenny. 2011. *Missing: Persons and Politics*. Ithaca: Cornell University Press.

Engels, Friedrich. 1969 (1845). *The Condition of the Working Class in England*. New York, NY: Panther.

Farmer, Paul. 1999. *Infections and Inequalities: The Modern Plagues* [Updated edition with a new preface]. Berkeley, CA: University of California Press.

February, Aaron. 2016. "Tent City: An Analysis of Honolulu's Homelessness." Master of Science in Urban Planning, Columbia University.

Ferrándiz, Francisco. 2011. "A Social Autopsy of Mass Grave Exhumations in Spain." *ISEGORIA* 45: 525–44.

———. 2013. "Exhuming the Defeated: Civil War Mass Graves in 21st-Century Spain." *American Ethnologist* 40, no. 1: 38–54. https://doi.org/10.1111/amet.12004

Fitzpatrick, Suzanne. 2005. "Explaining Homelessness: A Critical Realist Perspective." *Housing, Theory and Society* 22, no. 1: 1–17. https://doi.org/10.1080/14036090510034563

Galtung, Johan. 1969. "Violence, Peace, and Peace Research." *Journal of Peace Research* 6, no. 3: 167–91.

Goad, Gennifer. 2020. "Expanding Humanitarian Forensic Action: An Approach to U.S. Cold Cases." *Forensic Anthropology* 3, no. 1: 50–8.

Grisbaum, Gretchen A., and Douglas H. Ubelaker. 2001. *An Analysis of Forensic Anthropology Cases Submitted to the Smithsonian Institution by the Federal Bureau of Investigations from 1962 to 1994.* Smithsonian Contributions to Anthropology, 45. Washington, DC: Smithsonian Institution Press.

Groot, Shiloh, and Darrin Hodgetts. 2012. "Homemaking on the Streets and Beyond." *Community, Work & Family* 15, no. 3: 255–71. https://doi.org/10.1080/13668803.2012.657933

Haraway, Donna. 2016. *Staying with the Trouble: Making Kin in the Chthulucene.* Durham, NC: Duke University Press.

Hopwood, Judith. 2020. "The Narrative of Being Houseless: Lived Experiences of Cave Dwellers." Doctor of Philosophy thesis, School of Health and Society, University of Wollongong. https://ro.uow.edu.au/theses1/973

Hughes, Cris E., Chelsey Juarez, and An-Di Yim. 2021. "Forensic Anthropology Casework Performance: Assessing Accuracy and Trends for Biological Profile Estimates on a Comprehensive Sample of Identified Decedent Cases." *Journal of Forensic Sciences* 66, no. 5: 1602–16. https://doi.org/10.1111/1556-4029.14782

Johnson, David B., Neil Oyama, Loic LeMarchand, and Lynne Wilkens. 2004. "Native Hawaiians Mortality, Morbidity, and Lifestyle: Comparing Data from 1982, 1990, and 2000." *Pacific Health Dialog* 11, no. 2: 120–30.

Julien-Chinn, Francie J., and Mei Linn N. Park. 2021. "Understanding the Connection between the 'Āina, Strengths, and Houselessness among Previously Houseless Native Hawaiian and Micronesian Families." *Journal of Human Behavior in the Social Environment*: 1–12. https://doi.org/10.1080/10911359.2021.1914798

Kimmerle, Erin H., Anthony Falsetti, and Ann H. Ross. 2010. "Immigrants, Undocumented Workers, Runaways, Transients and the Homeless: Towards Contextual Identification among Unidentified Decedents." *Forensic Science Policy and Management* 1, no. 4: 178–86. https://doi.org/10.1080/19409041003636991

Klinenberg, Eric. 2002. *Heat Wave: A Social Autopsy of Disaster in Chicago.* Chicago, IL: University of Chicago Press.

Leong, Chris Sun. 1997. "'You Local or What?': An Exploration of Identity in Hawai'i." Doctoral Dissertation: The Union Institute.

Mallett, Shelley. 2004. "Understanding Home: A Critical Review of the Literature." *The Sociological Review* 52, no. 1: 62–89. https://doi.org/10.1111%2Fj.1467-954X.2004.00442.x

McDonell, Martin. 2014. "Houseless versus Homeless: An Exploratory Study of Native Hawaiian Beach Dwellers on O'ahu's West Coast." Doctoral Dissertation: The University of Utah.

Mello, Christy. 2017. "Aloha 'Āina: Homelessness, Learning Communities, and Social Justice." *Practicing Anthropology* 39, no. 4: 31–4. https://doi.org/10.17730/0888-4552.39.4.31

Mitchell, Don. 2003. *The Right to the City: Social Justice and the Fight for Public Space.* New York: The Guilford Press.

Mulligan, Jessica M., and Madeline Weil. 2022. "A Eulogy for Jane Robinson: A Social Autopsy of Uncare Policies." *Medical Anthropology Quarterly* 36, no. 1: 27–43. https://doi.org/10.1111/maq.12664

National Institute of Justice. n.d. "The NamUs Mission." Accessed March 29, 2022. https://namus.nij.ojp.gov/about#the-history-of-namus

National Law Center on Homelessness & Poverty. 2019. Housing Not Handcuffs: Ending the Criminalization of Homelessness in U.S. Cities. https://homelesslaw.org/wp-content/uploads/2019/12/HOUSING-NOT-HANDCUFFS-2019-FINAL.pdf

National Park Service. 2018. Hawai'i Island: Pu'uhonua o Hōnaunau National Historical Park. https://www.nps.gov/articles/puohonau.htm accessed February 19, 2022.

Naya, Seiji. 2007. "Income Distribution and Poverty Alleviation for the Native Hawaiian Community." *The Indian Economic Journal* 54, no. 4: 35–48. https://doi.org/10.1177%2F0019466220070403

Niheu, Kalamaoka'āina. 2014. "7. Pu'uhonua: Sanctuary and Struggle at Mākua." In *A Nation Rising*, edited by Noelani Goodyear-Kaopua, Ikaika Hussey, and Erin Kahunawaika'ala Wright, 161–79. Durham, NC: Duke University Press.

North, Carol S., Elizabeth M. Smith, and Edward L. Spitznagel. 1994. "Violence and the Homeless: An Epidemiologic Study of Victimization and Aggression." *Journal of Traumatic Stress* 7, no. 1: 95–110.

Partners in Care. 2020. *Partners in Care, O'ahu Continuum of Care, 2020 O'ahu Point in Time Count: Comprehensive Report.* https://static1.squarespace.com/static/5db76f1aadbeba4fb77280f1/t/5efa984a8ae4f774863509e8/1593481306526/PIC+2020+PIT+Count+Report+Final.pdf

Pukui, Mary Kawena., and Samuel H. Elbert. 1986. *Hawaiian Dictionary.* Honolulu, HI: University of Hawai'i Press.

Ritter, Nancy. 2007. "Missing Persons and Unidentified Remains: The Nation's Silent Mass Disaster." *National Institute of Justice Journal* 256: 2–7.

Rohrer, Judy. 2008. "Disrupting the 'Melting Pot': Racial Discourse in Hawai'i and the Naturalization of Haole." *Ethnic and Racial Studies* 31, no. 6: 1110–25. https://doi-org.ezproxy.library.unlv.edu/10.1080/01419870701682329

Rosa, John P. 2018. "'EH! WHERE YOU FROM?': Questions of Place, Race, and Identity in Contemporary Hawai'i." In *Beyond Ethnicity: New Politics of Race in Hawai'i*, edited by Camilla Fojas, Rudy P. Guevarra Jr., and Nitasha Tamar Sharma, 78–93. Honolulu: University of Hawai'i Press.

Rosenheck, Robert, Catherine Leda, Linda Frisman, and Peggy Gallup. 1997. "Homeless Mentally Ill Veterans: Race, Service Use, and Treatment Outcomes." *American Journal of Orthopsychiatry* 67, no. 4: 632–8. https://doi.org/10.1037/h0080260

Ross, Ann H., and Shanna E. Williams. 2021. "Ancestry Studies in Forensic Anthropology: Back on the Frontier of Racism." *Biology* 10, no. 7: 602. https://doi .org/10.3390/biology10070602

Shinn, Marybeth, Scott R. Brown, Brooke E. Spellman, Michelle Wood, Daniel Gubits, and Jill Khadduri. 2017. "Mismatch between Homeless Families and the Homelessness Service System." *Cityscape* 19, no. 3: 293–307.

Somerville, Peter. 1992. "Homelessness and the Meaning of Home: Rooflessness or Rootlessness?" *International Journal of Urban and Regional Research* 16, no. 4: 529–39. https://doi.org/10.1111/j.1468-2427.1992.tb00194.x

Spickard, Paul. 2018. "LOCAL HAOLE? Whites, Racial and Imperial Loyalties, and Membership in Hawai'i." In *Beyond Ethnicity: New Politics of Race in Hawai'i*, edited by Camilla Fojas, Rudy P. Guevarra Jr., and Nitasha Tamar Sharma, 178–92. Honolulu: University of Hawai'i Press. https://doi.org/10.1515 /9780824873523-012

Streinzer, Andreas. 2021. "Uncanny Companions: Kinship, Activism, and Public Health as Interdependent Modalities of Care Provision under Greek Austerity." *EtnoAntropologia* 9, no. 1: 101–18.

Stull, Kyra E., Eric J. Bartelink, Alexandra R. Klales, Gregory E. Berg, Michael W. Kenyhercz, Ericka N. L'Abbé, Matthew C. Go, Kyle McCormick, and Carlos Mariscal. 2021. "Commentary On: Bethard JD, DiGangi EA. Letter to the Editor-Moving beyond a Lost Cause: Forensic Anthropology and Ancestry Estimates in the United States." *J Forensic Sci.* 2020; 65, no. 5: 1791–2." *Journal of Forensic Sciences* 66, no. 1: 417–20. https://doi.org/10.1111/1556-4029.14616

Takaki, Ronald. 1984. *Pau Hana: Plantation Life and Labor in Hawai'i, 1835-1920.* University of Hawai'i Press.

Taschner, John. 2021. "Native Hawaiians' Disproportional Incarceration Rates Leading to Disproportional Jail Deaths." *Journal of Law in Society* 21, no. 1 (Winter): 93–115.

Terrell, Jessica. 2021. "How Do You Build a Community From Scratch? This Homeless Advocate is Trying." *Honolulu Civil Beat.* Accessed April 8, 2022. https://www.civilbeat.org/2021/09/how-do-you-build-a-community-from-scratch -this-homeless-advocate-is-trying/

Timmermans, Stefan, and Pamela J. Prickett. 2021. "The Social Autopsy." *Sociological Methods & Research* (August). https://doi.org/10.1177/00491241211036163

United States Census Bureau. 2020. *P1: Race. 2020 American Community Survey.* U.S. Census Bureau's American Community Survey Office. Retrieved from https:// data.census.gov/

Wood, James W., George R. Milner, Henry C. Harpending, Kenneth M. Weiss, Mark N. Cohen, Leslie E. Eisenberg, Dale L. Hutchinson et al. 1992. "The Osteological Paradox: Problems of Inferring Prehistoric Health from Skeletal Samples [and comments and reply]." *Current Anthropology* 33, no. 4: 343–70. https://doi.org/10 .1086/204084

Chapter 10

Identification of the Korean War Dead

Family Reference Samples at the Intersection of Race, Class, and Structural Vulnerability

Briana T. New, Paulina Domínguez Acosta,
Janet E. Finlayson, Amanda N. Friend,
Matthew C. Go, Amanda Hale, Sadé J. Johnson,
Devin N. Williams, and Jennie Jin

INTRODUCTION

Within the United States, axes of privilege, such as race, wealth, citizenship and immigration status, health, and mobility, among others, produce structural vulnerabilities that shape the demographics of missing persons and unidentified decedents (Beatrice and Soler 2016; Goad 2020; Hughes et al. 2017; Paulozzi et al. 2008; Soler et al. 2019; Soler and Beatrice 2018). The intersection of these factors often determines whether someone is counted on rosters of the missing, whether investigators can access their antemortem information, and whether family members are willing or able to help. Thus, the vulnerabilities that marginalize individuals in life continue to marginalize them in death. While it may be tempting to assume that the U.S. military culture of precision, preparedness, and thorough accounting, amidst vast resources of wealth and influence, spare military missing and unidentified service members from falling into identification pitfalls, axes of privilege still operate within this milieu.

In the context of forensic identification and parallel to determining what happened to an unidentified individual, locating a person's biological family is paramount for the identification of any missing person. If there are no antemortem records or genetic family reference samples (FRSs) available for comparison against the remains of unidentified decedents, the identification of missing persons may never move forward. Among U.S. military personnel, documentation, including the names and locations for next of kin, is meticulous during an individual's time of service. However, the more time that passes from a given conflict, the more likely it is that personnel records are lost, damaged, made obsolete, or discarded, and the more difficult it becomes to locate family members. Thus, among missing and unaccounted for service members from historic, twentieth-century conflicts (World War II [WWII], Korean War, among others), locating a family and obtaining FRSs in the twenty-first century can be difficult. Moreover, time is not the only challenge facing those investigators seeking FRSs for unaccounted for military personnel. Decades of changes in the U.S. sociopolitical context, perceptions toward governmental authority figures and genetic testing, and the complexity of the structural vulnerabilities faced by service members and their families merge to create a deeply complex, entangled situation. The nuanced effect of these factors on present-day identification processes is particularly evident among missing and unidentified service members from the U.S. Korean War. The U.S. armed forces that fought in the Korean War comprised individuals from different races, nationalities of origin, and economic positions (Bruscino 2010; Espiritu 2010; Flynn 1988; Kriner and Shen 2010, 2016; Lutz 2008; MacGregor 1981; Perri 2013). This diversity is unparalleled in any prior conflicts and provides an excellent vector for understanding the lasting effect of structural vulnerabilities on forensic identification.

At the Defense POW/MIA Accounting Agency (DPAA), the Korean War Identification Project (KWIP) is tasked with the identification of unaccounted for U.S. casualties from this conflict. The Korean War began on June 25, 1950 when the North Korea People's Army breached the 38th parallel division between communist-controlled North Korea and capitalist-controlled Republic of Korea (South Korea). In response, a coalition of forces under the banner of the United Nations (UN) deployed to aid in the defense of South Korea. Chief among those UN forces were U.S. military personnel comprising approximately 90 percent of the total forces (Fehrenbach 1963). The conflict claimed the lives of over 36,000 U.S. soldiers throughout the three-year war. The Korean Armistice Agreement was signed on July 27, 1953, instating a ceasefire, and permanently established the Korean Demilitarized Zone near the 38th parallel as the boundary between North Korea and South Korea.

While the majority of casualties were identified at the conclusion of the conflict, approximately 8,000 individuals remained unidentified until the DPAA and its predecessor agencies began additional identification efforts (Jin et al. 2014). With the introduction of DNA comparison in the early 2000s and the formation of KWIP in 2011, identifications steadily increased resulting in ~591 identifications as of February 2021 and ~7,569 remaining unresolved. Now, after a decade of KWIP identifications and tracking, trends are beginning to emerge among identified and unidentified service members that allow us to reflect on how we can improve the identification process. Here we explore the relationship between FRS availability and identification potential and discuss the intricacies and difficulties of obtaining FRSs. We utilize this framework to understand how intersectional structural vulnerabilities across race and class (e.g., socioeconomic status [SES], nationality, educational attainment) may influence the identification process for missing service members, and how these factors may eventually culminate in differential rates of identification.

Family Reference Samples and Identification of U.S. Korean War Dead

Identification efforts at the DPAA are led by anthropologists who function as skeletal experts as well as case managers that synthesize complex case information, including FRS availability, historical documentation, anthropological analysis, and material evidence, to make identification recommendations to the medical examiner (Taylor, New, and Tegtmeyer 2021). Rosters of possible matches are dictated by the recovery context of the remains, the loss location of the missing, and other historical information of import. As such, military war dead are considered "closed populations" wherein possible matches for unidentified decedents are restricted to known rosters of missing persons. However, DNA comparisons remain integral to the identification process because rosters of missing service members often still comprise thousands of men with similar biological profiles (i.e., younger men of average stature with no individuating physical characteristics).

The DPAA exclusively works in conjunction with the Armed Forces Medical Examiner System's Armed Forces DNA Identification Laboratory (AFMES-AFDIL) to process and store DNA samples, as well as to conduct DNA comparisons between military personnel and their FRSs. However, AFMES-AFDIL is not the agency responsible for locating family members to provide FRSs. Rather, the Service Casualty Office for every military branch of the service members are responsible for overseeing the FRS search, each with their own protocols, records, yearly quotas, and resources. In this process, DPAA anthropologists can request prioritization of an FRS search based on the likelihood that a set of unidentified remains belong to a service member who lacks an FRS type necessary for positively identifying that individual. However, this is the extent of involvement in the search for FRSs for anthropologists in this DPAA context. Because of this trilateral effort, KWIP has the largest percentage of FRS coverage of all DPAA identification efforts.

Mitochondrial DNA (mtDNA) is the genetic baseline for FRS comparison utilized by the DPAA due to the historic age and often poor condition of samples taken from a set of remains (Edson and Christensen 2015; Marshall et al. 2020; Taylor, New, and Tegtmeyer 2021). While autosomal DNA (auDNA) is utilized for baseline comparison in the traditional medicolegal context, the age and condition of samples can prevent reliable auDNA results from being obtained (Edson and Christensen 2015; Marshall et al. 2020). Thus, mtDNA provides robust, consistent results while also potentially further narrowing the rosters of missing service members (Jin et al. 2014). Individuals with a mtDNA FRS profile available for comparison that does not match the mtDNA profile of the remains, along with any other mismatched case information, can be excluded from consideration in an identification. Any additional exclusions or inclusions are further guided by auDNA and/or Y-chromosome DNA (yDNA) whenever possible. However, the availability of any of these DNA reference types for a given service member is dictated by the presence and participation of specific family members. For example, the daughter of a service member will be able to provide auDNA, but not mtDNA or yDNA; a brother will be able to provide all three systems of DNA for comparison; and a second maternal cousin will only be able to provide an mtDNA reference.

Whom the military branch is able to contact and who is willing to participate in the FRS process dictates what types of DNA are able to be compared to a given set of remains. A lack of any one of these FRS types can inhibit identification if other lines of evidence are not strong enough to support a positive identification. Twenty-first-century technology has eased some of the difficulty of locating the families of service members lost in historic conflicts. However, military personnel involved in FRS searches report numerous barriers to obtaining FRSs, such as name changes, commonality of family names, unknown family migration within and outside the United States, family member death, unwillingness to participate, and so on. The culmination of these factors has produced discernable patterns for FRS availability among identified and unidentified Korean War service members.

DISTRIBUTION OF IDENTIFIED AND UNIDENTIFIED U.S. KOREAN WAR CASUALTIES

To assess the distribution of FRS availability among Korean War dead, counts of resolved and unresolved individuals as of February 2021 were tabulated, subset by reported race, and additionally subset by FRS type. Due to extreme sample size differences, each subset is presented by proportion to improve the comparative analytical capacity between groups. To evaluate the statistical significance of observed differences in availability between groups, FRS availability was subsequently dichotomized into two categories: no FRS available and at least one FRS available. Pairwise Fisher's exact tests were then conducted between each group. While our research seeks to assess FRS availability among race and class, data on the SES of these service members are not available. Therefore, we highlight the distribution of FRS across race categories and discuss the results in the context of the intersectional vulnerabilities that service members and their families may face.

Historical records for Korean War casualties contain a range of different racial categories with varying degrees of specificity and consistency that are dependent on the documentation available and the observer who completed that documentation. Race documentation among historic military records is notoriously subjective (MacGregor 1981). Therefore, for the purpose of analytical consistency and to preserve anonymity where sample sizes are low, we have condensed the racial classification information from historical documentation (i.e., personnel files of unidentified Korean War dead) into the following groups: White, Black, Latin American, Asian/Pacific Islander, Native American or Alaska Native, and Other (table 10.1). The White grouping consists of individuals whose records state White or provide some indication of European ancestry. Similarly, the Black grouping consists of individuals whose records state Black or provide some indication of African ancestry. The Latin American grouping consists of individuals whose records indicate regional or ethnic association with Latin American countries such as Puerto Rico or Mexico. The Asian/Pacific Islander grouping consists of individuals whose records indicate regional or ethnic association with various East Asian, Southeast Asian, or Polynesian groups. The grouping of Native Americans or Alaska Natives consists of individuals whose records indicate Native American heritage through the

Table 10.1   Distribution of groups among all KWIP casualties with the total percentage resolved and unresolved per reported race as of February 2021

Reported Race	N	Frequency	Resolved	Unresolved
White	6922	84.83%	8%	92%
Black	822	10.07%	7%	93%
Latin American	271	3.32%	5%	95%
Asian/Pacific Islander	98	1.20%	4%	96%
Native American or Alaska Native	43	0.53%	10%	90%
Other	4	0.05%	0%	100%
Totals	8160	100%	7%	93%

racial classification of "Indian." Finally, the Other category consists of individuals whose records do not provide racial or regional classification information or are unique from the above groupings.

It is important to emphasize that while these groupings are our inter-pretations of the historical documentation available, these categorizations may not reflect how the individuals identified in life or how their families would identify them presently. Historically, race was prescribed by the inducting officer and had to fit into regulation-approved racial categories regardless of how an individual may have self-identified (MacGregor 1981). Moreover, inherent human variation and the possibility for "mixed-race" individuals were largely omitted in these historic contexts (Taylor, New, and Tegtmeyer 2021). For Korean War Latin American and Asian/ Pacific Islander groupings, racial classifications within the military docu-mentation often elaborate on the specific ethnic heritage (i.e., Mexican, Puerto Rican, Japanese, Hawaiian, Filipino, among others) of the indi-vidual whereas the same specificity is often not afforded to individuals categorized as White, Black, or Native American/Alaska Native. This is a well-documented phenomenon among military and government records that is still maintained today (Berg and Ta'ala 2015; Taylor, New, and Tegtmeyer 2021).

When looking at all unresolved and resolved casualties it is clear that all groups, except for White and Native American/Alaska Native, have pro-portionally less FRS coverage (table 10.2, figure 10.1). Among White and Native American/Alaska Native individuals, 91.4 percent and 97.67 percent, respectively, have at least one type of FRS available (mtDNA, yDNA, and/ or auDNA). However, Black individuals have only 75.06 percent cover-age, Latin American individuals have 80.07 percent coverage, Asian/Pacific Islander individuals have 79.59 percent coverage, and individuals in the Other group have only 25.00 percent coverage. Additionally, all groups range between 32 percent and 39 percent availability for all FRS types except Black (25.00%) and Other (0%). The variation of FRS availability between no FRS and all FRS types indicates that for nearly every group at least one family member was located and willing to give a DNA sample.

Pairwise Fisher's exact tests further corroborate the proportional trends observed above. There are statistically significant differences ($p < 0.05$) in the proportion of FRS availability (no FRS available versus at least one FRS available for comparison) between all pairwise comparisons except for White–Native American or Alaska Native ($p = 0.2041$), Asian/Pacific Islander–Latin American ($p = 0.9998$), Black–Latin American ($p = 0.1246$), and Black–Asian/Pacific Islander ($p = 0.4118$). The lack of significance among these pairwise comparisons is reflective of similar proportions in FRS availability discussed above.

Table 10.2 Distribution of FRS availability by FRS type and reported races for all unresolved and resolved KWIP casualties

Reported Race	No FRS (Any Type)	auDNA Only	yDNA Only	yDNA and auDNA	mtDNA Only	mtDNA and auDNA	mtDNA and yDNA	All FRS Types	Totals
White	8.60% (595)	0.56% (39)	2.21% (153)	1.36% (94)	18.33% (1269)	25.87% (1791)	3.38% (234)	39.69% (2747)	100% (6922)
Black	24.94% (205)	1.09% (9)	3.04% (25)	2.43% (20)	18.86% (155)	21.78% (179)	3.04% (25)	24.82% (204)	100% (822)
Latin American	19.93% (54)	0.74% (2)	1.11% (3)	2.95% (8)	10.33% (28)	23.62% (64)	4.80% (13)	36.53% (99)	100% (271)
Asian/Pacific Islander	20.41% (20)	0.00% (0)	2.04% (2)	4.08% (4)	12.24% (12)	20.41% (20)	3.06% (3)	37.76% (37)	100% (271)
Native American or Alaska Native	2.33% (1)	4.65% (2)	0.00% (0)	2.33% (1)	34.88% (15)	18.60% (8)	4.65% (2)	32.56% (14)	100% (98)
Other	75.00% (3)	0.00% (0)	0.00% (0)	0.00% (0)	25.00% (1)	0.00% (0)	0.00% (0)	0.00% (0)	100% (43)
Totals	10.75% (878)	0.64% (52)	2.24% (183)	1.56% (127)	18.14% (1480)	25.27% (2062)	3.39% (277)	38.00% (3101)	100% (8160)

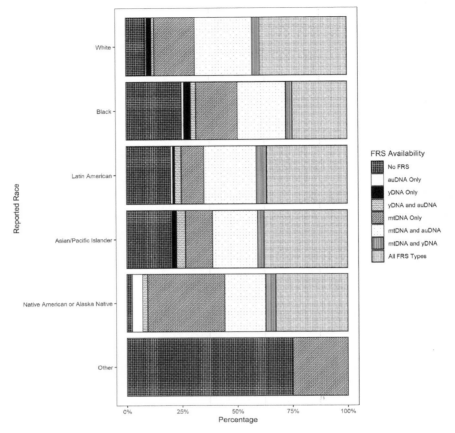

Figure 10.1   Combined proportions of FRS availability for all unresolved and resolved KWIP casualties by reported race. Credit: Briana T. New.

To further contextualize the effect that differences in FRS availability have on identification prospects we explored differences between resolved and unresolved casualties (tables 10.3–10.4, figure 10.2). Among resolved individuals it is rare for an identification to be made with no FRS available. Only 8.93 percent of the identified Black individuals and 5.07 percent of the identified White individuals had no FRS available for comparison. These identifications were only made possible through strong comparisons to antemortem records such as dental charts and/or radiographs, historical evidence, and anthropological analysis (D'Alonzo et al. 2017; Shiroma 2016a and b; Stephan et al. 2018). The majority of resolved casualties had all FRS types available (75.00% for Native Americans/Alaska Natives and Asians/Pacific Islanders, 37.5% for Black, and 45.22% for White) or mtDNA and auDNA (57.14% for Latin Americans) (table 10.3).

Table 10.3 Distribution of FRS availability by FRS type and reported races for all resolved KWIP casualties

Reported Race	No FRS (Any Type)	auDNA Only	yDNA Only	yDNA and auDNA	mtDNA Only	mtDNA and auDNA	mtDNA and yDNA	All FRS Types	Totals
White	5.07% (26)	0.00% (0)	0.58% (3)	0.00% (0)	15.01% (77)	29.04% (149)	5.07% (26)	45.22% (232)	100% (513)
Black	8.93% (5)	0.00% (0)	0.00% (0)	1.79% (1)	25.00% (14)	25.00% (14)	1.79% (1)	37.50% (21)	100% (56)
Latin American	0.00% (0)	0.00% (0)	0.00% (0)	0.00% (0)	21.43% (3)	57.14% (8)	0.00% (0)	21.43% (3)	100% (14)
Asian/Pacific Islander	0.00% (0)	0.00% (0)	0.00% (0)	0.00% (0)	0.00% (0)	25.00% (1)	0.00% (0)	75.00% (3)	100% (4)
Native American or Alaska Native	0.00% (0)	25.00% (1)	0.00% (0)	0.00% (0)	0.00% (0)	0.00% (0)	0.00% (0)	75.00% (3)	100% (4)
Other	– (0)	– (0)	– (0)	– (0)	– (0)	– (0)	– (0)	– (0)	– (0)
Totals	5.25% (31)	0.17% (1)	0.51 (3)	0.17% (1)	15.91% (94)	29.10% (172)	4.57% (27)	44.33% (262)	100% (591)

Table 10.4 Distribution of FRS availability by FRS type and reported races for all unresolved KWIP casualties.

Reported Race	No FRS (Any Type)	auDNA Only	yDNA Only	yDNA and auDNA	mtDNA Only	mtDNA and auDNA	mtDNA and yDNA	All FRS Types	Totals
White	8.88% (569)	0.61% (39)	2.34% (150)	1.47% (94)	18.60% (1192)	25.62% (1642)	3.25% (208)	39.24% (2515)	100% (6,409)
Black	26.11% (200)	1.17% (9)	3.26% (25)	2.48% (19)	18.41% (141)	21.54% (165)	3.13% (24)	23.89% (183)	100% (766)
Latin American	21.01% (54)	0.78% (2)	1.17% (3)	3.11% (8)	9.73% (25)	21.79% (56)	5.06% (13)	37.35% (96)	100% (257)
Asian/Pacific Islander	21.28% (20)	0.00% (0)	2.13% (2)	4.26% (4)	12.77% (12)	20.21% (19)	3.19% (3)	36.17% (34)	100% (94)
Native American or Alaska Native	2.56% (1)	2.56% (1)	0.00% (0)	2.56% (1)	38.46% (15)	20.51% (8)	5.13% (2)	28.21% (11)	100% (39)
Other	75.00% (3)	0.00% (0)	0.00% (0)	0.00% (0)	25.00% (1)	0.00% (0)	0.00% (0)	0.00% (0)	100% (4)
Totals	7.23% (847)	0.67% (51)	2.38% (180)	1.66% (126)	18.31% (1386)	24.97% (1890)	3.30% (250)	37.50% (2839)	100% (7569)

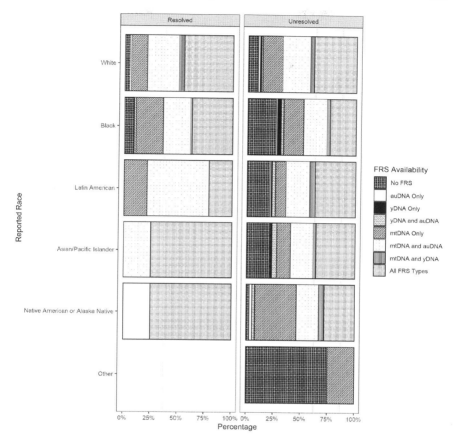

Figure 10.2   Differences in proportion of FRS availability between unresolved and resolved KWIP casualties by reported race. Credit: Briana T. New.

When looking among unresolved casualties, the proportional disparity in FRS availability becomes quite apparent (table 10.4, figure 10.2). Of all unresolved, only 8.88 percent of the White individuals and 2.56 percent of the Native Americans/Alaska Natives have no FRS available for comparison. In contrast, no FRSs are available for comparison for 21.01 percent of unresolved Latin American individuals, 21.28 percent of unresolved Asian/Pacific Islander individuals, 26.11 percent of unresolved Black individuals, and 75 percent of individuals in Other (though sample size is only 4 individuals for this group). Therefore, while overall FRS availability for the entire KWIP population appears to have good coverage among unresolved individuals, the same degree of coverage is not proportionally reflected at the group level. Our data demonstrates that FRSs are not equitably distributed across racial

categories in accordance with the proportion of the KWIP casualty population
that they encompass.

THE EFFECT OF STRUCTURAL
VULNERABILITIES ON FRS AVAILABILITY

Currently, positive identifications in the KWIP casualty population are generally equitably and proportionally distributed when subset by race such that no
group is disproportionally identified over other groups. This distribution suggests that, thus far, the identification of service members has not been biased
by differences in FRS availability among racial groupings. However, the FRS
distributions clearly demonstrate the importance of FRS availability for the
identification of these service members. While the identification process is
complex with many more factors than just FRS availability that contribute
to building a case for identification, the fact remains that identification of
an individual without at least one FRS is historically rare and unlikely to
move forward in the future. The DPAA has hundreds of Korean War remains
undergoing analysis that have yet to be identified because there are no consistent FRSs (i.e., FRS genetic profiles that match the genetic profile of the
remains), no matching antemortem records, and/or a strong enough case cannot yet be built to meet the burden of proof as set by the medical examiner
(see Taylor, New, and Tegtmeyer [2021] for a discussion on the burden of
proof). As more remains are disinterred or recovered, the disparities in FRS
availability across race will inevitably lead to inequitable identification proportions among the Korean War identified service members.

To proactively address this issue and provide the DPAA or other forensic
identification endeavors with the necessary tools for approaching disparities
in FRS availability, we mobilize structural vulnerability theory. *Structural
vulnerability* was formalized within medical anthropology as a concept that
builds upon the effects of structural violence while operationalizing the specific positionalities it produces on an individual or community (Quesada,
Hart, and Bourgois 2011). Structural violence systemically devalues human
lives and emphasizes the external forces that *act upon* the vulnerable in a
variety of ways (e.g., economically, politically, biologically) and ultimately
inhibits the agency of individuals (Farmer 2003, 2004; Galtung 1969;
Quesada, Hart, and Bourgois 2011; Soler and Beatrice 2018). As such, in
forensic identification contexts, structural violence is an apt framework for
contextualizing the ways in which the physical and the abstract forces of economics, politics, and so on, shape the lives and bodies of the structurally vulnerable (Beatrice and Soler 2016; Farmer 2003; Soler et al. 2019; Soler and
Beatrice 2018). However, in the context of obtaining Korean War FRSs, we

employ an understanding of structural vulnerabilities, similarly to Quesada, Hart, and Bourgois (2011), as a *positionality* in a hierarchical system that recognizes the forces of structural violence on groups but equally weighs its effect on the agency of individuals.

Structural violence produces the structural vulnerabilities that not only inhibit the choices available to someone, but also alter the form of personal agency in decision-making (Leatherman 2005; Quesada, Hart, and Bourgois 2011). For risk assessment in the medical field, understanding structural vulnerabilities is a helpful framework for removing bias and judgment in practitioners when someone does not seem to follow "rational" decision-making (Quesada, Hart, and Bourgois 2011). Similarly, when specifically addressing the embodied positionality of structural vulnerabilities in forensic identification, this framework is a powerful tool for understanding how the combined effects of structural violence and the positionality of structural vulnerabilities create conditions that cause certain individuals to arrive disproportionately among the missing and unidentified (Hughes et al. 2017). Furthermore, the structural vulnerabilities of the missing often extend to their families, impacting the types of choices available to them and the decision-making process that they undergo when working within medicolegal systems. In other words, we seek to balance the structures that shape a family's ability to provide FRSs with the process of decision-making by families who may be hesitant to participate in the DNA comparison process.

Within this framework we build a narrative that contextualizes the racial and class make-up of U.S. Korean War service members and, by extension, the racial and class distribution of family members who might contribute FRSs. Previously, this structural vulnerability approach has been employed to demonstrate the impact that intersectional positionality can have on the identification potential for U.S.-Mexico southern border forensic cases (Hughes et al. 2017; Soler et al. 2019); however, to our knowledge, the approach has not been explicitly used to understand the dual effects of structure and agency on obtaining FRSs for forensic identification endeavors in the context of military conflicts. This approach is especially important to consider in multiscale temporal contexts, such as historic conflicts or humanitarian contexts, where the form of structural forces acting upon the vulnerable shifts over time and alters the relationship between vulnerabilities and axes of privilege.

A More Diverse Fighting Force

To understand how the race and class distribution of missing and unidentified service members and their families in the twenty-first century impacts FRS availability, one must also understand the U.S. sociopolitical structure that shaped the race and class distribution of U.S. Korean War service members in the 1950s. The Korean War saw the most diverse fighting force in U.S. history up to that point, which comprised individuals from varying races, economic positions, and nations of origin (Bruscino 2010; Espiritu 2010; Flynn 1988; Kriner and Shen 2010, 2016; Lutz 2008; MacGregor 1981; Perri 2013). Standardized service records for military service members of this era often recorded their date of birth, location of birth, enlistment location, and race. Additional information might have included weight, health conditions, dental records, and/or treatments received while enlisted. However, beyond these basic individual characteristics, little documentation currently exists that documents the class of an individual. Class, as it is utilized in this chapter, defines the social stratification of individuals based on parameters of SES such as wealth distribution, educational attainment, and/or nationality. Therefore, we employ inference from historical documentation, legislation, and research on demographic trends within the armed forces to contextualize the vulnerabilities that shape the overall distribution of service members who died during this conflict. We emphasize the inextricable effects of race and class on the distribution of unidentified service members and the barriers that this positionality can produce for their families.

The diversification of the U.S. armed forces during the Korean War was aided by executive orders and legislation that instated desegregation policies for all military branches and allowed naturalization through years of military service (Espiritu 2010; Knight 1940; Lutz 2008; MacGregor 1981). While full desegregation of military units was not completed until after the conflict, the removal of segregation barriers increased racial quotas (i.e., limits to the number of enlisted individuals per racial group) within the armed forces which allowed the U.S. government to enlist or draft a larger number of non-White individuals (Espiritu 2010; Lutz 2008; MacGregor 1981). These expanded quotas increased enlistments of U.S. citizens (i.e., Black and Puerto Rican individuals), but they also enabled more Asian Americans (e.g., Japanese, Korean, Chinese), Pacific Islanders (e.g., Guamanian, Hawaiian), and other individuals from former U.S. territories (e.g., Filipinos), who were denied citizenship up to that point regardless of their place of birth, a pathway for obtaining citizenship through enlistment (Espiritu 2010; Rottman 2002). Thus, military service was particularly incentivized among Asians and Pacific Islanders who desired U.S. citizenship for themselves and their families (Espiritu 2010).

In addition to racial and nationality diversification, U.S. Korean War armed forces experienced enlistment biases toward individuals with less income and lower educational attainment (Flynn 1988; Kriner and Shen 2010, 2016; Perri 2013). In the Korean War era, the U.S. military was still a conscript force that relied on drafts to fill out the ranks, though the Selective Service only provided approximately 27 percent (1,529,539) of new service members during the Korean War (Selective Service System 2021). While the frequency of drafts and draft policies were continually evolving to meet the needs of the armed forces at a given moment, deferment policies allowed men currently enrolled in professional schools (e.g., medicine, dentistry), undergraduate or graduate programs, pending admission to a university, and/or with certain family dependent situations to defer their conscription (Flynn 1988; Kriner and Shen 2010, 2016; Perri 2013). This deferment policy was eventually extended to men in apprenticeship programs or industries that were necessary for U.S. defense; however, men with lower SES and less educational attainment who worked in non-defense-related industries were still disproportionately represented in military service because they were unable to defer their conscription (Flynn 1988; Kriner and Shen 2010, 2016; Perri 2013).

Additionally, the *Servicemen's Readjustment Act of 1944*, commonly known as the G.I. Bill, further incentivized military service following WWII by providing the possibility for increased educational attainment, which many voluntarily enlisting and enlisted men saw as an opportunity to improve their economic standing (Espiritu 2010; Turner and Bound 2003). Research has further demonstrated statistically significant, positively correlated higher casualties among men from lower-income areas with lower educational attainment (Kriner and Shen 2010, 2016). Higher casualty rates were not significant for race alone, but were also higher among communities with higher percentages of minority groups, which also tended to be lower-income communities (Kriner and Shen 2010). Importantly, SES was the greatest predictor of casualty status during the Korean War and subsequent conflicts (Kriner and Shen 2010). Moreover, the diversification of the U.S. military was largely restricted to lower-ranking positions, such as infantrymen, rather than officer positions (Bruscino 2010). Thus, individuals from lower SES and/or minority communities were disproportionally placed in the most hazardous combat roles. This means that the poor, regardless of race, suffered the most casualties, but minority communities still tended to be among the most economically disadvantaged communities in the overall U.S. population.

Thus, the relationships between lower SES and lower educational attainment, which are further still tied to race and nationality, are inextricable. The U.S. sociopolitical context of the Korean War era created more opportunities for people of color to be drafted, limited the chances of deferment for individuals with lower SES, incentivized voluntary enlistment through legislation that could improve upward mobility (i.e., the G.I. Bill and naturalization), and resulted in disproportionate casualties among the vulnerable. The historical context discussed here provides a temporal framework through which we can interpret FRS disparities across race and class. For example, any service member whose family were not U.S. citizens or resided outside the contiguous states and/or internationally inherently faced more substantial structural barriers to their identification in the 1950s. Service members with lower SES may not have had standard access to pre-service healthcare or dental care that could provide antemortem documentation for comparison against remains. These structural vulnerabilities that are produced by the 1950s historic context, in combination with vulnerabilities reinforced over time into the twenty-first century, may contribute to the distribution of absent or limited FRSs among the missing and unaccounted service members.

Barriers to DNA Contribution in the Twenty-First Century

Through ingenuity and persistence, KWIP has made tremendous strides in the identification of Korean War service members over the last decade. However, the identification processes for many other KWIP cases are paused because there are no matching genetic FRSs available at this time. As we have demonstrated, there are structural sociopolitical factors that produced the distribution of the Korean War casualty population across race and class. Therefore, if the service members of this era were more racially diverse and/or from lower income regions with less educational attainment, then we can surmise that their closest family members (e.g., mothers, fathers, siblings, children) were likely similarly positioned. How then can we mobilize this knowledge to understand the layered structural barriers that affect, and have affected for over seventy years, the families of those still lost?

Availability of FRSs is not simply inequitably distributed across groups for reasons unknown. First, the availability of FRS is predicated on the assumption that the family members can be located or are still alive. We would be remiss if we did not further acknowledge the effects of structural violence and vulnerabilities on the lifespan of family members for service members lost in historic contexts. Mortality research has repeatedly demonstrated that death rates and health disparities in the United States are strongly linked to income and education inequalities (Boing et al. 2020; Feldman et al. 1989; Henning-Smith et al. 2019; Jemal et al. 2008; Pappas et al. 1993; Steenland, Hu, and Walker 2004; Woolf and Schoomaker 2019). The relationship between income, or proxies to income such as occupation, and education are consistently strong predictors of premature mortality among White and Black communities (Boing et al. 2020; Cullen, Cummins, and Fuchs 2012; Feldman et al. 1989; Harper, MacLehose, and Kaufman 2014; Jemal et al. 2008; Pappas et al. 1993; Steenland, Hu, and Walker 2004). However, these health disparities and mortality trends are further impacted by factors such as immigration status and where in the United States an individual resides due to the convergence of different state and local policies, legislation, benefits, and more (Cullen, Cummins, and Fuchs 2012; Harper, MacLehose, and Kaufman 2014; Hastings et al. 2015; Henning-Smith et al. 2019; Krieger et al. 2014;

Winkleby and Cubbin 2003). For example, research indicates that immigrants tend to have longer life expectancies than their U.S-born counterparts, but when broken down by country of origin Chinese, Japanese, and Filipino immigrants are among those with higher mortality rates (Mehta et al. 2016; Singh and Miller 2004). Furthermore, when mortality rates are broken down regionally, county-level predictors and their ties to the demographic makeup of communities (i.e., SES, race, education, and so on.) are more salient predictors than large region-based (i.e., Western United States versus Southern United States) predictors (Boing et al. 2020; Cullen, Cummins, and Fuchs 2012; Henning-Smith et al. 2019; Woolf and Schoomaker 2019). Research on mortality trends from the perspective of forensic identification for unidentified decedents is still emerging, but the intersectional effect of the aforementioned factors significantly impacts who joins the ranks of the unidentified dead (Goad 2020; Hughes et al. 2017; Paulozzi et al. 2008; Reineke 2019; Soler and Beatrice 2018). Thus, structural violence and the vulnerabilities it produces do not only shape who remains to be identified among missing and unidentified service members from historic conflicts, they also significantly shape who is alive to participate in the FRS comparison process in the twenty-first century.

Inquiry into both the context of medical research as well as forensic investigation has identified patterns of personal and structural barriers for contributing DNA information to DNA databases among living members of structurally vulnerable communities (Dye et al. 2016; Farahany, Chodavadia, and Katsanis 2019; Katsanis 2020; Katsanis et al. 2018; Kim et al. 2011; Kim and Katsanis 2013; Kraft et al. 2018; Sanderson et al. 2017). In a survey of 13,000 people, willingness to extend broad consent for biobank research (i.e., DNA data that can be stored and anonymously utilized for research other than the initially consented to project) was most common among individuals with "self-identified white race, higher educational attainment, lower religiosity" while individuals with lower educational attainment, lower household incomes, and people of color were less willing to extend broad consent (Sanderson et al. 2017, 414). Recurrent areas of concern among focus groups include worries over cultural competency, such as language barriers, differences in cultural perspectives toward biological material, and the desire for a sense of comfortability and trust with researchers from their own communities (Dye et al. 2016; Kraft et al. 2018; Sanderson et al. 2017). Importantly, desires for cultural competency are intertwined with skepticism toward the trustworthiness and ethicality of genetic research/testing because of the histories of discrimination, exploitation, and abuses that medical research is steeped in among more structurally vulnerable communities (Bates and Harris 2004; Dye et al. 2016; Farahany, Chodavadia, and Katsanis 2019; Kraft et al. 2018; Park and Grayson 2008; Sanderson et al. 2017; Shavers,

Lynch, and Burmeister 2000). Moreover, desires for explicit communication of who is maintaining and managing the DNA data, as well as the consequences for misappropriation have been repeatedly expressed (Dye et al. 2016; Park and Grayson 2008; Sanderson et al. 2017).

More specifically in the context of forensic investigations and identifications, DNA collection is jurisdiction-specific and, as such, there are no national standardized practices for the explicit use of the DNA data procured for forensic investigative purposes or for obtaining family consent (Katsanis et al. 2018; Kim and Katsanis 2013). Compounded onto the concerns expressed in the context of genetic medical research are additional hesitancies produced by recent familial searching successes (i.e., the comparison of unidentified offender DNA to familial DNA databases in search of possible FRSs for the purposes of prosecution) as well as potential fears over incidental findings (i.e., previously undisclosed adoptions or familial discrepancies between purported father and/or sibling relationships) (Katsanis 2020; Kim et al. 2011; Parker, London, and Aronson 2013). Confusion over the DNA contribution process, unclear limitations to its use, and the unassuaged fears discussed above all impact the willingness or desire to contribute FRSs for DNA comparison. Each potential FRS donor has agency of choice when deciding whether to provide an FRS for comparison, but differences in structural vulnerabilities produce different experiences and levels of trust toward the systems surrounding the FRS collection process. These positionalities and experiences can make that contribution decision more complex among more vulnerable communities. As a result, some families may enact their agency of choice and refuse to contribute FRSs without clear mitigation of the barriers discussed above

In the Korean War context discussed here, not only are there proportionally greater casualties among individuals with lower SES and/or lower educational attainment, as well as people of color, but the general U.S. population similarly reflects those mortality rates through lower life expectancies. Moreover, individuals that live within this positionality typically discuss greater hesitancies toward providing DNA, whether for medical research or genetic comparison. Thus, the structural forces that acted upon the service members in the 1950s continued to act upon their families through life and partially influenced who is alive to contribute or who is willing to contribute an FRS in the twenty-first century. The data presented in this chapter demonstrate that the proportion of identifications for DPAA-identified Korean War service members is not inequitably skewed by race at this time. However, the proportion of FRSs available for unidentified service members is inequitably skewed by race. Furthermore, though our data cannot explicitly elaborate on class distributions for these specific individuals, our analysis situates FRS availability within the sociopolitical context of the Korean War with attention to intersectional class barriers that may further skew the ability or willingness to contribute FRS. Thus, as identifications move forward in this or any forensic identification context, analysts must not only consider the positionality of the unidentified remains in question, but also the effects of societally engrained, structural inequalities on the family members from which we seek references for DNA comparison.

CONCLUSION

The identification of U.S. service members is a distinct context in that there is a closed population of identification possibilities, and the vast resources of the U.S. military are available to pursue known FRSs. This context enabled us to highlight inequities in FRS availability and deconstruct the structural vulnerabilities that shape the distribution of those inequities. However, the lessons learned here can certainly extend outside of this Korean War context. Anthropologists working in coalition with medical examiner offices, in humanitarian endeavors, and in other medicolegal contexts are well positioned to apply similar analyses in understanding not just the remains under investigation, but the families on the other side of the process as well. As a discipline, anthropologists involved in human identification have long prioritized the scientific analysis of human remains. Similarly, critiques of the efficacy of this biologically centered approach typically attribute identification difficulties to inconsistencies produced by biological profile analyses. However, we emphasize that identification difficulties also source from the lack of appropriate FRSs for DNA comparison and, in a similar vein, family-provided antemortem records for the missing. These difficulties are often a product of the structural vulnerabilities similarly faced by the unidentified individual as well as their family members, and the personal agency that those family members may choose to employ because of the experiences produced by their positionality.

While we are only able to discuss vulnerabilities pertaining to race and, by extension, class, the impact of vulnerabilities extends to other demographics, such as the homeless population, sex workers, mentally ill, children, among others, that constitute the missing and the unidentified population of forensic cases (Goad 2020; Park and Grayson 2008). Our call to action is for a deeper investigation into the role that FRS availability plays in other forensic identification contexts and a proactive mitigation of these effects where possible. Anthropologists can help spearhead interdisciplinary endeavors by engaging advocacy groups and/or non-governmental organizations (NGOs) that can provide the family members of the missing with community-based support (Farahany, Chodavadia, and Katsanis 2019; Kim and Katsanis 2013; Koay and Sharp 2013). To facilitate this effort at the DPAA, multiple public and private partnerships have been established allowing for direct lines of communication between families and government officials. Establishing these lines of communication may assist in trust building among communities that express distrust of governmental, medical, and/or military intentions (Dye et al. 2016; Farahany, Chodavadia, and Katsanis 2019; Kim and Katsanis 2013; Koay and Sharp 2013; Kraft et al. 2018). Collaborating with advocacy groups and/or NGOs has already been successful in supporting medical genetic research as well as in aiding the identification of migrants who died in the humanitarian crisis along the U.S.-Mexico border (Koay and Sharp 2013; Reineke 2019; Soler et al. 2019; Spradley and Gocha 2020). As such, a deeper understanding of how FRS availability alters the identification potential of the missing, combined with community-based collaborations can work to prevent identification inequities among military service members and to meet identification inequities in other medicolegal contexts.

REFERENCES

Bates, Benjamin R., and Tina M. Harris. 2004. "The Tuskegee Study of Untreated Syphilis and Public Perceptions of Biomedical Research: A Focus Group Study." *Journal of the National Medical Association* 96 (8): 1051–64. https://www-ncbi-nlm-nih-gov/pmc/articles/PMC2568492/.

Beatrice, Jared S., and Angela Soler. 2016. "Skeletal Indicators of Stress: A Component of the Biocultural Profile of Undocumented Migrants in Southern Arizona." *Journal of Forensic Sciences* 61 (5): 1164–72. https://doi.org/10.1111/1556-4029.13131.

Berg, Gregory E., and Sabrina C. Ta'ala. 2015. "Biological Affinity in Medicolegal, Public, and Anthropological Contexts." In *Biological Affinity in Forensic Identification of Human Skeletal Remains: Beyond Black and White*, edited by Gregory E. Berg and Sabrina C. Ta'ala, 17–26. Boca Raton, FL: CRC Press. ISBN: 9781439815779.

Boing, Antonio Fernando, Alexandra Crispim Boing, Jack Cordes, Rockli Kim, and S. V. Subramanian. 2020. "Quantifying and Explaining Variation in Life Expectancy at Census Tract, County, and State Levels in the United States." *Proceedings of the National Academy of Sciences* 117 (30): 17688–94. https://doi.org/10.1073/pnas.2003719117.

Bruscino, Thomas A. 2010. "Minorities in the Military." In *A Companion to American Military History*, edited by James C. Bradford, 880–98. Oxford, UK: Wiley-Blackwell. https://doi.org/10.1002/9781444315066.ch58.

Cullen, Mark R., Clint Cummins, and Victor R. Fuchs. 2012. "Geographic and Racial Variation in Premature Mortality in the U.S.: Analyzing the Disparities." Edited by Joan A. Caylà. *PLoS ONE* 7 (4): e32930. https://doi.org/10.1371/journal.pone.0032930.

D'Alonzo, Susan S., Pierre Guyomarc'h, John E. Byrd, and Carl N. Stephan. 2017. "A Large-Sample Test of a Semi-Automated Clavicle Search Engine to Assist Skeletal Identification by Radiograph Comparison." *Journal of Forensic Sciences* 62 (1): 181–86. https://doi.org/10.1111/1556-4029.13221.

Dye, Timothy, Dongmei Li, Margaret Demment, Susan Groth, Diana Fernandez, Ann Dozier, and Jack Chang. 2016. "Sociocultural Variation in Attitudes toward Use of Genetic Information and Participation in Genetic Research by Race in the United States: Implications for Precision Medicine." *Journal of the American Medical Informatics Association* 23 (4): 782–86. https://doi.org/10.1093/jamia/ocv214.

Edson, Suni M., and Alexander F. Christensen. 2015. "The Use of DNA in the Identification of Degraded Human Skeletal Remains: A Basic Primer." In *Biological Affinity in Forensic Identification of Human Skeletal Remains: Beyond Black and White*, edited by Gregory E. Berg and Sabrina C. Ta'ala, 278–91. Boca Raton, FL: CRC Press. ISBN: 9781439815779.

Espiritu, Yen. 2010. *Filipino American Lives*. Philadelphia: Temple University Press. http://www.SLQ.eblib.com.au/patron/FullRecord.aspx?p=547415.

Farahany, Nita, Saheel Chodavadia, and Sara H. Katsanis. 2019. "Ethical Guidelines for DNA Testing in Migrant Family Reunification." *The American Journal of Bioethics* 19 (2): 4–7. https://doi.org/10.1080/15265161.2018.1556514.

Farmer, Paul. 2003. "Pathologies of Power: Health, Human Rights, and the New War on the Poor." *North American Dialogue* 6 (1): 1–4. https://doi.org/10.1525/nad.2003.6.1.1.

———. 2004. "An Anthropology of Structural Violence." *Current Anthropology* 45 (3): 305–25. https://doi.org/10.1086/382250.

Fehrenbach, T. R. 1963. *This Kind of War: A Study in Unpreparedness*. New York: McMillan. ISBN: 1574883348.

Feldman, Jacob J., Diane M. Makuc, Joel C. Kleinman, and Joan Cornoni-Huntley. 1989. "National Trends in Educational Differentials In Mortality." *American Journal of Epidemiology* 129 (5): 919–33. https://doi.org/10.1093/oxfordjournals.aje.a115225.

Flynn, George Q. 1988. "The Draft and College Deferments During the Korean War." *The Historian* 50 (3): 369–85. https://doi.org/10.1111/j.1540-6563.1988.tb00750.x.

Galtung, Johan. 1969. "Violence, Peace, and Peace Research." *Journal of Peace Research* 6 (3): 167–91. https://www.jstor.org/stable/422690.

Goad, Gennifer. 2020. "Expanding Humanitarian Forensic Action: An Approach to U.S. Cold Cases." *Forensic Anthropology* 3 (1): 50–58. https://doi.org/10.5744/fa.2020.1006.

Harper, Sam, Richard F. MacLehose, and Jay S. Kaufman. 2014. "Trends In The Black-White Life Expectancy Gap Among US States, 1990–2009." *Health Affairs* 33 (8): 1375–82. https://doi.org/10.1377/hlthaff.2013.1273.

Hastings, Katherine G., Powell O. Jose, Kristopher I. Kapphahn, Ariel T. H. Frank, Benjamin A. Goldstein, Caroline A. Thompson, Karen Eggleston, Mark R. Cullen, and Latha P. Palaniappan. 2015. "Leading Causes of Death among Asian American Subgroups (2003–2011)." Edited by Vishnu Chaturvedi. *PLOS ONE* 10 (4): e0124341. https://doi.org/10.1371/journal.pone.0124341.

Henning-Smith, Carrie E., Ashley M. Hernandez, Rachel R. Hardeman, Marizen R. Ramirez, and Katy Backes Kozhimannil. 2019. "Rural Counties With Majority Black Or Indigenous Populations Suffer The Highest Rates Of Premature Death In The US." *Health Affairs* 38 (12): 2019–26. https://doi.org/10.1377/hlthaff.2019 .00847.

Hughes, Cris E., Bridget F.B. Algee-Hewitt, Robin Reineke, Elizabeth Clausing, and Bruce E. Anderson. 2017. "Temporal Patterns of Mexican Migrant Genetic Ancestry: Implications for Identification: Migrant Ancestry and Identification Trends." *American Anthropologist* 119 (2): 193–208. https://doi.org/10.1111/aman .12845.

Jemal, Ahmedin, Elizabeth Ward, Robert N. Anderson, Taylor Murray, and Michael J. Thun. 2008. "Widening of Socioeconomic Inequalities in U.S. Death Rates, 1993–2001." Edited by Thorkild I. A. Sorensen. *PLoS ONE* 3 (5): e2181. https:// doi.org/10.1371/journal.pone.0002181.

Jin, Jennie, Ashley L. Burch, Carrie LeGarde, and Elizabeth Okrutny. 2014. "Chapter 19 - The Korea 208: A Large-Scale Commingling Case of American Remains from the Korean War." In *Commingled Human Remains*, edited by Bradley J. Adams and John E. Byrd, 407–23. San Diego: Academic Press. https://doi.org/10.1016/ B978-0-12-405889-7.00019-8.

Katsanis, Sara H. 2020. "Pedigrees and Perpetrators: Uses of DNA and Genealogy in Forensic Investigations." *Annual Review of Genomics and Human Genetics* 21 (1): 535–64. https://doi.org/10.1146/annurev-genom-111819-084213.

Katsanis, Sara H., Lindsey Snyder, Kelly Arnholt, and Amy Z. Mundorff. 2018. "Consent Process for US-Based Family Reference DNA Samples." *Forensic Science International: Genetics* 32 (January): 71–79. https://doi.org/10.1016/j .fsigen.2017.10.011.

Kim, Joyce, and Sara H. Katsanis. 2013. "Brave New World of Human-Rights DNA Collection." *Trends in Genetics: TIG* 29 (6): 329–32. https://doi.org/10.1016/j.tig .2013.04.002.

Kim, Joyce, Danny Mammo, Marni B. Siegel, and Sara H. Katsanis. 2011. "Policy Implications for Familial Searching." *Investigative Genetics* 2 (1): 22. https://doi .org/10.1186/2041-2223-2-22.

Knight, George S. 1940. "Nationality Act of 1940." *American Bar Association Journal* 26 (12): 938–40. https://www.jstor.org/stable/25712994.

Koay, Pei P., and Richard R. Sharp. 2013. "The Role of Patient Advocacy Organizations in Shaping Genomic Science." *Annual Review of Genomics and Human Genetics* 14 (1): 579–95. https://doi.org/10.1146/annurev-genom-091212 -153525.

Kraft, Stephanie A., Mildred K. Cho, Katherine Gillespie, Meghan Halley, Nina Varsava, Kelly E. Ormond, Harold S. Luft, Benjamin S. Wilfond, and Sandra Soo-Jin Lee. 2018. "Beyond Consent: Building Trusting Relationships With Diverse Populations in Precision Medicine Research." *The American Journal of Bioethics* 18 (4): 3–20. https://doi.org/10.1080/15265161.2018.1431322.

Krieger, Nancy, Anna Kosheleva, Pamela D. Waterman, Jarvis T. Chen, Jason Beckfield, and Mathew V. Kiang. 2014. "50-Year Trends in US Socioeconomic

Inequalities in Health: US-Born Black and White Americans, 1959–2008." *International Journal of Epidemiology* 43 (4): 1294–313. https://doi-org/10.1093/ije/dyu047.

Kriner, Douglas L., and Francis X. Shen. 2010. *The Casualty Gap: The Causes and Consequences of American Wartime Inequalities.* Oxford: Oxford University Press. ISBN: 9780199779826.

———. 2016. "Invisible Inequality: The Two Americas of Military Sacrifice." *Memphis Law Review* 46: 545–635.

Leatherman, Thomas. 2005. "A Space of Vulnerability in Poverty and Health: Political-Ecology and Biocultural Analysis." *Ethos* 33 (1): 46–70. https://doi.org/10.1525/eth.2005.33.1.046.

Lutz, Amy. 2008. "Who Joins the Military?: A Look at Race, Class, and Immigration Status." *Sociology* 36 (2): 167–88. https://www.jstor.org/stable/45292868.

MacGregor, Morris J. 1981. *Integration of the Armed Forces, 1940-1965.* Vol. 1. Government Printing Office.

Marshall, Charla, Rebecca Taylor, Kimberly Sturk-Andreaggi, Suzanne Barritt-Ross, Gregory E. Berg, and Timothy P. McMahon. 2020. "Mitochondrial DNA Haplogrouping to Assist with the Identification of Unknown Service Members from the World War II Battle of Tarawa." *Forensic Science International: Genetics* 47 (July): 102291. https://doi.org/10.1016/j.fsigen.2020.102291.

Mehta, Neil K., Irma T. Elo, Michal Engelman, Diane S. Lauderdale, and Bert M. Kestenbaum. 2016. "Life Expectancy Among U.S.-Born and Foreign-Born Older Adults in the United States: Estimates From Linked Social Security and Medicare Data." *Demography* 53 (4): 1109–34. https://doi.org/10.1007/s13524-016-0488-4.

Pappas, Gregory, Susan Queen, Wilbur Hadden, and Gail Fisher. 1993. "The Increasing Disparity in Mortality between Socioeconomic Groups in the United States, 1960 and 1986." *New England Journal of Medicine* 329 (2): 103–9. https://doi.org/10.1056/NEJM199307083290207.

Park, Stephanie S., and Mitchell H. Grayson. 2008. "Clinical Research: Protection of the 'Vulnerable'?" *Journal of Allergy and Clinical Immunology* 121 (5): 1103–7. https://doi.org/10.1016/j.jaci.2008.01.014.

Parker, Lisa S., Alex John London, and Jay D. Aronson. 2013. "Incidental Findings in the Use of DNA to Identify Human Remains: An Ethical Assessment." *Forensic Science International: Genetics* 7 (2): 221–29. https://doi.org/10.1016/j.fsigen.2012.10.002.

Paulozzi, Leonard J., Christine S. Cox, Dionne D. Williams, and Kurt B. Nolte. 2008. "John and Jane Doe: The Epidemiology of Unidentified Decedents." *Journal of Forensic Sciences* 53 (4): 922–27. https://doi.org/10.1111/j.1556-4029.2008.00769.x.

Perri, Timothy J. 2013. "The Evolution of Military Conscription in the United States." *The Independent Review*, no. 17: 429–39. https://www.jstor.org/stable/24563185.

Quesada, James, Laurie Kain Hart, and Philippe Bourgois. 2011. "Structural Vulnerability and Health: Latino Migrant Laborers in the United States." *Medical Anthropology* 30 (4): 339–62. https://doi.org/10.1080/01459740.2011.576725.

Reineke, Robin C. 2019. "Necroviolence and Postmortem Care along the U.S.-México Border." In *The Border and Its Bodies: The Embodiment of Risk Along the U.S.- México Line*, edited by Thomas E. Sheridan and Randall H. McGuire, 144–72. Tucson, AZ: University of Arizona Press. ISBN: 9780816540563.

Rottman, Gordon L. 2002. *World War II Pacific Island Guide: A Geo-Military Study*. Westport, CT: Greenwood Press. ISBN: 9780313313950.

Sanderson, Saskia C., Kyle B. Brothers, Nathanial D. Mercaldo, Ellen Wright Clayton, Armand H. Matheny Antommaria, Sharon A. Aufox, Murray H. Brilliant, Diego Campos, and David S. Carrell. 2017. "Public Attitudes toward Consent and Data Sharing in Biobank Research: A Large Multi-Site Experimental Survey in the US." *The American Journal of Human Genetics* 100 (3): 414–27. https://doi.org/10.1016/j.ajhg.2017.01.021.

Selective Service System. 2021. "Historical Timeline: Korean War." 2021. sss.gov/history-and-records/timeline.

Shavers, V. L., C. F. Lynch, and L. F. Burmeister. 2000. "Knowledge of the Tuskegee Study and Its Impact on the Willingness to Participate in Medical Research Studies." *Journal of the National Medical Association* 92 (12): 563–72. https://www.ncbi.nlm.nih.gov/pmc/articles/PMC2568333.

Shiroma, Calvin Y. 2016a. "A Comparison of Dental Chartings Performed at the Joint POW/MIA Accounting Command Central Identification Laboratory and the Kokura Central Identification Unit on Remains Identified from the Korean War." *Journal of Forensic Sciences* 61 (1): 59–67. https://doi.org/10.1111/1556-4029.12916.

———. 2016b. "A Retrospective Review of Forensic Odontology Reports Written by the Joint POW/MIA Accounting Command Central Identification Laboratory for Remains Identified from the Korean War." *Journal of Forensic Sciences* 61 (1): 68–75. https://doi.org/10.1111/1556-4029.12986.

Singh, Gopal K., and Barry A. Miller. 2004. "Health, Life Expectancy, and Mortality Patterns Among Immigrant Populations in the United States." *Canadian Journal of Public Health* 95 (3): I14–21. https://doi.org/10.1007/BF03403660.

Soler, Angela, and Jared S. Beatrice. 2018. "Expanding the Role of Forensic Anthropology in a Humanitarian Crisis: An Example from the USA-Mexico Border." In *Sociopolitics of Migrant Death and Repatriation*, edited by Krista E. Latham and Alyson J. O'Daniel, 115–28. Cham: Springer International Publishing. https://doi.org/10.1007/978-3-319-61866-1_9.

Soler, Angela, Robin C. Reineke, Jared S. Beatrice, and Bruce E. Anderson. 2019. "Embodied Suffering in the Remains of Undocumented Migrants." In *The Border and Its Bodies the Embodiment of Risk along the U.S.-México Line*, edited by Thomas E. Sheridan and Randall H. McGuire, 173–207. Tucson, AZ: University of Arizona Press. ISBN: 9780816540563.

Spradley, M. Katherine, and Timothy P. Gocha. 2020. "Migrant Deaths along the Texas/Mexico Border: A Collaborative Approach to Forensic Identification of Human Remains." In *Forensic Science and Humanitarian Action*, edited by Roberto C. Parra, Sara C. Zapico, and Douglas H. Ubelaker, 535–48. Wiley. https://doi.org/10.1002/9781119482062.ch34.

Steenland, Kyle, Sherry Hu, and James Walker. 2004. "All-Cause and Cause-Specific Mortality by Socioeconomic Status Among Employed Persons in 27 US States, 1984–1997." *American Journal of Public Health* 94 (6): 1037–42.

Stephan, Carl N., Susan S. D'Alonzo, Emily K. Wilson, Pierre Guyomarc'h, Gregory E. Berg, and John E. Byrd. 2018. "Skeletal Identification by Radiographic Comparison of the Cervicothoracic Region on Chest Radiographs." In *New Perspectives in Forensic Human Skeletal Identification*, 277–92. Elsevier. https://doi.org/10.1016/B978-0-12-805429-1.00024-7.

Taylor, Rebecca J., Briana T. New, and Caryn E. Tegtmeyer. 2021. "Navigating Identity: The Intersection of Social and Biological Identity from the WWII Battle of Tarawa." *Human Biology* 93 (2): 1–19. https://doi-org/10.13110/humanbiology.93.2.01.

Turner, Sarah, and John Bound. 2003. "Closing the Gap or Widening the Divide: The Effects of the G.I. Bill and World War II on the Educational Outcomes of Black Americans." *The Journal of Economic History* 63 (1): 145–77. https://doi.org/10.1017/S0022050703001761.

Winkleby, Marilyn A., and Catherine Cubbin. 2003. "Influence of Individual and Neighbourhood Socioeconomic Status on Mortality among Black, Mexican-American, and White Women and Men in the United States." *Journal of Epidemiology & Community Health* 57: 444–52. http://dx.doi.org/10.1136/jech.57.6.444.

Woolf, Steven H., and Heidi Schoomaker. 2019. "Life Expectancy and Mortality Rates in the United States, 1959-2017." *JAMA* 322 (20): 1996–2016. https://doi.org/10.1001/jama.2019.16932.

Chapter 11

A Multidisciplinary Perspective on the Role of Marginalization in the Identification of Opioid Users in Medicolegal Investigations

Janna M. Andronowski and Randi M. Depp

INTRODUCTION

The opioid epidemic began in the 1970s with heroin, a semisynthetic illicit opioid, that caused an alarming number of overdose deaths, particularly among African American communities in the United States (Hernandez et al. 2020; Alexander, Kiang, and Barbieri 2018). In the 1990s, misleading data from pharmaceutical companies regarding the addictive nature of opioid pain relievers led to subsequent overprescribing of both synthetic and semisynthetic opioid medications (National Institute on Drug Abuse 2020; Hernandez et al. 2020; Alexander, Kiang, and Barbieri 2018; Center for Disease Control and Prevention 2020). This signaled the beginning of the second wave of the opioid epidemic, which lasted from 1999 to approximately 2013, and was characterized by a drastic increase in opioid overdose deaths (OODs) and a significant shift in the demographics of OODs to include more European individuals (National Institute on Drug Abuse 2020; Hernandez et al. 2020; Alexander, Kiang, and Barbieri 2018). In 2013, non-prescription synthetic opioid-related deaths began to increase sharply, marking the beginning of the third and current wave of the epidemic (Hernandez et al. 2020; Alexander, Kiang, and Barbieri 2018; Center for Disease Control and Prevention 2020; Rudd et al. 2016a). The rapid increase in the use of synthetic opioids like fentanyl and its analogues (e.g., carfentanil) is especially concerning because they are 50–100 times more powerful than prescription opioids such as morphine (World Health Organization 2020; Salmond and Allread 2019). Such synthetic opioids are added to, or substituted for, illicit drugs to increase potency, often without the drug-user's knowledge or understanding of the associated dangers (World Health Organization 2020; United Nations Office on Drugs and Labor 2020; Salmond and Allread 2019; Rudd et al. 2016a). Illicitly manufactured fentanyl is created in clandestine laboratories without regulation; therefore, its composition and proportion of fentanyl analogues and potency varies widely (Daniulaityte et al. 2017). As a result, OODs due to fentanyl and fentanyl analogues are at a record high (United Nations Office on Drugs and Labor 2020).

Each year, over 70 percent of the 500,000 drug-related deaths worldwide are categorized as opioid-related (World Health Organization 2020). In 2018 alone, approximately 1.2 percent of the global population between fifteen and sixty-four years old used opioids in the past year (United Nations Office on Drugs and Labor 2020). The crisis is markedly more severe in North America, which had the highest average rate of opioid use at 3.6 percent in 2018 (United Nations Office on Drugs and Labor 2020). The United States has been the epicenter of this crisis, with nearly 500,000 OODs from 1999 to 2019 (Center for Disease Control and Prevention 2021). Of those individuals prescribed opioids to manage pain in the United States, approximately 21 to 29 percent misuse their prescription and 8 to 12 percent develop an opioid-use disorder (OUD) (National Institute on Drug Abuse 2020).

Opioid ODs in the United States spiked to a record high of nearly 50,000 in 2019 with nearly 73 percent of these deaths involving synthetic opioids, signaling that the third wave of the opioid epidemic is far from over (Center for Disease Control and Prevention 2021). For example, there was a 31 percent increase in drug ODs in the United States in 2020, more than 69,000 of which were OODs, demonstrating the dramatic impact of the COVID-19 pandemic on this marginalized group (Ahmad, Rossen, and Sutton 2021; Hedegaard et al. 2021). Ohio is consistently one of the states with the most overdose deaths per year, along with West Virginia, Maryland, New Hampshire, and Massachusetts (Hedegaard, Miniño, and Warner 2020; Rudd et al. 2016a). Fentanyl-related deaths have further rapidly increased across Ohio in recent years, echoing national and global trends (Peterson et al. 2016; Cuyahoga County Opiate Task Force 2018).

PROFILE OF THE OPIOID EPIDEMIC

Understanding the demographics of who is being affected by the opioid epidemic and which groups are most vulnerable is vital to allocating proper funding and resources for prevention and treatment programs and to combating the systemic problems feeding the epidemic itself (Daniulaityte et al. 2017; Rubin 2018). It is also critical to the scientific design of forensic anthropological research projects investigating the effects of opioids on the human skeleton as well as micro- and macroscopic methods for identifying unknown human skeletal remains. Research samples must be balanced and representative of the study population, including marginalized groups. This is especially critical because opioid users may be subjected to marginalization and social stigma due to their drug use. Moving forward, the accurate reporting of opioid-related overdoses and deaths must be implemented, but jurisdictional variation in toxicology testing may be causing significant underreporting (Daniulaityte et al. 2017; Peterson et al. 2016; Lowder et al. 2018; Rubin 2018). Mandatory, standardized toxicology testing that includes illicitly manufactured fentanyl and its analogues must be adopted (Daniulaityte et al. 2017; Peterson et al. 2016; Lowder et al. 2018; Rubin 2018). This includes skeletal remains, which have been successfully tested for opioids (Rubin 2018). Such data may assist with identification efforts and informing law enforcement of the individual's potential life history or key investigative findings (Rubin 2018). Additionally, an accurate portrayal of the opioid epidemic and risk factors for overdose will ensure the availability of social support and naloxone, a drug used to counteract opioid overdose (Daniulaityte et al. 2017; Peterson et al. 2016; Lowder et al. 2018). Such risk factors such as mental illness, poor health, substance abuse disorders, and traits that lead to social exclusion, among others, increase the likelihood for isolated deaths (Archer et al. 2005; van Draanen et al. 2020). This is important in a forensic anthropological context because the vast majority of OODs occur in isolation or within residences (Visconti et al. 2015; Siegler et al. 2014), often delaying the discovery of the decedent until later stages of decomposition (Archer et al. 2005).

The following sections outline trends in opioid-related decedent profiles as reported by anthropological researchers and healthcare and government authorities, as well as risk factors and marginalized groups with increased susceptibility to OOD. These trends are compared to existing data gathered by the Andronowski Lab from Northeast Ohio, one of five states with the highest overdose rates nationwide, to highlight both the difficulty and importance of obtaining samples representative of the study population (Andronowski and Depp 2022). Many of the risk factors overlap and interact.

Sex

As biological sex is typically reported in binary categories of male and female, only those data are outlined here. Future research and statistical reporting should incorporate intersex, transgender, and gender-variant identities. In both the United States and Canada, OOD decedents are most likely to be male (Hernandez et al. 2020; Salmond and Allread 2019; Daniulaityte et al. 2017; Ohio Department of Health 2019; Love et al. 2018; Miller et al.

2001; Sorg 2010; Sorg and Greenwald 2003; Al-Tayyib et al. 2017; Belzak and Halverson 2018; Rudd et al. 2016b; Rudd et al. 2016a). In Ohio, for example, males represent roughly half of all unintentional drug overdose deaths (Ohio Department of Health 2019), but account for more than two-thirds of the fentanyl-related overdose deaths (Daniulaityte et al. 2017; Peterson et al. 2016). Researchers have found that synthetic opioid use is most common among males, which makes them disproportionately vulnerable to surges in fentanyl lacing and substitution in the illicit opioid market (Hernandez et al. 2020).

Age

Although drug-user data is typically skewed toward younger age groups, OODs span adolescence to middle age and beyond (Sorg and Greenwald 2003; Al-Tayyib et al. 2017; Sorg 2010; Peterson et al. 2016; Miller et al. 2001; Hernandez et al. 2020; Gomes et al. 2018; Belzak and Halverson 2018; Rudd et al. 2016b; Rudd et al. 2016a). Consistently throughout the United States and Canada, the age group of twenty-five to forty years has the highest burden of OODs (Ohio Department of Health 2019; Peterson et al. 2016; Miller et al. 2001; Sorg 2010; Al-Tayyib et al. 2017; Belzak and Halverson 2018; Wilson et al. 2020; Rudd et al. 2016b). This may be the result of medical and recreational opioid use typically beginning during this time frame (Hernandez et al. 2020). Opioid ODs have generally increased across all age groups over the course of the epidemic (Gomes et al. 2018; Ohio Department of Health 2019; Sorg 2010; Rudd et al. 2016b), but there is a rapid and alarming increase in opioid-related deaths of middle-aged and older individuals (Gomes et al. 2018; Miller et al. 2001; Sorg 2010; Belzak and Halverson 2018; Rudd et al. 2016a). At the time of this writing, it remains unclear whether the increasing age of decedents is due to long-term opioid-users growing older or an increase in new opioid users in those age groups.

Ancestry

Following the movements toward equity in biological and forensic anthropology, an individual's population affinity is herein referred to as *ancestry* (DiGangi and Bethard 2021). Although racial terminology is common in medical, social, and governmental statistics, such outdated terms are grounded in colonialism and race science and do not accurately represent descriptions of biological populations (DiGangi and Bethard 2021). Instead, five groupings based on geographical heritage will be employed to characterize ancestry in the United States: African American, Asian, European, Indigenous, and Latinx.

Despite similar drug addiction rates across populations in the United States (Kreek 2011), different groups are not represented equally among OODs. In 2018, Europeans had the highest rate of overdose deaths in every opioid category, typically followed by Indigenous peoples and African Americans (Wilson et al. 2020). The Latinx and Asian populations are ranked fourth and fifth in the overdose death rate for all opioid categories, respectively (Wilson et al. 2020). It should be noted, however, that individuals from the Latinx, Asian, and Indigenous populations are frequently misclassified on death certificates, resulting in inconsistent reporting and underestimated death rates (Arias et al. 2016). Much of the literature reports that the majority of OODs from the second and third waves of the epidemic are of European descent and these trends direct media, political, research, and public attention toward European populations (Alexander, Kiang, and Barbieri 2018; Kline, Pan, and Hepler 2021; James and Jordan 2018), which has, over time, shaped Americans' understanding of a typical opioid user to be European (Sobotka and Stewart 2020). Yet, two groups are disproportionately affected by the opioid epidemic: African Americans (Kline, Pan, and Hepler 2021; Visconti et al. 2015; James and Jordan 2018; Furr-Holden et al. 2021) and Indigenous peoples (Tipps, Buzzard, and McDougall 2018; Joshi, Weiser, and Warren-Mears 2018).

In both the United States and Ohio, the OOD rate of African Americans has not only kept pace with that of Europeans but was similar to, or even locally surpassed, the European rate for approximately the last decade (Kline, Pan, and Hepler 2021; James and Jordan 2018; Furr-Holden et al. 2021). Localized data demonstrate trends in rural areas like Appalachia are not always mirrored in urban areas (Daniulaityte et al. 2017; Kline, Pan, and Hepler 2021; James and Jordan 2018). For example, in Washington D.C. in 2016, African Americans comprised approximately 48 percent of the population but accounted for more than 79 percent of the opioid-related deaths (James and Jordan 2018). An alarming increase in OODs has also been recorded among Indigenous populations for nearly two decades (Tipps, Buzzard, and McDougall 2018). Compared to national trends, Indigenous peoples are dying from opioid overdoses at nearly the same rate as Europeans, increasing from 2.9 to 13.9 per 100,000 from 1999 to 2016 (Tipps, Buzzard, and McDougall 2018). The problem is especially dire in the Pacific Northwest and Great Lakes regions (Tipps, Buzzard, and McDougall 2018; Joshi, Weiser, and Warren-Mears 2018). The opioid overdose mortality rate in Minnesota in 2016 was 47.6 per 100,000 for Indigenous peoples while only 7.3 for Europeans (Tipps, Buzzard, and McDougall 2018). In Washington from 2013 to 2015, Indigenous people experienced 2.7 times the OOD rate of Europeans and since 2001 this rate has increased faster than in Europeans (Joshi, Weiser, and Warren-Mears 2018). A review of death certificates in Washington found that the drug overdose death rate among Indigenous peoples was underestimated by 40 percent, indicating that the reality of the crisis is far worse than demonstrated by existing data (Joshi, Weiser, and Warren-Mears 2018).

Other Risk Factors and Marginalized Groups

Socioeconomic Instability, Housing Instability, and Education

Socioeconomic status and related variables (e.g., employment, financial stress, training, and opportunities) can be difficult to assess and measure because of the complexity of interactions among the various parameters (van Draanen et al. 2020). Poverty, unemployment, and insecure housing situations all have significant positive correlations with OODs while education level attained has an inverse correlation with OODs (van Draanen et al. 2020). Due to the limited documentation of these categories presented in medical and decedent profiles, these variables will not be discussed in depth here.

Incarceration

A high proportion of opioid users and decedents have been previously incarcerated (Peterson et al. 2016; Al-Tayyib et al. 2017; Belzak and Halverson 2018; van Draanen et al. 2020). The susceptibility to overdose increases immediately following release from incarceration (van Draanen et al. 2020; Ødegård et al. 2010) due to reduced drug tolerance following treatment or drug abstention for the period imprisoned (Peterson et al. 2016). The weeks immediately after release are the most vulnerable, with prior inmates at 12.7 times the risk for drug overdose than those not previously incarcerated (Ødegård et al. 2010; Binswanger et al. 2007). An increased risk for overdose further exists as the length of incarceration increases (Brinkley-Rubinstein et al. 2018; Ochoa et al. 2005; Seal et al. 2001). The rate of OODs among previously incarcerated individuals is approximately 13.5 per 100,000 and is more common among prior users (Belzak and Halverson 2018). In Ohio from 2013 to 2015, 10.3 percent of fentanyl-related fatality decedents had been incarcerated in the last thirty days (Peterson et al. 2016).

Health and Access to Healthcare

Access to health insurance is significantly correlated with lower opioid overdose rates (van Draanen et al. 2020). Fentanyl-related fatality decedents are less likely to have had access to healthcare or to have received an opioid or antidepressant prescription in the thirty days prior to death (Belzak and Halverson 2018). Physical illnesses, disabilities, chronic health conditions (e.g., hypertension, renal disease, diabetes), and acute injuries, including those that occur in the workplace, all place individuals at a higher risk for developing OUD or OOD (Salmond and Allread 2019; Sorg and Greenwald 2003; Cheng et al. 2013; Archer et al. 2005; Hasegawa et al. 2014; Feng, Iser, and Yang 2016; Nadpara et al. 2018). This is partially because experiencing pain drives individuals to seek relief, either through prescription opioids or other self-medicated means (Jalali et al. 2020). Opioid users are also at high risk for contracting blood-borne diseases such as HIV, Hepatitis B, and Hepatitis C, especially if they are intravenous drug users (Miller et al. 2001; Archer et al. 2005).

Mental Health

Mental health disorders are significant social factors that increase the risk of OOD (Sorg and Greenwald 2003). Depression and anxiety increase the risk for opioid overdose by three times (Salmond and Allread 2019) and a large portion of people with OUD or who have experienced an opioid overdose also have a mood or anxiety disorder (Jalali et al. 2020; Paulozzi et al. 2009; Cheng et al. 2013; Hasegawa et al. 2014; Nadpara et al. 2018). Mental health disorders or a history of traumatic events may further lead to social isolation (Archer et al. 2005), which can exacerbate the risks. In the United States, more than half of the opioids prescribed annually are given to adults with mental health disorders (Salmond and Allread 2019). The addictive nature of prescription opioids, high rates of OUD among individuals with mental health disorders, and large numbers of prescribed opioids is a frightening combination. Among fentanyl-related deaths from 2013 to 2015 in Ohio, for example, 25 percent of decedents had a documented mental health disorder (Peterson et al. 2016).

Gender Identity and Sexual Orientation

Unfortunately, both gender identity and sexual orientation are not frequently documented in research investigating OODs. This is despite members of lesbian, gay, bisexual, transgender, gender queer, intersex, and asexual (LGBTQIA+) communities being at an increased risk for opioid overdose (Ochoa et al. 2005; Seal et al. 2001; Jenkins et al. 2011; Ochoa et al. 2001). Individuals from these groups may experience more economic stress and social stigma, which can prevent access to resources and prospects to maintain their safety and well-being (Seal et al. 2001). It is vital that future studies include LGBTQIA+ communities in their sample groups and accurately document these factors for analysis.

Alcohol and Other Drug Use

Polysubstance use increases the risk for abusing opioids (Peterson et al. 2016; Jalali et al. 2020) and OODs occur most often when an individual has taken one or more non-opioid substances (Belzak and Halverson 2018; Marshall et al. 2019; Cheng et al. 2013). There has been a significant increase among intravenous drug users combining heroin and methamphetamines (Al-Tayyib et al. 2017). Alcohol and benzodiazepines, which are both depressants, frequently accompany OODs (Sherman, Cheng, and Kral 2007; Kerr et al. 2007; Siegler et al. 2014; Paulozzi et al. 2009; Marshall et al. 2019; Visconti et al. 2015; Cheng et al. 2013). In Ohio, for example, a high proportion of fentanyl-overdose deaths also involved heroin, cocaine, psychostimulants, natural or semi-synthetic opioids, and/or alcohol near the time of death (Ohio Department of Health 2019; Peterson et al. 2016). It must be noted, however, that the large increase in fentanyl lacing and substitution in the illicit drug market in recent years may be contributing to this trend.

Region

The rate of OODs in the United States varies by region and state. In 2018, the rate of all OODs was highest in the Northeast (22.8 per 100,000) followed by the Midwest (17.2), the South (13.5), and the West (8.3) (Wilson et al. 2020). In 2018, the five states with the highest age-adjusted rate of drug overdose death for all opioids were West Virginia (42.4 per 100,000), Maryland (33.7), New Hampshire (33.1), Ohio (29.6), and Massachusetts (29.3) (Wilson et al. 2020). The opioid mortality rates have increased in all regions, but especially in the Northeast and the South (Rudd et al. 2016b). There is also variation within states and at the county level.

The opioid epidemic is often considered to be a rural problem (Salmond and Allread 2019; Kline, Pan, and Hepler 2021; James and Jordan 2018; Schalkoff et al. 2020; Monnat 2019). Although the rate of OODs in rural counties has increased drastically in recent years (Meiman, Tomasallo, and Paulozzi 2015), the vast majority of OODs occur in urban and suburban communities (Daniulaityte et al. 2017; Kline, Pan, and Hepler 2021; Tipps, Buzzard, and McDougall 2018; Joshi, Weiser, and Warren-Mears 2018; Meiman, Tomasallo, and Paulozzi 2015). Variables other than county type may better explain these patterns. In Ohio, for example, the OOD rate is similar in urban counties (Kline, Pan, and Hepler 2021) and there are five concentrations of opioid-related deaths in urban sectors: Cleveland/Akron, Cincinnati, Columbus, Dayton, and Toledo (Rembert et al. 2017). Surprisingly, in 2016 only one of the top ten counties in Ohio with the highest OOD rate was located in one of the urban centers (Rembert et al. 2017). Hernandez and colleagues (2020) suggested that the epidemic is occurring in hotspots, which increase and localize the crisis like a positive feedback loop (Hernandez et al. 2020). They found that Southwestern Ohio had the greatest risk for OOD and includes nine counties with the highest OOD rate, eight of which are rural and one that encompasses the urban center of Dayton (Rembert et al. 2017; Hernandez et al. 2020). The region as a whole has a history of reduced access to jobs and education (Hernandez et al. 2020), which may be feeding the crisis. In addition, the severity of the opioid epidemic in Southwestern Ohio may be correlated to the high rate of opioid drug seizures in Ohio, Kentucky, and Indiana (Hernandez et al. 2020). This further indicates that drugs are more easily accessible in this region.

The above trends are reflected in the demographics of a selection of recent decedents included in ongoing bone histological research in the Andronowski Lab (outlined below). Decedents were categorized into four drug use groups: non-drug users (control), drug user (non-overdose death), overdose (non-OOD), and OODs (table 11.1). These data indicate a high rate of OODs (17%), an underrepresentation of non-European individuals, higher rates of previous incarceration, and documented mental health history. Although the Northeast region is not the epicenter of OODs in Ohio, it does contain the Cleveland/Akron urban concentration as well as rural counties for comparison. Kruskal-Wallis H tests were employed to demographic (sex, age, ancestry), health (chronic health condition, Hepatitis B+, Hepatitis C+, mental health disorder), and lifestyle (current and prior tobacco use, prior incarceration, LGBTQIA+ identity) variables versus the drug use groups. Current tobacco use ($p = 0.002$), prior incarceration ($p = 0.001$), LGBTQIA+ identity ($p = 0.020$), and Hepatitis C+ status ($p = 0.000$) were statistically significant parameters (Andronowski and Depp 2022). To extract significant effects for the above relationships, post-hoc pairwise comparisons with Dunn-Bonferroni corrections were conducted. All significant variables were statistically different between controls and OODs. Current tobacco use was also significantly different between controls and drug users. Prior incarceration, LGBTQIA+ identity, and Hepatitis C+ status were significantly different between drug users and OODs as well (Andronowski and Depp 2022). Ongoing bone specimen collection will increase sample size and create more balanced drug use groups, likely revealing further significant demographic, health, and lifestyle parameters.

IMPLICATIONS FOR FORENSIC ANTHROPOLOGY

Impact of Risk and Lifestyle Factors on the Human Skeleton

In a forensic anthropological context, it is important to consider the interacting nature of the above risk and lifestyle factors as they may influence the bone metabolism of opioid users and subsequent histological and macroscopic skeletal analyses. As such, focusing on a specific stimulus (e.g., opioid use) and its prolonged impact on bone formation and resorption should

Table 11.1 Demographic, health, and lifestyle variables of recent decedents in North-east Ohio. Variables that reached statistical significance ($p < 0.05$) are indicated by *

	Control	Drug User	Overdose (Non-OOD)	OOD	Total
Sample size (n)	24	23	36	17	100
Sex					
Male	15	14	21	13	63
Female	9	9	15	4	37
Ancestry					
African American	1	4	5	0	10
European	20	17	28	15	80
Latinx	3	2	3	2	10
Age					
10–19	1	1	0	0	2
20–29	3	3	10	6	22
30–39	8	3	7	5	23
40–49	4	7	12	4	27
50–59	8	8	7	2	25
60–69	0	1	0	0	1
Manner of Death					
Natural	18	9	6	0	33
Accident	5	11	24	17	57
Suicide	1	3	5	0	9
Unknown	0	0	1	0	1
Polysubstance Use at Death					
Yes	0	0	15	9	24
No	24	23	21	8	76
Chronic Health Condition					
Yes	19	16	22	7	64
No	5	7	14	10	36
Hepatitis B+	0	0	2	2	4
Hepatitis C+*	0	1	10	9	20
Mental Health Disorder					
Yes	8	9	17	8	42
No	16	14	19	9	58
Incarceration*					
In last 12 months	0	2	5	5	12
>1 year ago	0	1	5	4	10
No	24	20	26	8	78
LGBTQIA+*					
Yes	0	0	0	2	2
No	24	23	36	15	98
Tobacco Use					
Current*	9	14	30	15	68
Past	5	0	3	0	8

be considered in light of various confounding indirect effects of opioid use including physical activity regimes, caloric intake, hormonal factors, communicable disease through needle sharing, and length of time and severity of drug abuse (Karinen 2009; Clemens et al. 2007; Spalding 2006). For example, chronic alcohol use disrupts bone and mineral metabolism, and has been well-established to have deleterious effects on bone fragility and fracture risk (Turner 2000; Michael and Bengtson 2016). Histological evidence for decreased bone formation is supported by consistent clinical findings of reduced osteocalcin, a biochemical marker of bone formation (González-Reimers 2015; Turner 2000). Further forensic anthropological work has shown that drug abuse can further impact the products of bone remodeling (e.g., osteonal systems, Haversian canal diameter) using traditional bright-field microscopy (Karinen 2009). With the increase in opioid use and overdose throughout the COVID-19 pandemic (Center for Disease Control and Prevention 2021), it is critical that further research be conducted to delve into the mechanisms underlying opioid-induced bone pathology, how long deleterious effects last once opioid use has ceased, and the prolonged impact on the bone remodeling process that ultimately impacts bone morphology both microscopically and macroscopically.

The following sections will: 1) describe how opioid abuse may affect forensic anthropological analyses and subsequent human identification efforts, with a specific focus on age-at-death, and 2) highlight case studies from modern decedents with reported or suspected opioid abuse and associated gross skeletal irregularities.

Clinical Descriptors of Opioid-induced Bone Pathology

Forensic anthropologists often encounter OODs in their casework (Love et al. 2018; Sorg 2010; Sorg and Greenwald 2003), but data concerning how opioids affect their scientific methodologies is considerably lacking. In fact, although there is anecdotal evidence of opioid-induced bone changes in forensic casework, no published literature on the subject currently exists. Recent work, however, demonstrated that chronic alcohol abuse causes increased macroscopic bone porosity and an older gross appearance while reducing microscopic age predictions (Michael and Bengtson 2016).

In the clinical literature, chronic opioid exposure has been shown to induce osteoporotic-like effects and increase risk of bone fracture in documented users. There are three primary hypotheses that may explain the increased risk of bone fracture associated with opioid analgesics that impact both public health and interpretation of skeletal age-at-death indicators: 1) reduced bone mass caused by the inhibition of osteoblastic activity, 2) an increased risk of falls caused by sedation and/or dizziness, and 3) chronic opioid-induced hypogonadism (Brennan 2013; Coluzzi et al. 2015; Mattia, Di Bussolo, and Coluzzi 2012; Vestergaard, Rejnmark, and Mosekilde 2006). Opioid inhibition of osteoblast receptors results in lowered rates of bone formation and decreased bone mineral density (Mattia, Di Bussolo, and Coluzzi 2012). Opioid use also increases the risk of falls due to their sedative effects and the disruption of areas of the brain responsible for balance (Vestergaard, Rejnmark, and Mosekilde 2006). Opioids can further inhibit the release of luteinizing hormone (LH), follicle-stimulating hormone (FSH), and gonadotropin-releasing hormone (GnRH) in the pituitary gland (Boshra 2011). The lack of LH and GnRH limits the levels of androgens and estrogen, causing hypogonadism and disrupting menstrual cycles (Brennan 2013; Boshra 2011). Lastly, in a forensic context, violence-related bone trauma may be encountered that has been exacerbated by chronic opioid use and associated bone fragility. These clinically less visible and potentially adverse side effects remain understudied and underdiagnosed. Consequently, opioid-abuse comorbidities such as osteoporosis may be overlooked in clinical and autopsy contexts, leaving this source of skeletal trauma undiagnosed. In a field that requires methods that are accurate, precise, and have low error rates, such a knowledge gap may prevent the identification of unidentified human remains and accurate assessment of skeletal trauma.

Age-at-Death Estimation

Skeletal analyses can be approached at various hierarchical levels from the macroscopic to the histological. Bone's mineralized structure, combined with the products of cellular activity, becomes encrypted in the bone tissue allowing for the quantification of age-related changes to bone microarchitecture (Ahlqvist and Damsten 1969; Cho et al. 2002; Frost 1983; Kerley 1965; Kerley and Ubelaker 1978; Stout 1986; Stout and Gehlert 1982; Thompson 1979). Bone histological research within forensic anthropology has traditionally focused on the ability to accurately estimate age-at-death (Ahlqvist and Damsten 1969; Bouvier and Ubelaker 1977; Cho et al. 2002; Crowder 2005; Ericksen 1991; Kerley 1965; Pfeiffer 1992; Singh and Gunberg 1970; Stout 1986; Stout and Gehlert 1982; Stout and Paine 1992; Thompson 1979; Goliath, Stewart, and Stout 2016; Hauser et al. 1980; Maat et al. 2006; Yoshino et al. 1994; Kim et al. 2007; Pavón, Cucina, and Tiesler 2010; Lee et al. 2014; Streeter 2012; 2010), and differentiate nonhuman from human bone (Dominguez and Crowder 2012; Hillier and Bell 2007; Mulhern and Ubelaker 2012; Mulhern and Ubelaker 2001; 2003; Crescimanno and Stout 2012). Recent research has further emphasized method improvement and validation (Crowder 2005; Lagacé et al. 2019; Maggio and Franklin 2019;

Milenkovic et al. 2013; Kranioti et al. 2020; García-Donas et al. 2021), increasing accuracy and precision of current histological techniques (Crowder 2005; Crowder et al. 2022), and the error generated in applying such methods (Christensen et al. 2014; Christensen and Crowder 2009).

Current research offers an incomplete picture of the extent that advancing age explains the variability in histological structures used in microscopic methods, and further information is needed regarding descriptors of histological parameters from diverse populations. For example, investigating the influences of intrinsic life history variables such as biomechanical stressors, drug and alcohol use, disease, trauma, diet and nutrition, and hormones (e.g., vitamin D, estrogen) (Crowder 2005; Robling and Stout 2008; Ott et al. 2002; Pfeiffer et al. 2016; Beresheim et al. 2018) provide avenues for future research as their influences are not fully understood. Previous studies have shown that pathological conditions can affect bone remodeling and therefore age estimations (Karinen 2009; Paine and Brenton 2006; Cook, Molto, and Anderson 1988; Wu et al. 1970). Work by Karinen (2009) revealed that individuals who abuse methamphetamine were more likely to have their age underestimated when evaluated using histological criteria. The author found that known users were under-aged an average of 11.57 years compared to non-users (Karinen 2009). The recognition that low osteon counts are associated with substance abuse has serious implications for anthropologists attempting to employ age-at-death analyses based on the products of bone remodeling. This is an example of how chronic substance use induces accelerated bone resorption, destroying or distorting the remodeling products required for accurate age-at-death estimation. Further evidence of microstructural sources of inaccurate age-at-death estimates in opioid users include histologic variables such as osteon population density (OPD) which may be impacted when accelerated remodeling fully obscures older osteons and OPD reaches an asymptote that prevents older-age estimation (Pfeiffer 1992; Cho et al. 2002; Frost 1987; Stout, Porro, and Perotti 1996; Walker, Lovejoy, and Meindl 1994; Crowder and Pfeiffer 2010). Increased cortical porosity will further remove osteons and lower OPD, leading to the reporting of underestimated age-at-death (Pfeiffer 1992; Pfeiffer, Lazenby, and Chiang 1995). Endocortical porosity can further erode cortical area, thus increasing OPD and overestimating age-at-death (Pfeiffer et al. 2016). Reduced cortical areas are further less heterogeneous and increase sampling error (Frost 1969; Wu et al. 1970). Recent variables employed in forensic bone histological analyses including osteon area and osteon circularity may also be impacted due to either a reduced or increased response to higher mechanical strain on fragile bone (Hennig et al. 2015; Dominguez and Agnew 2016; Abbott, Trinkaus, and Burr 1996; van Oers et al. 2008; Keenan, Mears, and Skedros 2017). Further, osteon area may be reduced by the preferential removal of large osteons close to the OPD asymptote (Seeman 2013), and slight variations in osteon perimeter may cause significant variations in osteon circularity (Hennig et al. 2015; Lagacé et al. 2019; Maggio and Franklin 2019; Goliath, Stewart, and Stout 2016; Maggiano, Maggiano, and Cooper 2021).

Coupling bone histological outcomes with 3D imaging data, however, is providing a more intricate picture of bone biology and the impact of pathological conditions. Recent bone tissue research is expanding to include alternative 3D techniques (e.g., micro-CT, synchrotron micro-CT) that consider virtual histologic indicators of age, bone quality, and fragility to further explore the intrinsic properties of bone.

MICROSCOPIC EVIDENCE OF OPIOID-INDUCED BONE PATHOLOGY DETECTED VIA HIGH-RESOLUTION IMAGING

Experiments in the Andronowski Lab evaluated human rib and femoral bone microarchitecture from known heroin and fentanyl users and yielded compelling results consistent with the clinical literature (Andronowski, Davis, and Cole 2020). These skeletal sites were chosen as they are commonly used for bone histology research in biological anthropology (Frost 1969; Sedlin, Frost, and Villanueva 1963). The sixth rib, for example, has become a comprehensive quantitative standard for normal bone dynamics due to its rapid turnover and relatively invariable biomechanical environment among individuals (Tommerup et al. 2009). Rib specimens from documented opioid users and controls were surgically obtained through a collaboration with an American organ donation non-profit organization. Human anterior femoral specimens were procured from bone blocks of identified individuals with documented opioid use history and controls from a modern autopsy sample. Specimens were prepared for Synchrotron Radiation micro-Computed Tomography (SRμCT) imaging using a coring technique uniquely adapted for bone (Andronowski, Davis, and Holyoke 2020).

Proof-of-principle SRμCT experiments were conducted on anterior femoral bone microarchitecture on the BioMedical Imaging and Therapy Bend Magnet (BMIT-BM) beamline at the Canadian Light Source (CLS) national synchrotron facility (Wysokinski et al. 2015), equipped with a white beam microscope and a 5x objective lens. The experimental parameters included an exposure time of 30–35 ms, pixel size of 1.44 μm, 2-mm aluminum filter, 180° scan rotation, and a sample-to-detector distance of 5 cm. Each dataset comprised 2,500 tomographic images equating to a height of 3.084 mm.

Anterior femoral specimens included cores from known female heroin users (ages 24, 25, and 27 years old) and young female non-users (ages 21,

22, 23 years old) and elderly non-users (90 and 93 years old). Mid-shaft sixth rib micro-CT (μCT) scans were age-matched for known female opioid users (ages 24, 25, and 27 years old), a young female non-user (aged 21), and elderly female non-users (90, 93 years old). As per parameter definitions outlined by (Cooper et al. 2003), variables measured for cortical porosity included: percent porosity (Ct. Po, %), canal surface density (1/μm), pore connectivity density (1/mm³), pore density (1/mm³), mean and standard deviation of pore thickness (μm), and mean and standard deviation of pore separation (μm). Except for pore thickness and separation, these aggregate measurements were calculated as percentages of the Volume of Interest (VOI). The variables evaluated for osteocyte lacunae included: percent lacunar volume (Lc.V, %) and surface density (1/μm), lacunar population density (1/mm³), and mean/standard deviation of lacunar thickness (μm).

Datasets were reconstructed as image stacks of 32-bit grayscale TIFF slices via ufo-kit software (Vogelgesang et al. 2016). To extract and separate vascular canals and osteocyte lacunae from the reconstructions, a custom image processing workflow was designed for the ImageJ distribution FIJI (v. 1.53c, NIH) (Schindelin et al. 2012) and software packages DataViewer and CTAnalyser (v. 1.18.4.0, Bruker, Kontich, Belgium). Our image processing workflow included the following steps: 1) 3D orientation (DataViewer), 2) 2D pore and lacunar extraction (FIJI), 3) 3D vascular canal and lacunar differentiation (CT-Analyser), 4) 2D artifact removal (FIJI), 5) manual inspection (FIJI), and 6) 3D morphometry (CT-Analyser).

Our proof-of-principle results indicated that chronic opioid use induces osteoporotic-like effects and increased fracture risk in prolonged analgesic users that is consistent with the clinical literature (Hsu, Lin, and Kao 2019; Vestergaard, Rejnmark, and Mosekilde 2006; Boshra 2011). In the anterior femur, percent porosity of young drug users (4.32%–36.94%) and mean vascular pore thickness (54.34–354.69 μm) considerably exceeded young non-users (3.57%–6.84%; 50.03–68.94 μm; figure 11.1; table 11.2) and was more comparable to elderly non-users (18.03–18.18%; 143.07–239.29 μm). Osteocyte lacunar density (21,558–28,217 lacunae/mm³) and lacunar thickness (3.84–3.91 μm) of young drug users was decreased compared to young non-users (25,472–30,640 lacunae/mm³; 3.94–4.21 μm) and was more comparable to elderly non-users (18,838–21,058 lacunae/mm³; 3.73–3.88 μm; table 11.3). In young drug users, a decrease in osteocyte population density and lacunar thickness indicates further disruption to the osteocyte network. Such dysregulation of cellular activity will increase bone fragility and fracture risk, and makes prolonged opioid use an additional risk factor for early-onset osteoporosis.

In the rib, percent porosity of two out of three young drug users (4.17–6.31%) exceeded the young non-user (4.31%) and was more comparable

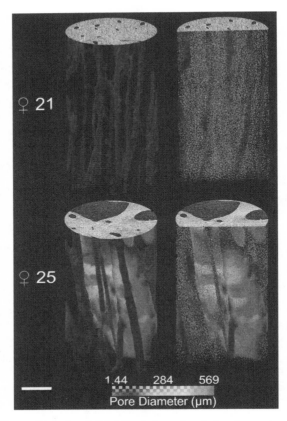

Figure 11.1   Three-dimensional SRμCT renders of anterior femoral cores, with a 2D slice demonstrating a single cross-section, from a healthy 21-year-old female and a 25-year-old female who was a known opioid user. These data sets were gathered on the BMIT-BM beamline at the Canadian Light Source. Osteocyte lacunae are visualized in gold. The color map denotes the diameter of vascular canals from 1.44 – 569 μm. Note the increased canal diameters in the known opioid user. Please refer to the eBook for the color version of Figure 11.1. Scale bar is 400 μm. Image courtesy of JM Andronowski.

to elderly non-users (7.36–16.71%; table 11.2). The ribs of both drug users and elderly non-users further displayed elevated cortical pore density and pore connectivity density (figure 11.2; table 11.2). One twenty-four-year-old drug user showed these patterns of bone loss in the rib, but not the matched anterior femur. Despite this, unusually high pore density and pore connectivity were observed in the femur, suggesting the formation of new pore systems. Such systems may converge into the large and exaggerated pores that were observed in the other drug users and could represent an example of early cellular responses to chronic drug use.

Table 11.2 Femoral and Rib Cortical Pore Morphometry

Age	Sex	Drug Status	Bone	Percent Porosity (%)	Canal Surface Density (1/μm)	Pore Conn. Density (1/mm³)	Pore Density (1/mm³)	Mean Pore Thickness (μm)	St. Dev. Pore Thickness (μm)	Mean Pore Separation (μm)	St. Dev. Pore Separation (μm)
21	F	Non-user	Femur	4.31	0.0034	10	4.11	50.03	17.11	307.56	79.04
22	F	Non-user	Femur	6.84	0.0039	10	2.36	68.94	19.07	320.39	88.91
23	F	Non-user	Femur	3.57	0.0026	10	3.88	57.67	20.45	376.70	91.56
24	F	User	Femur	4.32	0.0035	20	7.95	54.34	18.10	345.94	99.19
25	F	User	Femur	36.94	0.0061	10	2.99	354.69	174.15	278.08	105.59
27	F	User	Femur	9.81	0.0049	10	3.52	96.91	52.97	285.07	79.94
90	F	Non-user	Femur	18.18	0.0059	20	4.58	239.29	163.24	233.66	66.42
93	F	Non-user	Femur	18.03	0.0072	30	2.56	143.07	84.53	228.73	67.45
21	F	Non-user	Rib	4.17	0.0026	5814	6.54	123.84	99.53	391.91	119.90
24	F	User	Rib	6.31	0.0040	9692	17.38	99.72	79.98	390.32	121.62
25	F	User	Rib	7.37	0.0039	13771	14.53	130.71	87.47	344.83	115.94
27	F	User	Rib	3.81	0.0023	3619	4.56	123.68	89.88	319.26	103.81
90	F	Non-user	Rib	7.36	0.0055	45339	22.24	87.95	71.54	221.09	76.97
94	F	Non-user	Rib	16.71	0.0096	68368	34.09	116.01	98.50	188.10	70.08

All values adjusted for core volume

Table 11.3 Femoral Core Osteocyte Morphometry

Age	Sex	Drug Status	Percent Lacunar Volume (%)	Lacunar Surface Density (1/μm)	Lacunar Population Density (1/mm³)	Mean Lacunar Thickness (μm)	St. Dev. Lacunar Thickness (μm)
21	F	Non-user	0.99	0.0098	30640	4.21	1.48
22	F	Non-user	0.58	0.0066	29396	3.94	1.41
23	F	Non-user	0.69	0.0071	25472	4.07	1.44
24	F	User	0.77	0.0081	28217	3.91	1.40
25	F	User	0.62	0.0065	22378	3.94	1.40
27	F	User	0.66	0.0068	21558	3.84	1.42
90	F	Non-user	0.47	0.0052	21058	3.88	1.40
93	F	Non-user	0.50	0.0054	18838	3.73	1.34

All values adjusted for cortical volume (core volume – pore volume)

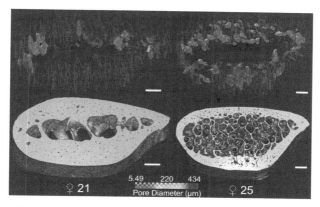

Figure 11.2 **Three-dimensional μCT renders of mid-shaft sixth ribs from a 25-year-old female who was a known opioid user and a healthy 21-year-old female.** The color map denotes vascular canal diameters of 5.49–434 μm. High pore density and connectivity, and increased porosity are evident in the opioid user. Please refer to the eBook for the color version of Figure 11.2. Scale bar is 1 mm. Image courtesy of JM Andronowski.

Our preliminary results suggested that chronic opioid use mimics age-associated bone loss, including increased cortical bone porosity, vascular pore thickness, and decreased pore separation (i.e., distance between pores). It is essential to note, however, that describing suspected opioid-related bone pathology is complex and concrete conclusions cannot be drawn from our small experimental sample. Thus, it is critical that we continue to collect and evaluate bone tissue specimens from a larger and more diverse group of known opioid users and controls. Bone tissue procurement for this project remains underway with an American organ procurement non-profit organization. Live animal experiments in the Andronowski Lab are further ongoing that seek to decipher the effects of chronic opioid exposure on bone remodeling without confounding physiological factors.

MACROSCOPIC INDICATORS OF OPIOID-INDUCED BONE PATHOLOGY: CASE STUDIES

As demonstrated above, the dynamics of bone maintenance are complex and critical to adult bone health. To offer further evidence related to drug-induced bone pathology, three case studies from the Mercyhurst Forensic Anthropology Laboratory (M-FAL) at Mercyhurst University, Erie, Pennsylvania with reported or suspected drug use were analyzed for macroscopic skeletal irregularities (table 11.4). Each decedent was a young European male; their identities were confirmed through DNA analysis of the skeletal remains. It is highly uncommon, however, to evaluate skeletal material and/or any remaining soft tissues for traces of narcotics. This limits the drug-related patient history and associated forensic evidence to informational interviews with family and/or law enforcement. Media reports following the positive identification of a decedent may include additional information from the next-of-kin or individuals in the community. Inaccurate, non-specific, and incomplete data regarding a decedent's drug-use history, however, may prevent beneficial patterns or conclusions from being detected through forensic casework. Standard toxicological analysis of skeletal remains and thorough drug use histories conducted by forensic laboratory personnel and law enforcement may alleviate these issues.

Skeletal pathological findings suspected to be linked to decedents' substance abuse history are explored here with the goal of highlighting the paucity of data concerning drug-related skeletal changes and their potential impact on macroscopic forensic anthropological analyses. Macroscopic observations of decedents A, B, and C revealed a range of porosity impacting various skeletal elements from each individual. For example, "pitting" defects, or regions of hypothesized increased bone resorption uncharacteristic of younger individuals, were consistently observed. In Decedent A, porosity was concentrated in the cranium, particularly the maxillae. Decedent B exhibited significant porosity across most recovered skeletal elements, most notably in the vertebrae, scapulae, proximal femora, and clavicles (figure 11.3). Decedent C presented with significant porosity of both clavicles that was concentrated along the inferior surface near the medial ends.

Of particular significance, all three decedents were observed to possess regions of extreme resorption and pitting along the inferior surface of the medial aspect of both clavicles (figure 11.4). The clavicle is the first bone

Table 11.4   Summary of Decedent Demographics and Skeletal Abnormalities noted during Forensic Anthropological Analyses by the Mercyhurst Forensic Anthropology Laboratory

Decedent	Sex	Age	Ancestry	Drug Use	Skeletal Pathology Observed
A	M	32	European	Reported long-term user	Porosity of the maxilla, overall poor dental health, resorptive defects on medial clavicles
B	M	19	European	Suspected user	Very porous skeleton overall, large resorptive defects on inferior medial clavicles, marked degeneration of vertebral bodies
C	M	19	European	Suspected user	Large resorptive defects on medial clavicles

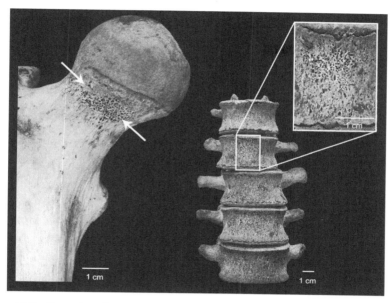

Figure 11.3   Examples of porosity and "pitting" located on anterior proximal surface of right femur (left) and anterior bodies of lumbar vertebrae (right) of decedent B. Porosity on the femoral neck is indicated by white arrows. One area of porosity on the second lumbar vertebra is indicated by the white box and magnified in the corresponding inset. Images courtesy of Dennis Dirkmaat.

to commence ossification and does so through endochondral and intramem-branous ossification with two primary centers of ossification (Cunningham, Scheuer, and Black 2016). It is also the last bone to complete ossification, typically in early adulthood, approximately between ages twenty and twenty-five (Cunningham, Scheuer, and Black 2016; Calixto et al. 2015). The medial epiphysis begins as a fragment of bone by ages sixteen to twenty-one and develops to cover the medial clavicular surface between ages twenty-four and twenty-nine (Cunningham, Scheuer, and Black 2016; Langley-Shirley and Jantz 2010). Complete epiphyseal fusion of the medial clavicle is not complete until approximately age twenty-two to thirty (Cunningham, Scheuer, and Black 2016; Langley-Shirley and Jantz 2010). Histological analysis of the postnatal development of the clavicle illustrates that the secondary ossification center of the medial clavicle may be present at the age of nineteen without evidence of growth and/or closure (Calixto et al. 2015). Research has further demonstrated a negative relationship between analgesics and opioids and pri-mary bone formation in fracture healing, but causality and mechanisms remain elusive (Richards, Graf, and Mashru 2017; Gerner and O'Connor 2008). Each decedent in our case study was known or suspected to have used drugs (e.g.,

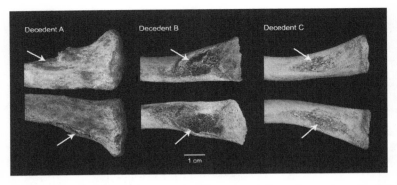

Figure 11.4   Irregularities with resorptive-like presentation observed on the inferior aspect of the left (above) and right (below) medial clavicles of decedents A, B, and C are indicated by white arrows. Images courtesy of Dennis Dirkmaat.

opioids) before or during the period of medial clavicle epiphyseal fusion, but the lack of data regarding the effects of opioids on primary bone formation precludes any conclusions about the resorptive-like defects observed in each case.

Future Directions

The anthropological assessment of such cases leaves us with many queries regarding the accuracy and bias of our current macroscopic and histologic methods and their efficacy when applied to suspected drug users. For example, 1) what are the identification implications for decedents with fragmentary or partial remains? and 2) how does drug use physiologically impact macroscopic and histological skeletal age-at-death indicators? Thus, we argue a call-to-action for expanding our knowledge, both clinically and anthropologically, regarding disruptions to the bone remodeling process by aiming to address the impacts of prolonged opioid use on bone turnover, and associated confounding indirect effects (e.g., caloric intake, hormonal factors, physical activity regimens, infectious disease processes). To begin addressing this goal, live animal studies in the Andronowski Lab employing a rabbit model system will further decipher the effects of chronic opioid use on bone remodeling without confounding physiological factors.

The implications moving forward are critical given that many sets of skeletal remains examined by forensic anthropologists come from marginalized backgrounds with substance-abuse issues and overall poor health. As such, current macroscopic and histologic aging methods developed on healthy cases may not be accurate for the analysis of such individuals. Until it is clear how gross and histological parameters are impacted by various physiological indicators and contribute to a successful age estimate, it will be difficult to hone such methods toward greater precision. The exploration of additional morphological features, such as the development of a clavicle resorption scoring protocol, may offer positive developments in the field.

CONCLUSION

The work presented here is culturally relevant and highly important as the misuse and addiction to prescription opioids (and illicit synthetic opioids) continues to be a serious public health crisis. As the opioid epidemic persists, it is critical that further research efforts be undertaken to understand the impacts on bone metabolism, macroscopic and microscopic skeletal age-at-death indicators, and social factors that may contribute to the persistence of unidentified substance users in forensic anthropological casework.

Forensic anthropologists are specifically challenged by the confounding effects of opioid use on age-at-death estimation and fracture assessment from bone tissue. Given all of the unknowns and scarce data available, it is clear that a considerable opportunity exists to characterize human opioid-related bone pathology, both on the macro- and micro-scales. Ongoing research in the Andronowski Lab will offer broader applications as we work toward identifying risk factors for opioid-induced osteoporotic bone fragility and fracture risk, which have both clinical and forensic applications. These new data will allow forensic anthropologists to better understand how chronic drug use can contribute to alterations of skeletal indicators commonly used in age-at-death estimation and beyond.

NOTE

1. Acknowledgments: Research described in this paper was performed at the BMIT facility at the Canadian Light Source, which is supported by the Canada Foundation for Innovation, Natural Sciences and Engineering Research Council of Canada, the University of Saskatchewan, the Government of Saskatchewan, Western Economic Diversification Canada, the National Research Council Canada, and the Canadian Institutes of Health Research. The authors sincerely thank Lifebanc Ohio's Surgical Organ and Recovery Coordinator (SORC) team headed by Tiffany Ake for assisting with bone specimen procurement. We also wish to thank our donors for their selfless gifts to research and science education—without whom this important research would not be possible.

REFERENCES

Abbott, Stephen, Erik Trinkaus, and David B. Burr. 1996. "Dynamic Bone Remodeling in Later Pleistocene Fossil Hominids." *American Journal of Physical Anthropology* 99 (4): 585–601. https://doi.org/10.1002/(SICI)1096-8644(199604)99:4<585::AID-AJPA5>3.0.CO;2-T.

Ahlqvist, J., and O. Damsten. 1969. "A Modification of Kerley's Method for the Microscopic Determination of Age in Human Bone." *Journal of Forensic Sciences* 14 (2): 205–12.

Ahmad, Farida B., Lauren M. Rossen, and Paul Sutton. 2021. "Provisional Drug Overdose Death Counts." National Center for Health Statistics. https://www.cdc.gov/nchs/nvss/vsrr/drug-overdose-data.htm.

Alexander, Monica J., Mathew V. Kiang, and Magali Barbieri. 2018. "Trends in Black and White Opioid Mortality in the United States, 1979–2015." *Epidemiology (Cambridge, Mass.)* 29 (5): 707–15. https://doi.org/10.1097/EDE.0000000000000858.

Al-Tayyib, Alia, Stephen Koester, Sig Langegger, and Lisa Raville. 2017. "Heroin and Methamphetamine Injection: An Emerging Drug Use Pattern." *Substance Use & Misuse* 52 (8): 1051–58. https://doi.org/10.1080/10826084.2016.1271432.

Andronowski, Janna M., and Randi M. Depp. 2022. "Assessing Opioid Exposure and Opioid Overdose Deaths in Skeletal Casework Through Collaboration with Organ Procurement Organizations." *Proceedings of the American Academy of Forensic Sciences* 48.

Andronowski, Janna M., Reed A. Davis, and Caleb W. Holyoke. 2020. "A Sectioning, Coring, and Image Processing Guide for High-Throughput Cortical Bone Sample Procurement and Analysis for Synchrotron Micro-CT." *Journal of Visualized Experiments*, no. 160 (June): e61081. https://doi.org/10.3791/61081.

Andronowski, Janna M., Reed A. Davis, and Mary E. Cole. 2020. "Investigating the Impact of Opioid Abuse on Intracortical Porosity and Bone Cellular Density: A Synchrotron-Radiation Micro-Computed Tomography Approach." *Proceedings of the American Academy of Forensic Sciences* 102.

Archer, Melanie S., Richard B. Bassed, Christopher A. Briggs, and Matthew J. Lynch. 2005. "Social Isolation and Delayed Discovery of Bodies in Houses: The Value of Forensic Pathology, Anthropology, Odontology and Entomology in the Medico-Legal Investigation." *Forensic Science International* 151 (2–3): 259–65. https://doi.org/10.1016/j.forsciint.2005.02.016.

Arias, Elizabeth, Heron, Melonie P., National Center for Health Statistics, Hakes, Jahn K., and National Longitudinal Mortality Study. 2016. "The Validity of Race and Hispanic-origin Reporting on Death Certificates in the United States: An Update." *Vital and Health Statistics* 2, no. 172: 1–21. https://stacks.cdc.gov/view/cdc/45533

Belzak, Lisa, and Jessica Halverson. 2018. "Evidence Synthesis - The Opioid Crisis in Canada: A National Perspective." *Health Promotion and Chronic Disease Prevention in Canada* 38 (6): 224–33. https://doi.org/10.24095/hpcdp.38.6.02.

Beresheim, Amy C., Susan K. Pfeiffer, Marc D. Grynpas, and Amanda Alblas. 2018. "Sex-Specific Patterns in Cortical and Trabecular Bone Microstructure in the Kirsten Skeletal Collection, South Africa." *American Journal of Human Biology* 30 (3): e23108. https://doi.org/10.1002/ajhb.23108.

Binswanger, Ingrid A., Marc F. Stern, Richard A. Deyo, Patrick J. Heagerty, Allen Cheadle, Joann G. Elmore, and Thomas D. Koepsell. 2007. "Release from Prison — A High Risk of Death for Former Inmates." *New England Journal of Medicine* 356 (2): 157–65. https://doi.org/10.1056/NEJMsa064115.

Boshra, Vivian. 2011. "Evaluation of Osteoporosis Risk Associated with Chronic Use of Morphine, Fentanyl and Tramadol in Adult Female Rats." *Current Drug Safety* 6 (3): 159–63. https://doi.org/10.2174/157488611797579267.

Bouvier, Marianne, and Douglas H. Ubelaker. 1977. "A Comparison of Two Methods for the Microscopic Determination of Age at Death." *American Journal of Physical Anthropology* 46 (3): 391–94. https://doi.org/10.1002/ajpa.1330460303.

Brennan, Michael J. 2013. "The Effect of Opioid Therapy on Endocrine Function." *The American Journal of Medicine*, Opioids in Chronic Pain: Evolving Best Practice Strategies 126 (3, Supplement 1): S12–18. https://doi.org/10.1016/j.amjmed.2012.12.001.

Brinkley-Rubinstein, Lauren, Alexandria Macmadu, Brandon D. L. Marshall, Andrew Heise, Shabbar I. Ranapurwala, Josiah D. Rich, and Traci C. Green. 2018. "Risk of Fentanyl-Involved Overdose among Those with Past Year Incarceration: Findings from a Recent Outbreak in 2014 and 2015." *Drug and Alcohol Dependence* 185 (April): 189–91. https://doi.org/10.1016/j.drugalcdep.2017.12.014.

Calixto, Luis Fernando, Rodrigo Penagos, Lina Jaramillo, María Lucia Guitierrez, and Diego Garzón-Alvarado. 2015. "A Histological Study of Postnatal Development of Clavicle Articular Ends." *Universitas Scientiarum* 20 (3): 361. https://doi.org/10.11144/Javeriana.SC20-3.ahso.

Center for Disease Control and Prevention. 2020. "Understanding the Epidemic." Opioid Overdose. March 19, 2020. https://www.cdc.gov/drugoverdose/epidemic/index.html.

———. 2021. "Drug Overdose Deaths." Opioid Overdose: Drug Overdose Deaths. 2021. https://www.cdc.gov/drugoverdose/data/statedeaths.html.

Cheng, Melissa, Brian Sauer, Erin Johnson, Christina Porucznik, and Kurt Hegmann. 2013. "Comparison of Opioid-Related Deaths by Work-Related Injury." *American Journal of Industrial Medicine* 56 (3): 308–16. https://doi.org/10.1002/ajim.22138.

Cho, Helen, Sam D. Stout, Richard W. Madsen, and Margaret A. Streeter. 2002. "Population-Specific Histological Age-Estimating Method: A Model for Known African-American and European-American Skeletal Remains." *Journal of Forensic Sciences* 47 (1): 12–18. http://doi.org/10.1520/JFS15199J.

Christensen, Angi M., and Christian M. Crowder. 2009. "Evidentiary Standards for Forensic Anthropology." *Journal of Forensic Sciences* 54 (6): 1211–16. https://doi.org/10.1111/j.1556-4029.2009.01176.x.

Christensen, Angi M., Christian M. Crowder, Stephen D. Ousley, and Max M. Houck. 2014. "Error and Its Meaning in Forensic Science." *Journal of Forensic Sciences* 59 (1): 123–26. https://doi.org/10.1111/1556-4029.12275.

Clemens, Kelly J., Iain S. McGregor, Glenn E. Hunt, and Jennifer L. Cornish. 2007. "MDMA, Methamphetamine and Their Combination: Possible Lessons for Party Drug Users from Recent Preclinical Research." *Drug and Alcohol Review* 26 (1): 9–15. https://doi.org/10.1080/09595230601036945.

Coluzzi, Flaminia, Joe Pergolizzi, Robert B. Raffa, and Consalvo Mattia. 2015. "The Unsolved Case of 'Bone-Impairing Analgesics': The Endocrine Effects of Opioids on Bone Metabolism." *Therapeutics and Clinical Risk Management* 11: 515–23. https://doi.org/10.2147/TCRM.S79409.

Cook, Megan, El Molto, and Colin Anderson. 1988. "Possible Case of Hyperparathyroidism in a Roman Period Skeleton from the Dakhleh Oasis, Egypt, Diagnosed Using Bone Histomorphometry." *American Journal of Physical Anthropology* 75 (1): 23–30. https://doi.org/10.1002/ajpa.1330750104.

Cooper, David M. L., Andrei L. Turinsky, Christoph W. Sensen, and Benedikt Hallgrímsson. 2003. "Quantitative 3D Analysis of the Canal Network in Cortical Bone by Micro-Computed Tomography." *Anatomical Record. Part B, New Anatomist* 274 (1): 169–79. https://doi.org/10.1002/ar.b.10024.

Crescimanno, Annamaria, and Sam D. Stout. 2012. "Differentiating Fragmented Human and Nonhuman Long Bone Using Osteon Circularity." *Journal of Forensic Sciences* 57 (2): 287–94. https://doi.org/10.1111/j.1556-4029.2011.01973.x.

Crowder, Christian M. 2005. "Evaluating the Use of Quantitative Bone Histology to Estimate Adult Age at Death." Ph.D. Dissertation, Toronto, Canada: University of Toronto.

Crowder, Christian M., and Susan K. Pfeiffer. 2010. "The Application of Cortical Bone Histomorphometry to Estimate Age-at-Death." In *Age Estimation of the Human Skeleton*, edited by Krista E. Latham and Michael Finnegan, 193–215. Springfield, OL: Charles C. Thomas.

Crowder, Christian M., Victoria M. Dominguez, Jarred Heinrich, Deborrah Pinto, and Sophia Mavroudas. 2022. "Analysis of Histomorphometric Variables: Proposal and Validation of Osteon Definitions." *Journal of Forensic Sciences* 67 (1): 80–91. https://doi.org/10.1111/1556-4029.14949.

Cunningham, Craig, Louise Scheuer, and Sue Black. 2016. *Developmental Juvenile Osteology*. Academic Press. https://www.elsevier.com/books/developmental-juvenile-osteology/cunningham/978-0-12-382106-5.

Cuyahoga County Opiate Task Force. 2018. "Opiate Collaborative – The Epidemic." The Epidemic. April 10, 2018. http://opiatecollaborative.cuyahogacounty.us/en-US/The-Epidemic.aspx.

Daniulaityte, Raminta, Matthew P. Juhascik, Kraig E. Strayer, Ioana E. Sizemore, Kent E. Harshbarger, Heather M. Antonides, and Robert R. Carlson. 2017. "Overdose Deaths Related to Fentanyl and Its Analogs — Ohio, January–February 2017." *MMWR. Morbidity and Mortality Weekly Report* 66 (34): 904–8. https://doi.org/10.15585/mmwr.mm6634a3.

DiGangi, Elizabeth A., and Jonathan D. Bethard. 2021. "Uncloaking a Lost Cause: Decolonizing Ancestry Estimation in the United States." *American Journal of Physical Anthropology* 175, no. 2: 422–36. https://doi.org/10.1002/ajpa.24212.

Dominguez, Victoria M., and Christian M. Crowder. 2012. "The Utility of Osteon Shape and Circularity for Differentiating Human and Non-Human Haversian Bone." *American Journal of Physical Anthropology* 149 (1): 84–91. https://doi.org /10.1002/ajpa.22097.

Dominguez, Victoria M., and Amanda M. Agnew. 2016. "Examination of Factors Potentially Influencing Osteon Size in the Human Rib." *Anatomical Record* 299 (3): 313–24. https://doi.org/10.1002/ar.23305.

Draanen, Jenna V., Christie Tsang, Sanjana Mitra, Mohammad Karamouzian, and Lindsey Richardson. 2020. "Socioeconomic Marginalization and Opioid-Related Overdose: A Systematic Review." *Drug and Alcohol Dependence* 214 (September): 108127. https://doi.org/10.1016/j.drugalcdep.2020.108127.

Ericksen, Mary F. 1991. "Histologic Estimation of Age at Death Using the Anterior Cortex of the Femur." *American Journal of Physical Anthropology* 84 (2): 171–79. https://doi.org/10.1002/ajpa.1330840207.

Feng, Jing, Joseph P. Iser, and Wei Yang. 2016. "Medical Encounters for Opioid-Related Intoxications in Southern Nevada: Sociodemographic and Clinical Correlates." *BMC Health Services Research* 16 (1): 438. https://doi.org/10.1186/ s12913-016-1692-z.

Frost, Harold M. 1969. "Tetracycline-Based Histological Analysis of Bone Remodeling." *Calcified Tissue Research* 3 (1): 211–37. https://doi.org/10.1007/BF02058664.

———. 1983. "The Skeletal Intermediary Organization." *Metabolic Bone Disease & Related Research* 4 (5): 281–90. https://doi.org/10.1016/s0221 -8747(83)80001-0.

———. 1987. "The Mechanostat – a Proposed Pathogenic Mechanism of Osteoporoses and the Bone Mass Effects of Mechanical and Nonmechanical Agents." *Bone and Mineral* 2 (2): 73–85.

Furr-Holden, Debra, Adam J. Milam, Ling Wang, and Richard Sadler. 2021. "African Americans Now Outpace Whites in Opioid-Involved Overdose Deaths: A Comparison of Temporal Trends from 1999 to 2018." *Addiction* 116 (3): 677–83. https://doi.org/10.1111/add.15233.

García-Donas, Julieta G., Andrea Bonicelli, Ashley R. Scholl, Caroline Lill, Robert R. Paine, and Elena F. Kranioti. 2021. "Rib Histomorphometry: A Reliability and Validation Study with a Critical Review of Histological Techniques for Forensic Age Estimation." *Legal Medicine* 49 (March): 101827. https://doi.org/10.1016/j .legalmed.2020.101827.

Gerner, Peter, and J. Patrick O'Connor. 2008. "Impact of Analgesia on Bone Fracture Healing." *Anesthesiology* 108 (3): 349–50. https://doi.org/10.1097/ALN .0b013e318164938c.

Goliath, Jesse R., Marissa C. Stewart, and Sam D. Stout. 2016. "Variation in Osteon Histomorphometrics and Their Impact on Age-at-Death Estimation in Older Individuals." *Forensic Science International* 262 (May): 282.e1–282.e6. https://doi .org/10.1016/j.forsciint.2016.02.053.

Gomes, Tara, Mina Tadrous, Muhammad M. Mamdani, J. Michael Paterson, and David N. Juurlink. 2018. "The Burden of Opioid-Related Mortality in the United States." *JAMA Network Open* 1 (2): e180217–e180217. https://doi.org/10.1001/jamanetworkopen.2018.0217.

González-Reimers, Emilio, Geraldine Quintero-Platt, Eva Rodríguez-Rodríguez, Antonio Martínez-Riera, Julio Alvisa-Negrín, and Francisco Santolaria-Fernández. 2015. "Bone Changes in Alcoholic Liver Disease." *World Journal of Hepatology* 7 (9): 1258. https://doi.org/10.4254/wjh.v7.i9.1258.

Hasegawa, Kohei, David F. M. Brown, Yusuke Tsugawa, and Carlos A. Camargo. 2014. "Epidemiology of Emergency Department Visits for Opioid Overdose: A Population-Based Study." *Mayo Clinic Proceedings* 89 (4): 462–71. https://doi.org/10.1016/j.mayocp.2013.12.008.

Hauser, R., D. Barres, M. Durigon, and L. Derobert. 1980. "[Identification using histomorphometry of the femur and tibia]." *Acta Medicinae Legalis Et Socialis* 30 (2): 91–97.

Hedegaard, Holly, Arialdi M. Miniño, and Margaret Warner. 2020. "Drug Overdose Deaths in the United States, 1999–2018." *NCHS Data Brief*, no. 356: 8. https://www.cdc.gov/nchs/products/databriefs/db356.htm.

Hedegaard, Holly, Arialdi M. Miniño, Merianne Rose Spencer, and Margaret Warner. 2021. "Drug Overdose Deaths in the United States, 1999–2020." *NCHS Data Brief* no. 428: 8. https://www.cdc.gov/nchs/products/databriefs/db428.htm

Hennig, Cheryl C., David L. Thomas, John G. Clement, and David M. L. Cooper. 2015. "Does 3D Orientation Account for Variation in Osteon Morphology Assessed by 2D Histology?" *Journal of Anatomy* 227 (4): 497–505. https://doi.org/10.1111/joa.12357.

Hernandez, Andres, Adam J. Branscum, Jingjing Li, Neil J. MacKinnon, Ana L. Hincapie, and Diego F. Cuadros. 2020. "Epidemiological and Geospatial Profile of the Prescription Opioid Crisis in Ohio, United States." *Scientific Reports* 10 (1): 4341. https://doi.org/10.1038/s41598-020-61281-y.

Hillier, Maria L., and Lynne S. Bell. 2007. "Differentiating Human Bone from Animal Bone: A Review of Histological Methods." *Journal of Forensic Sciences* 52 (2): 249–63. https://doi.org/10.1111/j.1556-4029.2006.00368.x.

Hsu, Wen-Yu, Cheng-Li Lin, and Chia-Hung Kao. 2019. "Association between Opioid Use Disorder and Fractures: A Population-based Study." *Addiction* 114 (11): 2008–15. https://doi.org/10.1111/add.14732.

Jalali, Mohammad S., Michael Botticelli, Rachael C. Hwang, Howard K. Koh, and R. Kathryn McHugh. 2020. "The Opioid Crisis: A Contextual, Social-Ecological Framework." *Health Research Policy and Systems* 18 (1): 87. https://doi.org/10.1186/s12961-020-00596-8.

James, Keturah, and Ayana Jordan. 2018. "The Opioid Crisis in Black Communities." *Journal of Law, Medicine & Ethics* 46 (2): 404–21. https://doi.org/10.1177/1073110518782949.

Jenkins, Lindsay M., Caleb J. Banta-Green, Charles Maynard, Susan Kingston, Michael Hanrahan, Joseph O. Merrill, and Phillip O. Coffin. 2011. "Risk Factors for Nonfatal Overdose at Seattle-Area Syringe Exchanges." *Journal of Urban Health* 88 (1): 118–28. https://doi.org/10.1007/s11524-010-9525-6.

Joshi, Sujata, Thomas Weiser, and Victoria Warren-Mears. 2018. "Drug, Opioid-Involved, and Heroin-Involved Overdose Deaths Among American Indians and Alaska Natives — Washington, 1999–2015." *Morbidity and Mortality Weekly Report* 67 (50): 1384–87. https://doi.org/10.15585/mmwr.mm6750a2.

Karinen, Robert C. 2009. "Histomorphometry of the Human Rib Cortex in Methamphetamine Users." Master's Thesis, Boise State University. http://scholarworks.boisestate.edu/cgi/viewcontent.cgi?article=1076&context=td.

Keenan, Kendra E., Chad S. Mears, and John G. Skedros. 2017. "Utility of Osteon Circularity for Determining Species and Interpreting Load History in Primates and Nonprimates." *American Journal of Physical Anthropology* 162 (4): 657–81. https://doi.org/10.1002/ajpa.23154.

Kerley, Ellis R. 1965. "The Microscopic Determination of Age in Human Bone." *American Journal of Physical Anthropology* 23 (2): 149–63. https://doi.org/10.1002/ajpa.1330230215.

Kerley, Ellis R., and Douglas H. Ubelaker. 1978. "Revisions in Microscopic Method of Estimating Age at Death in Human Cortical Bone." *American Journal of Physical Anthropology* 49 (4): 545–46. https://doi.org/10.1002/ajpa.1330490414.

Kerr, Thomas, Nadia Fairbairn, Mark Tyndall, David Marsh, Kathy Li, Julio Montaner, and Evan Wood. 2007. "Predictors of Non-Fatal Overdose among a Cohort of Polysubstance-Using Injection Drug Users." *Drug and Alcohol Dependence* 87 (1): 39–45. https://doi.org/10.1016/j.drugalcdep.2006.07.009.

Kim, Yi-Suk, Deog-Im Kim, Ddae-Kyoon Park, Je-Hoon Lee, Nak-Eun Chung, Won-Tae Lee, and Seung-Ho Han. 2007. "Assessment of Histomorphological Features of the Sternal End of the Fourth Rib for Age Estimation in Koreans*." *Journal of Forensic Sciences* 52 (6): 1237–42. https://doi.org/10.1111/j.1556-4029.2007.00566.x.

Kline, David, Yuhan Pan, and Staci A. Hepler. 2021. "Spatiotemporal Trends in Opioid Overdose Deaths by Race for Counties in Ohio." *Epidemiology* 32 (2): 295–302. https://doi.org/10.1097/EDE.0000000000001299.

Kranioti, Elena F., Effrosyni Michopoulou, Konstantina Tsiminikaki, Andrea Bonicelli, Michalis Kalochristianakis, Bledar Xhemali, Robert R. Paine, and Julieta G. García-Donas. 2020. "Bone Histomorphometry of the Clavicle in a Forensic Sample from Albania." *Forensic Science International* 313 (August): 110335. https://doi.org/10.1016/j.forsciint.2020.110335.

Kreek, Mary J. 2011. "Extreme Marginalization: Addiction and Other Mental Health Disorders, Stigma, and Imprisonment." *Annals of the New York Academy of Sciences* 1231 (August): 65–72. https://doi.org/10.1111/j.1749-6632.2011.06152.x.

Lagacé, Frédérique, Emeline Verna, Pascal Adalian, Eric Baccino, and Laurent Martrille. 2019. "Testing the Accuracy of a New Histomorphometric Method for Age-at-Death Estimation." *Forensic Science International* 296 (March): 48–52. https://doi.org/10.1016/j.forsciint.2019.01.020.

Langley-Shirley, Natalie, and Richard L. Jantz. 2010. "A Bayesian Approach to Age Estimation in Modern Americans from the Clavicle." *Journal of Forensic Sciences* 55 (3): 571–83. https://doi.org/10.1111/j.1556-4029.2010.01089.x.

Lee, U-Young, Go-Un Jung, Seung-Gyu Choi, and Yi-Suk Kim. 2014. "Anthropological Age Estimation with Bone Histomorphometry from the Human Clavicle." *The Anthropologist* 17 (3): 929–36. https://doi.org/10.1080/09720073 .2014.11891509.

Love, Sara A., Jessica Lelinski, Julie Kloss, Owen Middleton, and Fred S. Apple. 2018. "Heroin-Related Deaths from the Hennepin County Medical Examiner's Office from 2004 Through 2015." *Journal of Forensic Sciences* 63 (1): 191–94. https://doi.org/10.1111/1556-4029.13511.

Lowder, Evan M., Bradley R. Ray, Philip Huynh, Alfarena Ballew, and Dennis P. Watson. 2018. "Identifying Unreported Opioid Deaths Through Toxicology Data and Vital Records Linkage: Case Study in Marion County, Indiana, 2011–2016." *American Journal of Public Health* 108 (12): 1682–87. https://doi.org/10.2105/ AJPH.2018.304683.

Maat, George J. R., Ann Maes, M. Job Aarents, and Nico J. D. Nagelkerke. 2006. "Histological Age Prediction from the Femur in a Contemporary Dutch Sample." *Journal of Forensic Sciences* 51 (2): 230–37. https://doi.org/10.1111/j.1556-4029 .2006.00062.x.

Maggiano, Isabel S., Corey M. Maggiano, and David M. L. Cooper. 2021. "Osteon Circularity and Longitudinal Morphology: Quantitative and Qualitative Three-Dimensional Perspectives on Human Haversian Systems." *Micron* 140 (January): 102955. https://doi.org/10.1016/j.micron.2020.102955.

Maggio, Ariane, and Daniel Franklin. 2019. "Histomorphometric Age Estimation from the Femoral Cortex: A Test of Three Methods in an Australian Population." *Forensic Science International* 303 (October): 109950. https://doi.org/10.1016/j .forsciint.2019.109950.

Marshall, John R., Stephen F. Gassner, Craig L. Anderson, Richelle J. Cooper, Shahram Lotfipour, and Bharath Chakravarthy. 2019. "Socioeconomic and Geographical Disparities in Prescription and Illicit Opioid-Related Overdose Deaths in Orange County, California, from 2010–2014." *Substance Abuse* 40 (1): 80–86. https://doi.org/10.1080/08897077.2018.1442899.

Mattia, Consalvo, Eleonora Di Bussolo, and Flaminia Coluzzi. 2012. "Non-Analgesic Effects of Opioids: The Interaction of Opioids with Bone and Joints." *Current Pharmaceutical Design* 18 (37): 6005–9. https://doi.org/10.2174 /138161212803582487.

Meiman, Jon, Carrie Tomasallo, and Leonard Paulozzi. 2015. "Trends and Characteristics of Heroin Overdoses in Wisconsin, 2003–2012." *Drug and Alcohol Dependence* 152 (July): 177–84. https://doi.org/10.1016/j.drugalcdep.2015.04 .002.

Michael, Amy R., and Jennifer D. Bengtson. 2016. "Chronic Alcoholism and Bone Remodeling Processes: Caveats and Considerations for the Forensic Anthropologist." *Journal of Forensic and Legal Medicine* 38 (February): 87–92. https://doi.org/10.1016/j.jflm.2015.11.022.

Milenkovic, Petar, Ksenija Djukic, Danijela Djonic, Petar Milovanovic, and Marija Djuric. 2013. "Skeletal Age Estimation Based on Medial Clavicle-a Test of the

Method Reliability." *International Journal of Legal Medicine* 127 (3): 667–76. https://doi.org/10.1007/s00414-012-0791-6.

Miller, Carl L., Keith J. Chan, Anita Palepu, Mark Tyndall, Evan Wood, Robert Hogg, and Michael V. O'Shaughnessy. 2001. "Socio-Demographic Profile and Hiv and Hepatitis C Prevalence Among Persons Who Died of a Drug Overdose." *Addiction Research & Theory* 9 (5): 459–70. https://doi.org/10.3109/16066350109141764.

Monnat, Shannon M. 2019. "The Contributions of Socioeconomic and Opioid Supply Factors to U.S. Drug Mortality Rates: Urban-Rural and within-Rural Differences." *Journal of Rural Studies* 68 (May): 319–35. https://doi.org/10.1016/j.jrurstud.2018.12.004.

Mulhern, Dawn M., and Douglas H. Ubelaker. 2001. "Differences in Osteon Banding between Human and Nonhuman Bone." *Journal of Forensic Sciences* 46 (2): 220–22. https://doi.org/10.1520/JFS14952J.

———. 2003. "Histologic Examination of Bone Development in Juvenile Chimpanzees." *American Journal of Physical Anthropology* 122 (2): 127–33. https://doi.org/10.1002/ajpa.10294.

———. 2012. "Differentiating Human from Nonhuman Bone Microstructure." In *Bone Histology: An Anthropological Perspective*, edited by Christian M. Crowder and Sam D. Stout. Boca Ranton, FL: CRC Press.

Nadpara, Pramit A., Andrew R. Joyce, E. Lenn Murrelle, Nathan W. Carroll, Norman V. Carroll, Marie Barnard, and Barbara K. Zedler. 2018. "Risk Factors for Serious Prescription Opioid-Induced Respiratory Depression or Overdose: Comparison of Commercially Insured and Veterans Health Affairs Populations." *Pain Medicine* 19 (1): 79–96. https://doi.org/10.1093/pm/pnx038.

National Institute on Drug Abuse. 2020. "Opioid Overdose Crisis." Opioid Overdose Crisis. May 27, 2020. https://www.drugabuse.gov/drug-topics/opioids/opioid-overdose-crisis.

Ochoa, Kristen C., Peter J. Davidson, Jennifer L. Evans, Judith A. Hahn, Kimberly Page-Shafer, and Andrew R. Moss. 2005. "Heroin Overdose among Young Injection Drug Users in San Francisco." *Drug and Alcohol Dependence* 80 (3): 297–302. https://doi.org/10.1016/j.drugalcdep.2005.04.012.

Ochoa, Kristen C., Judith A. Hahn, Karen H. Seal, and Andrew R. Moss. 2001. "Overdosing among Young Injection Drug Users in San Francisco." *Addictive Behaviors* 26 (3): 453–60. https://doi.org/10.1016/S0306-4603(00)00115-5.

Ødegård, Einar, Ellen J. Amundsen, Knut Boe Kielland, and Ragnar Kristoffersen. 2010. "The Contribution of Imprisonment and Release to Fatal Overdose among a Cohort of Norwegian Drug Abusers." *Addiction Research & Theory* 18 (1): 51–58. https://doi.org/10.3109/16066350902818851.

Ohio Department of Health. 2019. "Ohio Drug Overdose Data: General Findings." https://odh.ohio.gov/wps/portal/gov/odh/know-our-programs/violence-injury-pre-vention-program/media/2019+ohio+drug+overdose+report.

Ott, Susan M., Anna Oleksik, Yili Lu, Kristine Harper, and Paul Lips. 2002. "Bone Histomorphometric and Biochemical Marker Results of a 2-Year Placebo-Controlled Trial of Raloxifene in Postmenopausal Women." *Journal of Bone and Mineral Research* 17 (2): 341–48. https://doi.org/10.1359/jbmr.2002.17.2.341.

Paine, Robert R., and Barrett P. Brenton. 2006. "Dietary Health Does Affect Histological Age Assessment: An Evaluation of the Stout and Paine (1992) Age Estimation Equation Using Secondary Osteons from the Rib." *Journal of Forensic Sciences* 51 (3): 489–92. https://doi.org/10.1111/j.1556-4029.2006.00118.x.

Paulozzi, Leonard J., Joseph E. Logan, Aron J. Hall, Edna McKinstry, James A. Kaplan, and Alexander E. Crosby. 2009. "A Comparison of Drug Overdose Deaths Involving Methadone and Other Opioid Analgesics in West Virginia." *Addiction* 104 (9): 1541–48. https://doi.org/10.1111/j.1360-0443.2009.02650.x.

Pavón, Margarita Valencia, Andrea Cucina, and Vera Tiesler. 2010. "New Formulas to Estimate Age at Death in Maya Populations Using Histomorphological Changes in the Fourth Human Rib." *Journal of Forensic Sciences* 55 (2): 473–77. https://doi.org/10.1111/j.1556-4029.2009.01265.x.

Peterson, Alexis, R. Matthew Gladden, Chris Delcher, Erica Spies, Amanda Garcia-Williams, Yanning Wang, John Halpin, Jon Zibbell, Carolyn Lullo McCarty, Jolene DeFiore-Hyrmer, et al. 2016. "Increases in Fentanyl-Related Overdose Deaths — Florida and Ohio, 2013–2015." *Morbidity and Mortality Weekly Report* 65 (33): 844–49. http://dx.doi.org/10.15585/mmwr.mm6533a3.

Pfeiffer, Susan K. 1992. "Cortical Bone Age Estimates from Historically Known Adults." *Zeitschrift Fur Morphologie Und Anthropologie* 79 (1): 1–10.

Pfeiffer, Susan K., Jarred Heinrich, Amy Beresheim, and Mandi Alblas. 2016. "Cortical Bone Histomorphology of Known-Age Skeletons from the Kirsten Collection, Stellenbosch University, South Africa." *American Journal of Physical Anthropology* 160 (1): 137–47. https://doi.org/10.1002/ajpa.22951.

Pfeiffer, Susan K., Richard Lazenby, and James Chiang. 1995. "Brief Communication: Cortical Remodeling Data Are Affected by Sampling Location." *American Journal of Physical Anthropology* 96 (1): 89–92. https://doi.org/10.1002/ajpa.1330960110.

Rembert, Mark, Michael Betz, Bo Feng, and Mark Partridge. 2017. "Taking Measure of Ohio's Opioid Crisis." *Ohio State University. Department of Agricultural, Environmental, and Development Economics* 27.

Richards, Christopher J., Kenneth W. Graf, and Rakesh P. Mashru. 2017. "The Effect of Opioids, Alcohol, and Nonsteroidal Anti-Inflammatory Drugs on Fracture Union." *Orthopedic Clinics* 48 (4): 433–43. https://doi.org/10.1016/j.ocl.2017.06.002.

Robling, Alexander G., and Sam D. Stout. 2008. "Histomorphometry of Human Cortical Bone: Applications to Age Estimation." In *Biological Anthropology of the Human Skeleton*, edited by M. Anne Katzenberg and Shelley R. Saunders, 149–82. Hoboken, NJ: John Wiley & Sons, Inc. https://doi.org/10.1002/9780470245842.ch5.

Rubin, Katie M. 2018. "The Current State and Future Directions of Skeletal Toxicology: Forensic and Humanitarian Implications of a Proposed Model for the in Vivo Incorporation of Drugs into the Human Skeleton." *Forensic Science International* 289 (August): 419–28. https://doi.org/10.1016/j.forsciint.2018.06.024.

Rudd, Rose A., Noah Aleshire, Jon E. Zibbell, and R. Matthew Gladden. 2016a. "Increases in Drug and Opioid Overdose Deaths—United States, 2000–2014." *American Journal of Transplantation* 16 (4): 1323–27. https://doi.org/10.1111/ajt.13776.

Rudd, Rose A., Puja Seth, Felicita David, and Lawrence Scholl. 2016b. "Increases in Drug and Opioid-Involved Overdose Deaths - United States, 2010-2015." *MMWR: Morbidity & Mortality Weekly Report* 65 (50/51): 1445–52. https://doi.org/10.15585/mmwr.mm655051e1.

Salmond, Susan, and Virginia Allread. 2019. "A Population Health Approach to America's Opioid Epidemic." *Orthopedic Nursing* 38 (2): 95–108. https://doi.org/10.1097/NOR.0000000000000521.

Schalkoff, Christine A., Kathryn E. Lancaster, Bradley N. Gaynes, Vivian Wang, Brian W. Pence, William C. Miller, and Vivian F. Go. 2020. "The Opioid and Related Drug Epidemics in Rural Appalachia: A Systematic Review of Populations Affected, Risk Factors, and Infectious Diseases." *Substance Abuse* 41 (1): 35–69. https://doi.org/10.1080/08897077.2019.1635555.

Schindelin, Johannes, Arganda-Carreras, Ignacio, Frise, Erwin, Kaynig, Verena, Longair, Mark, Pietzsch, Tobias, Preibisch, Stephan, et al. 2012. "Fiji: An Open-Source Platform for Biological-Image Analysis." *Nature Methods* 9 (7): 676–82. https://doi.org/10.1038/nmeth.2019.

Seal, Karen H., Alex H. Kral, Lauren Gee, Lisa D. Moore, Ricky N. Bluthenthal, Jennifer Lorvick, and Brian R. Edlin. 2001. "Predictors and Prevention of Nonfatal Overdose Among Street-Recruited Injection Heroin Users in the San Francisco Bay Area, 1998-1999." *American Journal of Public Health* 91 (11): 1842–46.

Sedlin, Elias D., Harold M. Frost, and A. Villanueva. 1963. "The Eleventh Rib Biopsy In The Study Of Metabolic Bone Disease." *Henry Ford Hosp Med Bull* 11 (2): 217–19.

Seeman, Ego. 2013. "Age- and Menopause-Related Bone Loss Compromise Cortical and Trabecular Microstructure." *The Journals of Gerontology: Series A* 68 (10): 1218–25. https://doi.org/10.1093/gerona/glt071.

Sherman, Susan G., Yingkai Cheng, and Alexander H. Kral. 2007. "Prevalence and Correlates of Opiate Overdose among Young Injection Drug Users in a Large U.S. City." *Drug and Alcohol Dependence* 88 (2–3): 182–87. https://doi.org/10.1016/j.drugalcdep.2006.10.006.

Siegler, Anne, Ellenie Tuazon, Daniella Bradley O'Brien, and Denise Paone. 2014. "Unintentional Opioid Overdose Deaths in New York City, 2005–2010: A Place-Based Approach to Reduce Risk." *International Journal of Drug Policy* 25 (3): 569–74. https://doi.org/10.1016/j.drugpo.2013.10.015.

Singh, Inder Jit, and D. L. Gunberg. 1970. "Estimation of Age at Death in Human Males from Quantitative Histology of Bone Fragments." *American Journal of Physical Anthropology* 33 (3): 373–81. https://doi.org/10.1002/ajpa.1330330311.

Sobotka, Tagart C., and Sheridan A. Stewart. 2020. "Stereotyping and the Opioid Epidemic: A Conjoint Analysis." *Social Science & Medicine* 255 (June): 113018. https://doi.org/10.1016/j.socscimed.2020.113018.

Sorg, Marcella H. 2010. "Drug-Induced Deaths in Maine 1997-2008, with Estimates for 2009." *Anthropology Faculty Scholarship* 20: 1–42.

Sorg, Marcella H., and Margaret Greenwald. 2003. "Patterns of Drug-Related Mortality in Maine, 1997-2002." *Maine Policy Review* 12 (1): 84–96.

Spalding, Frank. 2006. *Methamphetamine: The Dangers of Crystal Meth.* 1st ed. Drug Abuse and Society. New York: The Rosen Publishing Group, Inc.

Stout, Sam D. 1986. "The Use of Bone Histomorphometry in Skeletal Identification: The Case of Francisco Pizarro." *Journal of Forensic Sciences* 31 (1): 296–300. https://doi.org/10.1520/JFS11886J.

Stout, Sam D., and Sarah J. Gehlert. 1982. "Effects of Field Size When Using Kerley's Histological Method for Determination of Age at Death." *American Journal of Physical Anthropology* 58 (2): 123–25. https://doi.org/10.1002/ajpa.1330580203.

Stout, Sam D., and Robert R. Paine. 1992. "Brief Communication: Histological Age Estimation Using Rib and Clavicle." *American Journal of Physical Anthropology* 87 (1): 111–15. https://doi.org/10.1002/ajpa.1330870110.

Stout, Sam D., Marcello A. Porro, and Beatrice Perotti. 1996. "Brief Communication: A Test and Correction of the Clavicle Method of Stout and Paine for Histological Age Estimation of Skeletal Remains." *American Journal of Physical Anthropology* 100 (1): 139–42. https://doi.org/10.1002/(SICI)1096-8644(199605)100:1<139::AID-AJPA12>3.0.CO;2-1.

Streeter, Margaret. 2010. "A Four-Stage Method of Age at Death Estimation for Use in the Subadult Rib Cortex." *Journal of Forensic Sciences* 55 (4): 1019–24. https://doi.org/10.1111/j.1556-4029.2010.01396.x.

———. 2012. "The Determination of Age in Subadult from the Rib Cortical Microstructure." In *Forensic Microscopy for Skeletal Tissues,* edited by Lynne S. Bell, 101–8. Totowa, NJ: Humana. https://doi.org/10.1007/978-1-61779-977-8_6.

Thompson, D. D. 1979. "Core Technique in the Determination of Age at Death in Skeletons." *Journal of Forensic Sciences* 24 (4): 902–15.

Tipps, Robin T., Gregory T. Buzzard, and John A. McDougall. 2018. "The Opioid Epidemic in Indian Country." *Journal of Law, Medicine & Ethics* 46 (2): 422–36. https://doi.org/10.1177/1073110518782950.

Tommerup, Lorri, Diane Raab, Thomas Crenshaw, and Everett Smith. 2009. "Does Weight-Bearing Exercise Affect Non-Weight-Bearing Bone?" *Journal of Bone and Mineral Research* 8 (9): 1053–58. https://doi.org/10.1002/jbmr.5650080905.

Turner, Russell T. 2000. "Skeletal Response to Alcohol." *Alcoholism: Clinical and Experimental Research* 24 (11): 1693–701. https://doi.org/10.1111/j.1530-0277.2000.tb01971.x.

United Nations Office on Drugs and Labor. 2020. *World Drug Report.* Vol. Booklet 2. S.l.: United Nations. https://wdr.unodc.org/wdr2020/index2020.html.

van Oers, René. F. M., Ronald Ruimerman, Bert van Rietbergen, Peter A. J. Hilbers, and Rik Huiskes. 2008. "Relating Osteon Diameter to Strain." *Bone* 43 (3): 476–82. https://doi.org/10.1016/j.bone.2008.05.015.

Vestergaard, Peter, Lars Rejnmark, and L. Mosekilde. 2006. "Fracture Risk Associated with the Use of Morphine and Opiates." *Journal of Internal Medicine* 260 (1): 76–87. https://doi.org/10.1111/j.1365-2796.2006.01667.x.

Visconti, Adam J., Glenn-Milo Santos, Nikolas P. Lemos, Catherine Burke, and Phillip O Coffin. 2015. "Opioid Overdose Deaths in the City and County of San Francisco: Prevalence, Distribution, and Disparities." *Journal of Urban Health* 92 (4): 758–72. https://doi.org/10.1007/s11524-015-9967-y.

Vogelgesang, Matthias, Tomas Farago, Thilo F. Morgeneyer, Lukas Helfen, Tomy dos Santos Rolo, Anton Myagotin, and Tilo Baumbach. 2016. "Real-Time Image-Content-Based Beamline Control for Smart 4D X-Ray Imaging." *Journal of Synchrotron Radiation* 23 (5): 1254–63. https://doi.org/10.1107/S1600577516010195.

Walker, Robert A., C. Owen Lovejoy, and Richard S. Meindl. 1994. "Histomorphological and Geometric Properties of Human Femoral Cortex in Individuals over 50: Implications for Histomorphological Determination of Age-at-Death." *American Journal of Human Biology* 6 (5): 659–67. https://doi.org/10.1002/ajhb.1310060515.

Wilson, Nana, Kariisa, Mbabazi, Seth, Puja, Smith, Herschel IV, and Nicole L. Davis. 2020. "Drug and Opioid-Involved Overdose Deaths – United States, 2017–2018." *MMWR: Morbidity and Mortality Weekly Report* 69 (11): 290–7. http://dx.doi.org/10.15585/mmwr.mm6911a4.

World Health Organization. 2020. "Opioid Overdose." World Health Organization Newsroom. August 28, 2020. https://www.who.int/news-room/fact-sheets/detail/opioid-overdose.

Wu, K., K. E. Schubeck, Harold M. Frost, and A. Villanueva. 1970. "Haversian Bone Formation Rates Determined by a New Method in a Mastodon, and in Human Diabetes Mellitus and Osteoporosis." *Calcified Tissue Research* 6 (1): 204–19. https://doi.org/10.1007/BF02196201.

Wysokinski, Tomasz W., Dean Chapman, Gregg Adams, Michel Renier, Pekka Suortti, and William Thomlinson. 2015. "Beamlines of the Biomedical Imaging and Therapy Facility at the Canadian Light Source – Part 3." *Nuclear Instruments and Methods in Physics Research Section A: Accelerators, Spectrometers, Detectors and Associated Equipment* 775 (March): 1–4. https://doi.org/10.1016/j.nima.2014.11.088.

Yoshino, Mineo, Kazuhiko Imaizumi, Sachio Miyasaka, and Sueshige Seta. 1994. "Histological Estimation of Age at Death Using Microradiographs of Humeral Compact Bone." *Forensic Science International* 64 (2–3): 191–98. https://doi.org/10.1016/0379-0738(94)90231-3.

Index

dental stigma, 4–7; as additional layer of violence, 22–23
desaparecidos, 129, 136
Detroit Future City (DFC), 210
deviance: categorizations of, 96, 97; constructions of, 96; labeling of, 100; language, 98–100; legitimization, 99; normative expectations, 97; process of, *95*; raciolinguistic perspective, 99; social positionality across social dimensions, 97–98
direct political violence, 128–29; forensic anthropological evidence of, 136
direct violence, 4
disability, 151–55; and Camp Fire fatalities, 163–64, **164**; medical model of, 151–52; pre-fire census and, 159–60; social model of, 152
disaster anthropology, 155
disasters, 155–56
dismemberments, 72, 86n6
disorders of sex development (DSD), 182
drug intervention, 221–22
drug-related deaths, 282
drug user, 98
DSD. *See* disorders of sex development (DSD)

Ecuadorian Indigenous communities, 25
embodiment, 129; health outcomes and mechanisms of, 129–31
equality, definition of, 108
Equipo Colombiano Interdisciplinario de Trabajo Forense y Asistencia Psicosocial (EQUITAS), 78
equity, 108
equity-based approach, 108–10
eugenics, 125
everyday violence, 127–28; forensic anthropological evidence of, 134–35
expressive violence, xxvii

facial feminization surgeries (FFS), 184, 192

FACTS. *See* Forensic Anthropology Center at Texas State University (FACTS)
FADAMA. *See* Forensic Anthropology Database for Assessing Methods Accuracy (FADAMA)
false positives, 75, 80
family/intimate partner violence, 187
family reference samples (FRSs), 255–57; of U.S. Korean War dead, 257–58
family reference samples (FRSs) availability, xxxiii, 270; structural vulnerabilities effect on, 266–73; U.S. Korean War dead, differences in, 262, **263–64**, *265*, 265–66
Farmer, Paul, xxv, 22, 82, 85, 138, 215, 232
FBC. *See* Forensic Border Coalition (FBC)
fentanyl-related fatality decedents, 286
FFS. *See* facial feminization surgeries (FFS)
force majeure, 46
forensically significant burials, *52*, 54
forensic anthropological evidence: of direct political violence, 136; of everyday violence, 134–35; of resilience, 137; of structural violence, 133–34; of symbolic violence, 135–36; of weathering, 136–37
forensic anthropologists, 3, 140; complicit in intersectional violence, 190–92; effects of opioid use, 303; perspective to conflict, 67; shifting role of, 58–60
forensic anthropology, xi, xiii; cases, 232; in Colombia, 76–78; in Latin America, 75–76; opioid use, implications for, 289, 291–94; potential for structural violence, 123; specialization within, xiv
Forensic Anthropology Center at Texas State University (FACTS), 43

power, 72–73
power-sharing compromise, 67
pre-fire CFCs, 161
presumed migrant decedents, 54–57
Prevention through Deterrence, 39,
    47, 48, 58; border enforcement
    strategies, xv
prison industrial complex, 45
prolonged stress responses, 130
Pueblo Bello massacre, 84

racism, xxvii, 5, 126
refugee, 46
region, rate of OODs, 288–89
resilience, 132; forensic anthropological
    evidence of, 137
resource scarcity, 107–8
return of investment (ROI), 107–8
rheumatoid arthritis, 219, *220*
Right to Know, 40, 58
Rutas del Conflicto, 72, 73

Sanford, Victoria, 73, 85
Scheper-Hughes, Nancy, xiv, 123, 127,
    128
scurvy, 218, 219, *219*
Search Unit for Disappeared Persons,
    77
Security Police, 77
self-directed violence, 186, 187
Servicemen's Readjustment Act (1944),
    269
sex, 176; chromosome aneuploidies,
    181; hormones, 182; opioid
    epidemic, 283–84
sex-gender distinction, xvi
sexism, 126
sexual assault, 128–29
sexual orientation, opioid overdose, 287
silent mass disaster, xiii, 93, 111
Snow, Clyde, xi, 102
social autopsy, xiv, 232; of Hawai'i. *See*
    Hawai'i, social autopsy
Social Darwinism, 125
social epidemiologists, 123

social epidemiology, 123–24; relevant
    theories from, 125–32; shared goals
    and history of, 124–25
social inequality, 126
social inequity, 138
social isolation: causes and effects of,
    154; defined as, 153–54
social language, 98–99
social marginalization: acute and
    chronic stressors of, 122; forensic
    anthropological evidence of, 133–37
social model of disability, 152
social stigma, 94, 101
South Texas: burial sites for unidentified
    decedents in, 59; current death
    management practices in, 41;
    exhumation findings, 51–58, *52,
    53*; federal/state support for death
    management in, 48; jurisdictional
    system in, 49; migrant deaths at, 38;
    prevention effects through deterrence
    in, 42–44; systems of inaction, 47–49
South Texas Human Rights Center
    (STHRC), 43, 60
"state violence by proxy," 85
Stephen, Lynn, 38, 39
STHRC. *See* South Texas Human
    Rights Center (STHRC)
stigma: defined as, 94; process of, 94,
    95; toward missing and unidentified
    persons, 102; types of, 94–95
stigmatization, 94; of older adults, 153
stigmatized biologies, 5
Stop the Robberies and Enjoy Safe
    Streets (STRESS) Program, 209
structural inequity, 129–30
structural violence, xiii, xv, 3–7,
    47, 126–27, 187, 190, 215, 267,
    271; application of, 3; biology of
    poverty and osteology of, 205–8;
    central elements of, xxv; forensic
    anthropological evidence of, 133–34;
    oral pathologies as, 19–22; and
    victimology, 81–86
structural violence theory, 205, 232

About the Editors

Jennifer F. Byrnes (PhD, SUNY at Buffalo, 2015) is a biological anthropologist who has experience and training in both bioarchaeology and forensic anthropology. She is a diplomate of the American Board of Forensic Anthropology (No. 144). In 2017, she edited a volume titled *Bioarchaeology of Impairment and Disability: Theoretical, Ethnohistorical, and Methodological Perspectives*. She has published bioarchaeological and forensic anthropology research in both edited volumes and journals. She was a forensic anthropology consultant for four years for the City & County of Honolulu Office of the Medical Examiner. She currently consults for the Clark County Office of the Coroner/Medical Examiner.

Iván Sandoval-Cervantes (PhD, University of Oregon, 2016) is a cultural anthropologist from Ciudad Juárez, Mexico. His monograph *Oaxaca in Motion: An Ethnography of Internal, Transnational, and Return Migration* (University of Texas Press, 2022) documents his findings on internal and transnational migration in Mexico and in the United States. He has also published his work in *American Anthropologist*, *Journal of Latin American and Caribbean Anthropology*, and the *Journal of Ethnic and Migration Studies*. Sandoval-Cervantes is currently working on a new project in which he will analyze how different forms of violence are framed and resisted through different forms of activism in Mexico and in Latin America.

About the Contributors

Janna M. Andronowski is an assistant professor of clinical anatomy in the Division of BioMedical Sciences, Faculty of Medicine, at Memorial University of Newfoundland and the forensic anthropologist for the province of Newfoundland and Labrador at the Office of the Chief Medical Examiner in St. John's, NL. She received her BA and BSc from Simon Fraser University, MSc from the University of Toronto, PhD from the University of Tennessee, Knoxville, and was a postdoctoral fellow in the Department of Anatomy, Physiology, and Pharmacology at the University of Saskatchewan. Andronowski has more than ten years of experience working in forensic science-based laboratories (e.g., the Forensic Anthropology Unit at the Office of Chief Medical Examiner in New York City, Simon Fraser University's Centre for Forensic Research, and the Forensic Anthropology Center at the University of Tennessee, Knoxville). Her research focuses on the high-resolution 3D imaging of bone microarchitecture and the study of bone adaptation, quality, and fragility associated with substance abuse. Andronowski is a regular user at the Canadian Light Source synchrotron (Biomedical Imaging and Therapy beamlines) and primarily makes use of computed tomography.

Jared S. Beatrice earned his PhD in physical anthropology from Michigan State University. Beatrice is currently an associate professor in the Department of Sociology and Anthropology at the College of New Jersey. In addition to conducting research on the skeletal evidence for structural violence in undocumented migrants, Beatrice has conducted bioarchaeological fieldwork in Albania, Greece, and Italy and is currently working on a historic cemetery from Philadelphia.

William R. Belcher received his PhD in anthropology from the University of Wisconsin-Madison in 1998 and has been a board-certified forensic anthropologist (No. 66) since 2003. Between 1998 and 2019, Belcher served as a forensic anthropologist with the Department of Defense's Defense POW/MIA Accounting Agency (DPAA) (and its predecessors), with the last decade as supervisory anthropologist and deputy director of the DPAA-Hawaii Laboratory. Since his retirement from the Department of Defense in 2019, he has served as an associate professor in anthropology at the University of Nebraska-Lincoln, School of Global Integrative Studies. Belcher has more than sixty-five national and international journals and edited volume publications in forensic anthropology, faunal analysis/archaeology, and 3D assessment of forensic contexts. Belcher currently consults for the Department of Defense, the Lancaster County (Nebraska) Sheriff's Office, the Nebraska State Patrol, History Nebraska, the Nebraska Museum, and various Nebraska county coroner's offices.

Cate E. Bird is the missing persons and forensic advisor for the International Committee of the Red Cross (ICRC) Regional Delegation for the United States and Canada. Her work focuses on the humanitarian consequences of armed conflict and migration, including local, national, and international mechanisms to search for and identify missing persons. Cate received her PhD in anthropology from Michigan State University in 2013.

Jason D. P. Bird is an associate professor and chair of the Department of Social Work at Rutgers University—Newark. His areas of research include health and social disparities and resilience among LGBT populations, the impact of stigma on health risk behavior and health-related outcomes for gay men and men who have sex with men, and teaching empathy as a part of social work pedagogy. He is an affiliated member of the Rutgers Center for Gender and Sexuality, Law, and Policy and the Rutgers Health Disparities and Health Promotion Working Group. Jason received his PhD in social work from the University of Chicago in 2009.

Zoë Crossland is professor of anthropology and director of the Center for Archaeology at Columbia University. Her research, informed by a Peircean semeiotic perspective, deals with the historical archaeology of Madagascar, and with evidential practices around human remains. She is co-editor with Rosemary Joyce of *Disturbing Bodies: Anthropological Perspectives on Forensic Archaeology* (2015) and coauthor with Annia Cherryson and Sarah Tarlow of *A Fine and Private Place: The Archaeology of Death and Burial in Post-medieval Britain and Ireland* (2012).

Randi M. Depp is a PhD student in the Integrated Bioscience program at the University of Akron. She received a MSc in forensic anthropology from Mercyhurst University, a BS in Biology from Cleveland State University, and a BS in forensic science from the University of Findlay. Her research investigates taphonomy and bone biomechanics and seeks to improve methods for estimating the postmortem interval and interpreting trauma in forensic anthropological casework.

Elizabeth A. DiGangi is an associate professor of anthropology at Binghamton University. She received her PhD in biological anthropology from the University of Tennessee, Knoxville.

Paulina Domínguez Acosta is a forensic anthropology research associate with SNA International supporting the DPAA in Hawaii, as part of the Korean War Identification Project. She received her MA in biological anthropology from Texas State University, where she analyzed craniomorphological variations between northern, central, and southern regions of Mexico using geometric morphometric data. Paulina has completed internships at the Office of the Medical Examiner at El Paso, TX, Operation Identification (OpID), and the Forensic Anthropology Center at Texas State University (FACTS).

Janet E. Finlayson earned her PhD in anthropology from the University of Florida. Finlayson is currently a forensic anthropologist at the DPAA in Hawaii.

Amanda N. Friend is a forensic anthropologist for SNA International in support of the DPAA in Hawaii. She earned her BA in anthropology from Miami University and her MA and PhD in anthropology from the University of Florida.

Matthew C. Go is a forensic anthropologist working at the DPAA in Hawaii. He earned his MA and PhD in anthropology from the University of Illinois at Urbana-Champaign, and his BA (hons.) in archaeology with a minor in biological sciences and certificate in forensic studies from Simon Fraser University. Matthew's regional focus has been advancing both the research and practice of forensic anthropology in the Philippines and is the first and only Filipino to be certified by the American Board of Forensic Anthropology (No. 154). At the DPAA, he is a member of the Korean War Identification Project, which represents the largest and most complex assemblage of commingled human remains within the agency's purview. Ancillary interests include human anatomy, bioarchaeology, ecological and evolutionary biology, and entomology.

Amanda Hale is a forensic anthropologist with SNA International supporting the DPAA in Hawaii. Amanda received her MA in bioarchaeology in 2012 from North Carolina State University. Amanda spent nine years working with the North Carolina Human Identification and Forensic Analysis Laboratory as an analyst, case coordinator, and laboratory manager. She began her PhD in 2014 and is currently a PhD candidate in Biological Sciences, Ecology and Evolution at NC State and hopes to graduate in August 2022.

Jaxson D. Haug is an anthropology PhD student at Southern Methodist University and a medicolegal death investigator for the Dallas County Medical Examiner. He received his BA from California State University (CSU), Chico (2016) in anthropology and criminal justice and his MA from CSU, Los Angeles (2020) in biological anthropology. He has spent time as a forensic anthropology intern at medical examiner's offices in Clark County, Los Angeles County, Dallas County, and Tarrant County. His research has largely focused on ethics and inclusion of methods for sex- and gender-diverse casework in forensic anthropology.

Allison Hutson is a recent graduate from the University of West Florida with her MA in anthropology and is currently expanding her research skills in data analytics in the professional sphere. She received a BA in history and anthropology from Flagler College, and her interests include the intersection of inequality and burial practices, historic cemetery demography and preservation, and mortuary archaeology.

Jennie Jin has a PhD in anthropology from the Pennsylvania State University. After leading the Korean War Identification Project at the DPAA for eleven years, Jin became the special projects manager supervising a wide variety of projects from WWII, Korea, and Vietnam.

Sadé J. Johnson was a forensic anthropology postgraduate research associate with SNA International supporting the DPAA in Hawaii. Johnson received her BA in anthropology from the University at Albany, State University of New York. She earned her MA in biological anthropology with a focus in human skeletal biology from New York University. Her MA thesis comparatively analyzed different techniques for sampling dentin powder for mitochondrial DNA testing.

Molly A. Kaplan earned her MA and is a PhD candidate in the applied anthropology program at Texas State University. She is a doctoral research assistant for OpID, which seeks to locate, identify, and return unidentified migrant decedents to their families. Her research focuses on improving medicolegal death investigation of long-term unidentified persons and mitigating the migrant death crisis at the U.S.-Mexico border. As a former consultant researcher for the Argentine Forensic Anthropology Team (EAAF), she remains an active member of the Forensic Border Coalition (FBC), which seeks to assist families of missing migrants through casework and applied research.

Jaymelee J. Kim is a four-field anthropologist who earned a graduate certificate in linguistics, a graduate certificate in disasters, displacement, and human rights, and a PhD in anthropology from the University of Tennessee. Currently, she is an associate professor of forensic sciences at the University of Findlay and a forensic anthropologist for the Wayne County Medical Examiner's Office in Detroit, Michigan. Her research interests include structural violence, human rights, human trafficking, transitional justice, missing and unidentified persons, and forensic anthropology ethics and capacity building; research and consulting sites include the United States, Canada, and Uganda.

Meredith G. Marten is a medical anthropologist, and assistant professor of anthropology at the University of West Florida. Her primary research interests include equity in access to HIV and maternal health services in East Africa, focusing on how volatility in donor aid and health policy affects the well-being of women living in poverty. She has an MPH in international health and development from Tulane University, and a PhD in anthropology from the University of Florida.

Daniel E. Martínez is an associate professor in the School of Sociology and a co-director of the Binational Migration Institute at the University of Arizona. His research and teaching interests include race and ethnicity, undocumented immigration, and criminology. He is particularly interested in the social and legal criminalization of undocumented migration. Martínez has also conducted extensive research on deportations and undocumented border crosser deaths along the U.S.-Mexico border. He is a co-principal investigator of the Migrant Border Crossing Study, a Ford Foundation-funded research project that examines recently deported undocumented Mexican migrants' experiences crossing the U.S.-Mexico border and residing in the United States.

Chloe P. McDaneld is the laboratory manager for OpID at Texas State University. She received her MA in anthropology from Texas State University in 2016.

Samuel Mijal received his BS in anthropology in 2015 from Arizona State University. He is currently pursuing his MA in anthropology from CSU, Chico.

Mariah E. Moe is a PhD candidate in the applied anthropology program at Texas State University. She received her MA in anthropology from the University of Nevada, Las Vegas, and her BS in anthropology with a focus on human biology from the University of Arizona. Her dissertation aims to improve methods of grave detection through a combination of predictive modeling, ground penetrating radar, and drone-mounted infrared imagery. This research is being conducted in South Texas in the search for the unmarked graves of presumed migrants who perished while attempting to cross the U.S.-Mexico border.

Megan K. Moore received her PhD from the University of Tennessee, Knoxville, and is a diplomate of the American Board of Forensic Anthropology (No. 140). She is an associate professor in the Department of Sociology, Anthropology, and Criminology at Eastern Michigan University. She is a forensic anthropology consultant for Wayne, Washtenaw, and Monroe Counties Medical Examiners' Offices in Southeastern Michigan. Additionally, she has worked as a forensic anthropology consultant for the Physicians for Human Rights in Cyprus and the International Criminal Investigative Training Assistance Program through the U.S. DOJ in Colombia.

Briana T. New is a PhD student at the University of Nevada, Reno. She received her MA in biological anthropology from Texas State University and then worked as a forensic anthropologist for SNA International in support of the DPAA in Hawaii for three years.

Enrique Plasencia is currently a graduate student at the University of West Florida pursuing his MA in anthropology and received his BA in anthropology from the University of Florida in 2019, graduating cum laude. His research interests include techniques of forensic identification of remains of Latin American and Caribbean migrants found along U.S. international borders, development of international networks that provide a vital link between families of missing migrants and forensic practitioners, the implementation of biocultural approaches to forensic anthropology, and the embodiment of systemic social inequality in the remains of decedents of vulnerable populations.

Daniela Santamaria Vargas is an anthropologist from Colombia with a MA in biomedical anthropology from Binghamton University. She has an interest in human rights violations, forensic anthropology, Colombia and the post-conflict, and public health. She has participated in research projects back in Colombia with the National Institute of Legal Medicine and Forensic Sciences. Her internship as an undergraduate was with the Unit for the Attention and Integral Reparation of the Victims in her home country of Colombia.

Courtney C. Siegert graduated from the University of Texas in 2010 with her BA in anthropology with a focus in archaeology, and from Texas State University in 2016 with her MA in anthropology with a focus in biological anthropology. Since 2015, she has worked with OpID. Courtney is currently pursuing her PhD in applied anthropology at Texas State University where she continues to work with OpID. Her doctoral research focuses on understanding human variation through skeletally derived data and improving methods of estimating geographic origin and population affinity in a forensic setting.

Angela Soler earned her PhD in physical anthropology from Michigan State University. Soler is currently a board-certified forensic anthropologist at the New York City Office of Chief Medical Examiner. Prior to working in New York City, Soler completed a postdoctoral position at the Pima County Office of the Medical Examiner in Tucson, Arizona. Soler's research focuses on the identification of unknown persons in the U.S. medicolegal system and documentation of the skeletal evidence for structural violence in undocumented migrants.

M. Kate Spradley received her PhD in anthropology from the University of Tennessee, Knoxville. She is currently a professor at Texas State University.

Taylor Walkup is currently a graduate student at the University of West Florida pursuing her MA in anthropology. She received her BA in anthropology and history from the University of Florida in 2019 and has been accepted to the University of Tennessee's Biological Anthropology PhD program beginning Fall 2022.

P. Willey received his PhD in anthropology from the University of Tennessee, Knoxville. He taught at CSU Chico for more than twenty-five years, and on retirement in 2017, he became professor emeritus.

Devin N. Williams is a postgraduate research associate at the DPAA. She currently assists with the accounting of unidentified servicemen from the Korean War. She received her BS in anthropology and evolutionary/ecology biology from the University of Tennessee and her MA in applied anthropology from the University of South Florida (USF). During her tenure at USF, she supported operations at the Florida Institute of Forensic Anthropology and Applied Science (IFAAS) through search and recovery, cemetery exhumations, decomposition research, analysis of human remains and material evidence, and leading public outreach initiatives and interactive field trips.

Allysha P. Winburn is an assistant professor of anthropology at the University of West Florida and the forensic anthropologist for the Alabama Department of Forensic Sciences and Florida's District 1 Medical Examiner. A registered professional archaeologist and diplomate of the American Board of Forensic Anthropology (No. 136), she holds degrees from Yale (BA, archaeological studies), New York University (MA, anthropology), and the University of Florida (PhD, anthropology).

Katharine C. Woollen received her MSc in biological anthropology from Illinois State University. She is a current bioarchaeology and forensic anthropology PhD student at the University of Nevada, Las Vegas. Her research emphasizes the importance of recognizing the historical and contemporary social and societal pressures that lead to excess death rates of marginalized and at-risk individuals.